Prescribing Medicines for Children: From drug development to practical administration

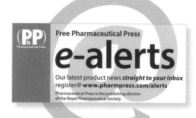

Prescribing Medicines for Children: From drug development to practical administration

Edited by
Dr Charlotte Barker MA, BM BCh, MRCPCH
NIHR Academic Clinical Fellow in Paediatrics, UCL Great Ormond Street Institute
of Child Health, London, UK
Honorary Research Fellow in the Paediatric Infectious Diseases Research Group,
St George's, University of London, UK

Professor Mark Turner PhD, DRCOG, MRCP(UK), MRCPCH,
FFPM (Hon)
Professor of Neonatology and Research Delivery, University of Liverpool, UK
Honorary Consultant Neonatologist, Liverpool Women's NHS Foundation Trust,
Liverpool, UK

Professor Mike Sharland CBE, MD, FRCPCH
Professor of Paediatric Infectious Diseases, St George's, University of London, UK
Honorary Consultant at St George's University Hospitals NHS Foundation Trust,
London, UK

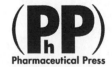

Pharmaceutical Press

Published by the Pharmaceutical Press

66-68 East Smithfield, London E1W 1AW, UK

© Pharmaceutical Press 2019

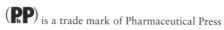 is a trade mark of Pharmaceutical Press

Pharmaceutical Press is the publishing division of the Royal Pharmaceutical Society

First published 2019

Typeset by SPi Global, Chennai, India
Printed in Great Britain by TJ International, Padstow, Cornwall

ISBN 9780857111357

A catalogue record for this book is available from the British Library.

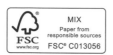

MIX
Paper from
responsible sources
FSC® C013056

Contents

Foreword

This excellent new text, *Prescribing Medicines for Children,* covers a broad range of important topics in paediatric therapeutics, ranging from the principles of clinical pharmacology in children through to medication safety and drug development. The clinical section draws on expert knowledge to improve prescribing in a variety of general and specialist settings in paediatrics. We particularly value the international nature of the authorship, illustrating how the principles that underlie the use of medicines for children are applicable globally.

This book will be a useful adjunct to standard paediatric textbooks and formularies such as the *British National Formulary for Children* (BNFC). It will enable clinicians, pharmacists and non-medical prescribers to improve their understanding of the optimum use of medicines in infants and children. The chapters are clear and concise and emphasise aspects of pharmacology and therapeutics that are relevant to clinical practice. The text will also be useful to those revising for MRCPCH examinations and other postgraduate qualifications, as well as to senior clinicians and pharmacists wishing to widen and update their knowledge.

The editors are keen to hear from readers with ideas for future editions, so if you have suggestions please do contact them.

Professor Neena Modi, President of the Royal College of Paediatrics and Child Health

Dr Helen Sammons, Chair of the RCPCH Joint Medicines Committee

Prescribing Medicines for Children: Preface

This handbook on medicines for children complements the *British National Formulary for Children* (BNFC) and will facilitate translation of essential pharmacological principles into good prescribing practice. The overall aim of the text is to promote safe and effective prescribing in paediatrics. This includes how to avoid medication errors and adverse drug reactions in children, and harnesses the expertise of paediatricians and pharmacists with extensive experience in the field. The variation in prescribing habits between countries has been considered when developing the text, which benefits from an international authorship and focuses on shared principles that underpin rational prescribing in paediatrics and neonatology.

The target readership comprises all professionals who prescribe for children in any context. This includes doctors working in paediatrics or neonatology (training grades and consultants), GPs, pharmacists and specialist nurse prescribers.

The development of this book was made possible by Global Research in Paediatrics (GRiP), www.grip-network.org/index.php/cms/en/home, which was an EU-funded network of scientists aiming to stimulate and facilitate the development and safe use of medicines in children. GRiP enabled creation of a leading research network in the field of paediatric clinical pharmacology.

It is hoped that this book will contribute to the lasting legacy of GRiP in promoting enhanced understanding of paediatric clinical pharmacology, with the ultimate aim of improving the safety and efficacy of medicines for children across the globe.

Topical content of the book

The chapter content is divided into two sections:

Part I provides concise educational material relating to paediatric pharmacology and optimising how medicines are developed and prescribed for children.

Part II contains the clinical prescribing areas. These chapters map principally to the content of the BNFC and relevant paediatric subspecialties. The chapters each focus on the key issues in prescribing for the respective clinical specialty or context. This section is intended to be useful for regular consultation, to support safe, effective prescribing for children/neonates in each subspecialty context.

The book does not discuss the components of a basic prescription, as it is anticipated that readers will have acquired this information from elsewhere, such as in the BNFC itself or via other resources.[1-4]

Acknowledgements

We are immensely grateful to the many contributors, editorial board members and expert reviewers, as well as Mary Simpson and the publishing team at Pharmaceutical Press, for their time and support in developing this book. We also extend special thanks to both Hana Tabusa and Jennifer Stuart, from the Paediatric Infectious Diseases Research Group at St George's, University of London, for their invaluable help.

The research leading to these results has received funding from the European Union's Seventh Framework Programme for Research, Technological Development and Demonstration under grant agreement no. 261060 (Global Research in Paediatrics – GRiP network of excellence), which funded Dr Charlotte Barker as a Clinical Research Fellow at St George's, University of London. Dr Barker also received funding from the National Institute for Health Research as an Academic Clinical Fellow in Paediatrics (NIHR ACF-2016-18-016).

The development of this book and the GRiP project were both supported by PENTA-ID, the Paediatric European Network for Treatment of AIDS and Infectious Diseases (penta-id.org) and the PENTA Foundation.

Corresponding with the editors

We would be delighted to hear from readers who have suggestions for additions or improvements to future editions of this book. Comments can be sent to Dr Charlotte Barker by email to um4c@sgul.ac.uk

Disclaimer

The views and opinions expressed in this book are those of the authors and do not necessarily reflect the official policy of the authors' institutions, funders or the editorial board.

In particular, any drug dosing recommendations within the text should be considered with appropriate reference to the relevant manufacturer's summary of product characteristics (SmPC), in conjunction with other appropriate and up-to-date literature, including local and national paediatric prescribing guidelines and formularies.

Responsibility for the appropriate use of medicines lies solely with the individual health professional. Further to appropriate prescribing, it is also expected that pharmacists or other suitably trained paediatric healthcare professionals will counsel patients and carers when necessary, providing written information where appropriate.[5]

References

1   Aronson JK *et al*. A prescription for better prescribing. *BMJ* 2006; 333(7566): 459–460.
2   Morkane CM, Binns KG, Coleman JJ. The medic's guide to prescribing: Prescribing for children. *Student BMJ* 2007; 15: 293–336
3   Royal College of Paediatrics and Child Health. Paediatric Prescribing Principles - eLearning. Available at: https://www.rcpch.ac.uk/resources/paediatric-prescribing-principles-online-learning [last accessed 15 May 2019].
4   Paediatric SCRIPT eLearning programme. Available at: www.safeprescriber.org/paediatric/ [last accessed 15 May 2019].
5   Medicines for Children. Information leaflets. Available at: https://www.medicinesfor children.org.uk/search-for-a-leaflet [last accessed 15 May 2019].

Editors

Professor Mike Sharland CBE, MD, FRCPCH

Professor Mike Sharland is a Professor of Paediatric Infectious Diseases at St George's, University of London, and Honorary Consultant at St George's University Hospitals NHS Foundation Trust. He has developed the Paediatric Infectious Diseases Unit at St George's into a recognised Centre of Excellence for clinical care, postgraduate training and research.

Professor Sharland previously chaired the UK Department of Health's Expert Advisory Committee on Antimicrobial Prescribing, Resistance and Healthcare Associated Infection (APRHAI). He is a paediatric advisor on antimicrobials for the World Health Organization and the European Centre for Disease Prevention and Control (ECDC). He is a vice chair of PENTA-ID, the Paediatric European Network for Treatment of AIDS and Infectious Diseases, which is the European Medicines Agency level 1 recognised clinical trials network on antimicrobials.

Professor Sharland has a longstanding interest in developing the evidence base for the use of paediatric antimicrobials. This work ranges from pharmacokinetic and pharmacodynamic studies to investigating clinical outcomes and safety. He has developed a clear research strategy using both cohort studies and clinical trials to improve the evidence base for antimicrobial prescribing. He has an interest in policy initiatives to reduce the burden of antimicrobial resistance (AMR) and has been closely involved in the implementation of the National AMR Strategy in the UK.

Professor Sharland was Lead Scientist for St George's, University of London, within the Global Research in Paediatrics (GRiP) Network.

Professor Mark Turner DRCOG, MRCP(UK), MRCPCH, FFPM (Hon)

Professor Mark Turner is Professor of Neonatology and Research Delivery at the University of Liverpool and Honorary Consultant Neonatologist at Liverpool Women's NHS Foundation Trust.

Professor Turner's research focuses on improving the access of babies and children to high quality medicines through rational drug development. He has particular experience in early phase drug development in premature neonates. He promotes efficient research delivery through the integration of the design and conduct of clinical trials by aligning the content and processes of trials across multiple institutions.

He was co-coordinator of the GRiP project and is currently Chair of the European Network of Paediatric Research at the European Medicines Agency, European Co-director of the International Neonatal Consortium and Co-coordinator of conect4children (c4c), an IMI2-funded project to develop a paediatric clinical research network involving 19 European countries.

Dr Charlotte Barker MA, BM BCh, MRCPCH

Dr Charlotte Barker is an NIHR Academic Clinical Fellow in Paediatrics at the UCL Great Ormond Street Institute of Child Health and Honorary Research Fellow in the Paediatric Infectious Diseases Research Group at St George's, University of London. Her current research is focused on paediatric antimicrobial population pharmacokinetics and the application of quantitative pharmacological techniques for evidence-based dose optimization strategies in clinical practice. She was previously the GRiP Clinical Research Fellow at St George's, University of London, where she coordinated the NAPPA study (Neonatal and Paediatric Pharmacokinetics of Antimicrobials), evaluating new methodologies in paediatric pharmacokinetic study design.

Contributors

Assunta Albanese
Department of Paediatrics, St George's University Hospitals NHS Foundation Trust, London, UK

Ali Al-Hashimi
Alder Hey Children's NHS Foundation Trust, Liverpool, UK

Ali Al-Khattawi
Aston Pharmacy School, Aston University, Birmingham, UK

Karel Allegaert
Department of Development and Regeneration, KU Leuven, Belgium, and Department of Paediatrics, Division of Neonatology, Erasmus MC, Sophia Children's Hospital, Rotterdam, The Netherlands

Annagrazia Altavilla
Espace Ethique Méditerranéen/Paca-Corse AP-HM Marseille, Marseille, France

Mark Anderson
Department of Paediatric Medicine, Newcastle upon Tyne NHS Foundation Trust, Newcastle, UK

Heather Bagley
Institute of Translational Medicine, University of Liverpool, Liverpool, UK

Eileen Baildam
Rheumatology Department, Alder Hey Children's NHS Foundation Trust, and University of Liverpool, Liverpool, UK

Catrin E Barker
Pharmacy Department, Alder Hey Children's NHS Foundation Trust, Liverpool, UK

Eric Bellissant
Clinical Pharmacology Department and Inserm 1414 Clinical Investigation Center, Rennes 1 University, and Rennes University Hospital, Rennes, France

Julia Bielicki

University Children's Hospital Basel, Basel, Switzerland, and Paediatric Infectious Diseases Research Group, Institute for Infection and Immunity, St George's, University of London, London, UK

Jill Bloom

Pharmacy Department, Moorfields Eye Hospital NHS Foundation Trust, London, UK

Efe Bolton

Department of Pharmacy, St George's University Hospitals NHS Foundation Trust, London, UK

Steve Bowhay

Pharmacy Department, Royal Hospital for Children, Glasgow, UK

Neil A Caldwell

Wirral University Teaching Hospital NHS Foundation Trust, Wirral, and Liverpool John Moores University, Liverpool, UK

Adriana Ceci

Gianni Benzi Pharmacological Research Foundation/Consorzio Valutazioni Biologiche e Farmacologiche, Bari, Italy

Jo Challands

The Royal London Hospital, Barts Health NHS Trust, London, UK

Robyn Challinor

Patient representative

Catherine Chiron

INSERM, Université Paris Descartes, Paris, France

Imti Choonara

Division of Child Health, Derby, University of Nottingham, Derby, UK

Nanna Christiansen

The Royal London Hospital, Barts Health NHS Trust, London, UK

Barbara Cochrane

Dietetic Department, Royal Hospital for Children, Glasgow, UK

Sharon Conroy

School of Medicine, University of Nottingham, Nottingham, UK

Katherine Cooper

Alder Hey Children's NHS Foundation Trust, Liverpool, UK

Karlien Cransberg

Department of Pediatrics, Erasmus MC University Medical Center, Sophia Children's Hospital, Rotterdam, The Netherlands

Noel Cranswick

Australian Paediatric Pharmacology Research Unit, Royal Children's Hospital, Murdoch Children's Research Institute, and Department of Pharmacology, University of Melbourne, Melbourne, Australia

Octavio Aragon Cuevas

Alder Hey Children's NHS Foundation Trust, Liverpool, UK

Annegret Dahlmann-Noor
   Moorfields Eye Hospital NHS Foundation Trust, London, UK
Caroline Davison
   Department of Paediatric Intensive Care, St George's University Hospitals
   NHS Foundation Trust, London, UK
Carine de Beaufort
   DECCP/CH de Luxembourg, Luxembourg, University of Luxembourg
   LCSB, Belval, Luxembourg; and Free University of Brussels, Belgium
Tiphaine de Beaumais
   Service de Pharmacologie Clinique Pédiatrique, Hôpital Universitaire
   Robert Debré, Paris, France
Huib de Jong
   Department of Pediatric Nephrology, Erasmus MC University Medical
   Center, Sophia Children's Hospital, Rotterdam, The Netherlands
Saskia N de Wildt
   Department of Pharmacology and Toxicology, Radboud University,
   Nijmegen, and Intensive Care and Department of Pediatric Surgery,
   Erasmus MC University Medical Center, Sophia Children's Hospital,
   Rotterdam, The Netherlands
Thomas Dennison
   Aston University, Birmingham, UK
Sujata Edate
   St George's University Hospitals NHS Foundation Trust, London, UK
Elizabeth Evans
   Alder Hey Children's NHS Foundation Trust, Liverpool, UK
Saul Faust
   NIHR Wellcome Trust Clinical Research Facility, University of
   Southampton, Southampton, UK
Helena Fonseca
   Department of Paediatrics, Adolescent Division, Hospital de Santa
   Maria/Faculty of Medicine, University of Lisbon, Lisbon, Portugal
Andy Fox
   Pharmacy Department, University Hospital Southampton NHS Founda-
   tion Trust, Southampton, UK
Edward Gaynor
   Department of Paediatrics, John Radcliffe Hospital, Oxford University
   Hospitals NHS Foundation Trust, Oxford, UK
Diane Gbesemete
   University of Southampton Hospital, Southampton NHS Foundation
   Trust, Southampton, UK
Niharendu Ghara
   Department of Haematology, Great Ormond Street Hospital for Children
   NHS Foundation Trust, London, UK

Lisa Gibb
Great Ormond Street Hospital for Children NHS Foundation Trust, London, UK

Andy Gray
Division of Pharmacology, University of KwaZulu-Natal, Durban, South Africa

Amanda Gwee
Department of Paediatrics, University of Melbourne, and Department of General Medicine, Royal Children's Hospital Melbourne, and Infectious Diseases & Microbiology group, Murdoch Children's Research Institute, Melbourne, Australia

Emily Harrop
Helen & Douglas House, and Oxford University Hospitals NHS Foundation Trust, Oxford, UK

Fauziah Hashmi
Moorfields Eye Hospital NHS Foundation Trust, London, UK

Daniel B Hawcutt
NIHR Alder Hey Clinical Research Facility, Alder Hey Children's NHS Foundation Trust, and Department of Women's and Children's Health, University of Liverpool, Liverpool, UK

Jennifer Haylor (Gray)
University Hospitals Bristol NHS Foundation Trust, Bristol, UK

Paul Heath
Paediatric Infectious Diseases Research Group, Institute for Infection and Immunity, St George's, University of London, London, UK

Michèle Hennekam
Department of Paediatric Dermatology, Sophia Children's Hospital, Erasmus University Medical Center Rotterdam, and Youth Health Care Rijnmond, Rotterdam, The Netherlands

Tara-eileen Hopmans
Department of Paediatric Dermatology, Sophia Children's Hospital, Erasmus University Medical Center Rotterdam, and Department of Psychiatry, University Medical Center Groningen, Groningen, The Netherlands

Kalle Hoppu
Poison Information Centre, Hospital District of Helsinki and Uusimaa, and Department of Paediatrics and Clinical Pharmacology, University of Helsinki, Helsinki, Finland

Lucy Howarth
Department of Paediatrics, John Radcliffe Hospital, Oxford University Hospitals NHS Foundation Trust, Oxford, UK

Shinya Ito
Clinical Pharmacology and Toxicology, The Hospital for Sick Children and University of Toronto, Toronto, Canada

Evelyne Jacqz-Aigrain
Department of Pediatric Pharmacology and Pharmacogenetics, APHP/Paris Diderot University, Paris, France

Prakash Jeena
Department of Paediatrics & Child Health, University of KwaZulu-Natal, Durban, South Africa

Gregory L Kearns
Arkansas Children's Research Institute, and University of Arkansas for Medical Sciences, Arkansas, USA

Niina Kleiber
Department of General Pediatrics and Clinical Pharmacology Unit, CHU Sainte-Justine, Montreal, Canada, and Intensive Care Department of Pediatric Surgery, Erasmus MC University Medical Center, Sophia Children's Hospital, Rotterdam, The Netherlands

Nigel Klein
Infection, Immunology and Inflammation, UCL Great Ormond Street Institute of Child Health, London, UK

Jana Lass
Department of Microbiology, Faculty of Medicine, University of Tartu, Tartu, Estonia

Warren Lenney
Faculty of Medicine and Health Sciences, Keele University, Staffordshire, and Glaxo Smith Kline Respiratory Franchise, GSK House, London, UK

Katherine Leonard
Department of Paediatric Cardiology, University Hospitals Bristol NHS Foundation Trust, Bristol, UK

Yves Liem
Department of Clinical Pharmacy, Wilhelmina Children's Hospital, University Medical Center Utrecht, Utrecht, The Netherlands

Alice Lo
Paediatrics and Women's Health, The Royal London Hospital, Barts Health NHS Trust, London, UK

Andrew Long
Great Ormond Street Hospital for Children NHS Foundation Trust, London, UK

Rebecca Lundin
PENTA Foundation, Padova, Italy

Andy Lunn
Children's Renal and Urology Unit, Nottingham University Hospitals NHS Trust, Nottingham, UK

Irja Lutsar
Department of Microbiology, Faculty of Medicine, University of Tartu, Tartu, Estonia

Djalila Mekahli
Department of Pediatric Nephrology and Organ Transplantation, University Hospital Leuven, Leuven, Belgium

Afzal R Mohammed
Aston Pharmacy School, School of Life and Health Sciences, Aston University, Birmingham, UK

Georgi Nellis
University of Tartu, Tartu, Estonia

Antje Neubert
Department of Paediatrics and Adolescent Medicine, University Hospital Erlangen, Erlangen, Germany

Atieno Ojoo
Formerly, Kenyatta National Hospital and Gertrude's Children's Hospital, Nairobi, Kenya

Catherine O'Sullivan
Paediatric Infectious Diseases Research Group, Institute for Infection and Immunity, St George's, University of London, London, UK

Kathryn Parker
Holland Bloorview Children's Rehabilitation Hospital and Centre for Interprofessional Education, University of Toronto, Toronto, Canada

Suzanne Pasmans
Department of Paediatric Dermatology, Erasmus University Medical Center, Sophia Children's Hospital, Rotterdam, The Netherlands

Stephane Paulus
Alder Hey Children's NHS Foundation Trust, Liverpool, UK

Barry Pizer
Alder Hey Children's NHS Foundation Trust, and University of Liverpool, Liverpool, UK

Gérard Pons
Department of Paediatric Clinical Pharmacology, Université Paris Descartes, Paris, France

Jenny Preston
Institute of Translational Medicine, University of Liverpool, Liverpool, UK

Catherine Prichard
Parent representative

Oliver J Rackham
Wirral University Teaching Hospital NHS Foundation Trust, Wirral, UK

Michael J Rieder
Department of Paediatrics, Physiology and Pharmacology and Medicine, Western University, Ontario, Canada

Agnès Saint-Raymond
European Medicines Agency, London, UK

Helen Sammons
North Devon District Hospital, Northern Devon Healthcare NHS Trust, Barnstaple, and University of Nottingham, Nottingham, UK

Sunil Sampath
Alder Hey Children's NHS Foundation Trust, Liverpool, UK

Bernd Schwahn
Manchester Centre for Genomic Medicine, St Mary's Hospital, Manchester, UK

Ravi K Sharma
Ear, Nose and Throat Department, Alder Hey Children's NHS Foundation Trust, Liverpool, UK

Ulrike Sigg
The Royal London Hospital, Barts Health NHS Trust, London, UK

Elizabeth Starkey
Derbyshire Children's Hospital, Derby, UK

Simon Stones
Academic Unit of Adult, Child and Mental Health Nursing, Faculty of Medicine and Health, University of Leeds, Leeds, UK

Robin Sunderland
Department of Paediatric Anaesthesia, St George's University Hospitals NHS Foundation Trust, London, UK

Susan Tansey
IQVIA, Therapeutic Strategy and Science Unit, Reading, UK

Mark Taranto
Great Ormond Street Hospital for Children NHS Foundation Trust, London, UK

Hugo Braga Tavares
Adolescent Medicine Unit, Centro Hospitalar de Vila Nova de Gaia/Espinho, Porto, Portugal

David Terry
Pharmacy Academic Practice Unit, Aston University, Birmingham, UK

Robert Tulloh
Department of Paediatric Cardiology, University Hospitals Bristol NHS Foundation Trust, and University of Bristol, Bristol, UK

Kristel Van Calsteren
Department of Obstetrics & Gynaecology, University Hospital Gasthuisberg, and Department of Development and Regeneration, Catholic University Leuven, Leuven, Belgium

John N van den Anker
Division of Clinical Pharmacology, Children's National Medical Center, Washington DC, USA, Division of Paediatric Pharmacology and Pharmacometrics, University of Basel Children's Hospital, Basel, Switzerland, and Intensive Care and Department of Pediatric Surgery, Erasmus MC, Sophia Children's Hospital, Rotterdam, the Netherlands

Teun van Gelder
Erasmus MC University Medical Center, Rotterdam, The Netherlands
Casey Vaughan
Alder Hey Children's NHS Foundation Trust, Liverpool, UK
Nicholas Webb
Royal Manchester Children's Hospital and NIHR Manchester Clinical Research Facility, Manchester, UK
Andrew Wignell
Department of Pharmacy, Nottingham University Hospitals NHS Trust, Nottingham, UK
Wei Zhao
Shandong University, Jinan, China
Sarah Zohar
French National Institute of Health and Medical Research (Inserm), Paris, France

Editorial board members

Karel Allegaert
KU Leuven, Belgium, and Erasmus MC, Rotterdam, The Netherlands
Charlotte Barker
St George's, University of London, and UCL Great Ormond Street Institute of Child Health, London, UK
Mati Berkovitch
Tel Aviv Sourasky Medical Center, Tel Aviv, Israel
Adriana Ceci
Gianni Benzi Pharmacological Research Foundation/Consorzio Valutazioni Biologiche e Farmacologiche, Italy
Saskia N de Wildt
Radboud University, Nijmegen, The Netherlands
Carlo Giaquinto
University of Padova, Padova, Italy
Evelyne Jacqz-Aigrain
Department of Pediatric Pharmacology and Pharmacogenetics, APHP/Paris Diderot University, Paris, France
Betty Kalikstad
University of Oslo, Institute of Clinical Medicine, Rikshospitalet, Oslo, Norway
Warren Lenney
Institute for Science & Technology in Medicine, Keele University, Keele, UK
Irja Lutsar
University of Tartu, Tartu, Estonia
Tony Nunn
University of Liverpool and Liverpool John Moores University, Liverpool, UK
Gérard Pons
University Paris Descartes, Paris, France

PART I

1

General principles of paediatric clinical pharmacology

JN van den Anker and K Allegaert

Introduction

A rational approach to determine a safe and effective dose in an individual child necessitates understanding the pharmacokinetic (PK) and pharmacodynamic (PD) properties of a given compound, in combination with the clinical characteristics of that unique child. Developmental pharmacology includes: (i) PK, representing the mathematical description of the drug concentration–time profile; (ii) PD, describing the relationship between a given concentration and the extent of a specific response (e.g. blood pressure, analgesia, fever reduction); and (iii) how PK/PD change with physiological growth and development.

The learning objectives of this chapter are:

- to understand the key processes of pharmacokinetics: absorption, distribution, metabolism and elimination
- to know the meaning of key PK parameters: volume of distribution and clearance
- to understand that multiple maturational, disease and treatment related differences result in differences in PK and PD in children compared with adults.

The two most important parameters, or so-called primary parameters, of the PK of most drugs are the volume of distribution (V_d) and clearance (CL). V_d can be defined as a proportionality constant that links the amount of drug administered to the measured plasma concentration (chapter 4). Clearance is a measure of drug elimination, and represents the volume of blood or plasma from which a given drug is completely removed per unit of time (hours or minutes). Clearance is through metabolism (chapter 5) and/or excretion (chapter 6). The combination of V_d and CL is reflected in the still commonly used elimination half-life ($t_{1/2}$). This means that a prolonged elimination half-life can be explained by either reduced clearance or increased distribution volume. Whereas drugs administered by the intravenous route are completely available to the systemic circulation, absorption (rate and extent) also matters when other routes (e.g. enteral, subcutaneous) are considered (chapter 3).

All these consecutive PK processes (absorption, distribution, metabolism, elimination; ADME) display maturation. The rate of maturation of these ADME processes is most pronounced in the first two years of life. Developmental PD explores the maturational concentration–effect profile and is explained by, e.g., the ontogeny of receptor expression or activation, or maturational physiology (chapter 7).

Related to both (PK/PD), better understanding of the underlying biological mechanisms and their ontogeny enables explanation (and prediction) of drug actions in the individual patient. However, at this moment, the impact of maturational PK has been studied in much more detail than the impact of maturational PD.

Maturational pharmacology: children are not small adults

Absorption: following oral drug administration, absorption displays extensive maturation because of gastrointestinal ontogeny (e.g. anatomy, motility, drug transporters, drug metabolism), but non-enteral routes (e.g. cutaneous, inhalation, muscular size and circulation) also display maturation. Examples of the impact of maturational changes on absorption are provided in Table 1 (chapter 3).

Distribution: although a theoretical volume, the distribution volume depends on physical (e.g. extra- and intracellular water, lipophilic or water soluble compound, ionisation and protein binding) and physiological (protein binding, tissue uptake, permeation to deep compartments) processes. Consequently, the distribution volume is also driven by maturational changes and disease characteristics (chapter 4).

Metabolism: the phenotypic drug metabolising capacity is affected by multiple covariates. Besides growth and maturation, co-morbidities, environmental issues and/or pharmacogenetics can explain inter-individual variability (chapter 5).

Excretion: the most relevant route of drug excretion is the renal route, both through glomerular filtration rate and renal tubular transport. These processes do not mature simultaneously (chapter 6).

Developmental PD: explores the maturational concentration–effect profile (chapter 7).

Specific characteristics of pharmacotherapy and drug evaluation in children

Unlicensed and off-label drug use in children

The treatment of children with medical products is of critical importance for their outcome and quality of life.[1] Despite this relevance, it is still common practice in children to use medicines outside their market authorisation ('off label'). Roughly half of drug use in children is off label, and this is even more pronounced in hospital settings and neonates. Although it is obvious that – in line with the legal initiatives and a paradigm shift in the ethics (from 'it is unethical to perform studies in children' to 'it is unethical not to perform studies in children') – knowledge of pharmacotherapy in children has accumulated significantly.

Drug formulations for children

Besides active ingredients, formulations can also result in unanticipated changes in efficacy or safety. The development of formulations for children should be guided by evidence-based information. Specific issues related to paediatric formulations are the need for dose flexibility, the suitability of a given dosage form (e.g. palatability, size) in children, or excipients (an excipient is a natural or synthetic substance formulated alongside the active ingredient of a medication). Again, neonates and infants are a specific subpopulation of interest. Until tailored formulations receive market authorisation, compounding practices for paediatric drug formulations should be evaluated to guarantee correct dosing, product stability, and safety, and to support pharmacists in their practices.

Adverse drug reactions, drug toxicity and pharmacovigilance

Drug therapy is a powerful tool to improve outcome, but there is a need to improve paediatric pharmacotherapy through tailored prevention and management of adverse drug reactions (ADRs) (see also chapter 10 and chapter 11).[2] The toxicity of many drugs is different in children to that documented in adults, and can be explained by specific aspects of developmental pharmacokinetics (e.g. valproate toxicity in infants due to isoenzyme specific maturation; chloramphenicol resulting in grey baby syndrome because of impaired glucuronidation; competitive protein binding with hyperbilirubinaemia; percutaneous unintended absorption). Pharmacovigilance to prevent ADRs also needs to be tailored to children. Specific aspects in children are prevention strategies for drug prescription and administration errors (e.g. formulation, bedside manipulation, access), detection through laboratory signalling or clinical outlier data (e.g. reference laboratory values), assessment through algorithm scoring (e.g. Naranjo or population specific), as well as understanding of the developmental toxicology (e.g. covariates, developmental pharmacology) to avoid re-occurrence and to develop guidelines through, e.g., targeted pharmacovigilance (e.g. visual field defects and vigabatrin).

Modelling and simulation

Quantitative pharmacology and pharmacometrics through modelling and simulation is a powerful tool to improve the quality and the feasibility of clinical studies and to avoid conventional PK studies. At best, such pharmacometric programmes integrate already available information through either mechanism-based PK or physiologically based PK. Model-based approaches aim to describe more accurately the age-related factors influencing drug disposition and response in paediatric patients.

Biomarkers in paediatrics

Despite the frequent utilisation of biomarkers in medical practice to assess the effects of drugs, there is only limited information about and validation of biomarkers in paediatric drug trials and pharmacotherapy. Biomarkers assumed to be efficacious in adults are simply extrapolated to the paediatric clinical setting, without considering that the pathogenesis can be different in children, while ontogeny may also affect disease evolution and therapeutic responses.

Conclusions

Developmental PK hereby represents the mathematical description of the concentration–time profile. All consecutive PK processes (ADME) display maturation. PD describes the relationship between a given concentration and the extent of a specific response.

The two most important parameters of the PK are the volume of distribution (V_d) and clearance (CL). V_d can be defined as a proportionality constant that links the amount of drug administered to the measured plasma concentration. CL represents the volume of blood or plasma from which a given drug is completely removed per unit of time.

Specific characteristics of pharmacotherapy and drug evaluation in children include unlicensed and off-label drug use in children, drug formulations, paediatric adverse drug reactions, drug toxicity and pharmacovigilance, paediatric modelling and simulation, and the use of biomarkers in paediatrics.[3]

References

1 Ito S. Children: are we doing enough? *Clin Pharm Ther* 2015; 98: 222–224.
2 Ferro A. Paediatric prescribing: why children are not small adults. *Br J Clin Pharmacol* 2015; 79: 351–353.
3 Macleod SM. A quarter century of progress in paediatric clinical pharmacology: a personal view. *Br J Clin Pharmacol* 2016; 81(2): 228–234.

2

Pharmacokinetics: an overview

E Jacqz-Aigrain

Introduction

Pharmacokinetics (PK) is defined as the impact of the body on the drug. It is a global description of the disposition of the drug and quantifies changes in the amount of drug in the body with time. PK is dependent upon drug characteristics (molecular weight, acid dissociation constant (p*Ka*) and ionisation) and drug–patient interactions.[1]

The learning objectives of this chapter are:

➢ to recognise key PK parameters
➢ to become familiar with different types of PK analysis: non-parametric, parametric and model-based approaches
➢ to be aware of the benefits of model-based methods for analysing paediatric PK data.

Pharmacokinetic parameters

In a PK study, whatever the methods (classical rich PK or population PK analysis, each discussed below), the aim is to determine key PK parameters in order to describe and quantify drug disposition:

T_{max}: time to reach the maximum concentration
C_{max}: maximum concentration
AUC (area under the (concentration–time) curve): measure of exposure, reflecting the amount of drug that reaches the central compartment (where it is usually measured)
Clearance: a measure of drug elimination from the body.

The total clearance is the sum of all clearances, as the drug may be cleared by metabolism by the liver, the lungs, excretion through the kidneys, the skin, and so on.

Clearance, depending on AUC, is a measure of drug elimination. It is easily calculated from the area under the curve, using the following equation:

$$CL = D/AUC$$

D is the amount of drug, in the central compartment. D should be corrected by the factor (F) measuring bioavailability in case of non-intravenous administrations (oral, intramuscular, etc.), as the equation measures the clearance of the available drug.

Many factors may affect a drug. For a given drug, clearance is dependent on pathways of elimination – renal, hepatic or both. This explains that renal impairment, affecting clearance, requires dosage adjustments based on the degree of impairment (chapter 47). It is acknowledged that in adults, reduction of creatinine clearance to $60\,mL/min/1.73\,m^2$ requires adjustment of renally excreted drugs. Hepatic clearance is dependent on two variables: hepatic blood flow and extraction coefficient (a measure of enzyme metabolic capacity). In children, renal and hepatic clearances vary widely with age, explaining the major differences in PK parameters in paediatric patients compared with adults. Changes with development and age result in a low renal clearance adjusted to weight, compared to adults, in neonates (particularly if premature), that increases in the first month of life. Similarly, hepatic clearance is low at birth because of immaturity. Enzyme activities increase independently after birth, reaching levels that may be above adult levels in infants and children, before then decreasing to reach adult levels.

Volume of distribution is an artificial, non-physiological volume quantifying the equilibrium between the central and peripheral compartments:

$$Vd = D/C0$$

D is the dose.

C0 is the concentration at the time of administration, and usually extrapolated to the time of intravenous administration (origin on the concentration–time curve).

Half-life

Elimination half-life is the time taken for the amount (or concentration) of the drug to halve. If the time to halve the amount (or concentration) is constant, then drug elimination is almost complete after five half-lives (after one half-life, 50% of the drug is eliminated; after two half-lives, 75%; after three, four, five half-lives, 85.5, 93.75 and 96.875%, respectively).

These PK parameters are revisited in the related chapters that follow.

Description of a pharmacokinetic curve

Drug concentrations are usually measured in the vascular space and reported as a concentration (Y axis) versus time (X axis) curve. The shape of the curve is dependent upon the route of administration (intravenously or orally in most cases) and the drug disposition within the body.

Routes of administration

After intravenous administration, the total amount of the drug dose reaches the vascular space and, in the absence of an absorption phase, concentrations decrease from a maximum concentration, as the drug is distributed and eliminated by metabolism and excretion. Although simultaneous, these two phases can be identified and separated on the curve, as distribution is rapid with an initial deep decrease in concentrations, while metabolism results in a slower decrease and flatter slope.

After oral administration, the time for absorption is illustrated by an initial increase of drug concentrations (absorption phase). The amount of drug reaching the central compartment is frequently lower than the dose taken by the patient, as part of it may be lost before reaching the vascular space by the first-pass effect.

Compartment models

PK data can be described using compartmental models.[2] The simplest model is a one compartment open model (see Figure 1): the body is analysed as one homogeneous volume, with immediate distribution and equilibrium of the drug throughout the body, and the concentration decreases in an exponential manner against time. For most drugs, the disposition is more complex and a two-compartment model is frequently the best model to fit the concentration–time points, with a bi-exponential decrease in concentrations versus time.

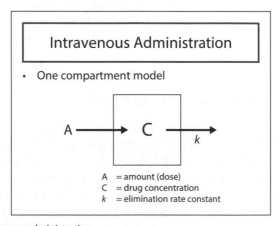

Figure 1 Intravenous administration

First or zero order pharmacokinetics

If PK is first order, the amount of drug absorbed (oral route) and eliminated (whatever the route: metabolised by the liver and/or cleared by the kidneys) is proportional to the amount of drug present. By contrast, in zero order kinetics the amount of drug absorbed or eliminated is constant, whatever the amount of drug present.

Analysis of classical (rich) pharmacokinetic data

Non-parametric analysis

Non-parametric analysis allows calculation of individual PK parameters, based on the concentrations measured at different time points and reported on the PK curve for one individual, without any initial assumption about drug disposition. This analysis does not require any hypothesis about how the drug is distributed, i.e. whether the drug is distributed in a unique compartment or multiple compartments (meaning that the body can be described as a unique compartment or multiple compartments).

The data required are: time of drug administration and dose, multiple drug concentrations and corresponding time after administration. Such information allows the following to be determined by inspection of the PK curve: the maximum concentration (C_{max}) and time to reach it after administration (T_{max}). The area under the concentration versus time curve from drug administration (T0) to last measured concentration (T) (AUC0-T) is calculated by the trapezoidal rule (addition of the trapezoid areas between two consecutive concentration–time points). This area can also be extrapolated to infinity.

Parametric analysis – modelling

Modelling is a mathematical approach to analysing drug disposition. One to multiple compartments can be tested, assuming that the body is made of either one or multiple compartments. The endpoint is to be able to select the best mathematical equation that will describe the observed concentration versus time curve.

Population pharmacokinetic analysis

During drug development, initial studies are conducted in healthy adult volunteers and then in sick adult patients with the disease of interest. For methodological and ethical reasons, historically most drugs were not studied in children, as the number of samples and blood volumes to be taken were too high. As a consequence, drugs were – and are still – used off label, particularly in the youngest patients, and administered with an empirical determination of dosage regimen extrapolated from adult data using body weight. However, the so-called 'trial and error' method fails to identify covariates with an impact on drug disposition and is associated with a high risk of under- or over-dosing, potentially causing limited efficacy or adverse drug reactions in paediatric patients.

The population approach is very different from the classical approach, as the number of patients studied is higher (to reflect the target population), but the number of samples is limited per patient (from one to two to three, usually).

The population analysis requires samples from many patients from different age groups (from neonates to adolescents), although the exact number needed cannot be calculated using a simple equation and it is dependent on the drug and the associated PK variability. Initially, routine therapeutic drug monitoring concentrations were used for many population studies. It is, however, possible now to conduct a population PK study of a new drug, embedded in the initial phase of an efficacy–safety study, in order to adapt the dosage regimen, initially selected by modelling – extrapolation from adults, older age groups or even animal or juvenile animal data. Such methods allow quantification of the PK parameters in the population of patients studied, but also identification and quantification of the clinical and biological factors (covariates) influencing these parameters.[3]

A population PK analysis follows different steps: 1) the first step aims at selecting the best model for residual variability, i.e. the model associated with the lowest error between the observed and model-predicted concentration. Residual variability quantifies all possible errors affecting the measured concentrations: error in dose, sampling time, drug measurement. 2) The second step is to identify all major covariates that affect drug disposition. In children, factors such as age, weight, associated therapies, disease and disease state, biological parameters of renal and hepatic functions, etc., are important; all these variables should be collected during paediatric PK studies and tested. In paediatric patients, there is a positive correlation between age and weight, and it might be difficult, particularly in neonates, to differentiate the potential impact of size and maturation on drug disposition.[4] Indeed, when renal function is considered, gestational age (size), postnatal age (maturation) and post menstrual age should ideally all be tested.

The theory of allometry, used to predict drug disposition, indicates that clearance is related to weight with a power of 0.75 as a correcting factor, while volume is linearly related to size.[5]

Advantages and limitations of the two approaches

In the classical approach, parameters are calculated for each individual, and precision requires numerous samples per participant (usually from 7–8 to 12 or more). Mean and variability of the PK parameters are reported in the study group of at least six to seven individuals and cannot, of course, be used to describe drug PK in populations or individuals who differ from the initial study group by age, disease or other factors.

In contrast, the model-based approach is based on a limited number of samples taken in numerous subjects. In addition, the mathematical equation to describe the PK curve includes significant covariates and allows dosing to be adapted to predict the impact of changing doses on drug disposition in real patient populations.

Conclusions

This chapter has introduced PK parameters and two key methods of PK analysis: non-parametric approaches (the traditional approaches), which require large numbers of samples per patient, in contrast to model-based approaches (including population PK and physiologically based PK), which require larger numbers of patients but fewer samples per patient. Model-based approaches are particularly beneficial in paediatric studies, which often only obtain a few PK samples per patient. These analytical methods are used to estimate the key PK parameters outlined above, which are important in designing and optimising dosing regimens for patients.

References

1 Benet LZ, Zia-Amirhosseini P. Basic principles of pharmacokinetics. *Toxicol Pathol* 1995; 23: 115–123.
2 Fan J, de Lannoy IA. Pharmacokinetics. *Biochem Pharmacol* 2014; 87: 93–120.
3 Anderson BJ *et al*. Population clinical pharmacology of children: modelling covariate effects. *Eur J Pediatr* 2006; 165: 819–829.
4 Anderson BJ, Holford NH. Mechanism-based concepts of size and maturity in pharmacokinetics. *Ann Rev Pharmacol Toxicol* 2008; 48: 303–332.
5 Holford NH. A size standard for pharmacokinetics. *Clin Pharmacokinet* 1996; 30: 329–332.

3

Drug absorption

K Allegaert and SN de Wildt

Introduction

Pharmacokinetics aims to describe the relationship between a given drug dosage and a drug concentration–time profile. This mathematical description is in essence based on the distribution and subsequent clearance of any drug (either through metabolism or primary elimination). However, when an extravascular route is used, absorption precedes distribution and clearance. Absorption reflects and quantifies the ability of a specific formulation to overcome or cross barriers (e.g. chemical, physical, mechanical, biological) to reach the systemic circulation.

The learning objectives of this chapter are:

> to know the key factors affecting oral and non-oral absorption of drugs in children
> to understand developmental, disease and environmental covariates of bioavailability
> to recognise the link between absorption and clinically relevant observations, since maturational absorption relates to effects or side-effects of specific formulations administered to children.

Formulations and absorption: background

Most commonly, paediatric pharmacotherapy is based on oral formulations. By convention, bioavailability (F) is quantified by comparing the area under the concentration–time curve following the extravascular administration (AUC_{ev}) with the AUC following intravenous administration (AUC_{iv}). The ratio (AUC_{ev}/AUC_{iv}) provides the F estimate. The anticipated absorption or bioavailability throughout the gastrointestinal tract relates to both patient specific characteristics (e.g. maturational changes, morbidity characteristics) as well as to external aspects (e.g. formulation, nutrition, co-medication).[1] Other frequently used extravascular routes in children are transcutaneous, rectal, intramuscular, buccal, inhalational, or topical ophthalmic, while also 'deep' compartment like intra-articular or intravitreal injected formulations may have absorption to the systemic circulation. All these routes also display absorption characteristics that are both formulation as well as patient dependent, including maturational changes.[2]

Oral

Following oral administration of a given formulation, absorption shows extensive maturation because both the gastrointestinal anatomy and function evolve throughout childhood.[3] These maturational changes can be observed throughout the gastrointestinal tract, starting with swallowing, through to saliva production and composition, development of oesophageal motor complexes, gastric changes (e.g. capacity, pH, motor activity), and changes in the duodenum, pancreas and bile (e.g. pH, enzymes, motor activity, bile salts), intestines (e.g. length and surface, motility, drug metabolising enzymes and drug transporters, permeability, microbiome) and colon (e.g. transit time, microbiome). Illustrations of the impact of these maturational changes on drug disposition for specific compounds are provided (Table 1).

Swallowing will transfer food or liquids from the oral cavity to the oesophagus, and this capacity will to a large extent drive the formulations considered in children (e.g. syrup, suspension or mini-tablets compared with regular tablets). The use of a nasogastric tube may result in adherence to the plastic tubing or obstruction.

Gastric pH is a relevant factor for determining the stability of a formulation passing through the stomach, because the low gastric pH acts as a chemical protective barrier to the outside world. The mean gastric pH in the first hour(s) after birth is neutral, with a subsequent decline to acidity. Since gastric pH also depends on the frequency and type of feeding, the median pH remains elevated in neonates.

Gastric emptying appears delayed in early infancy, but also depends on the type of feeding, with faster emptying for human milk compared with formula feeding, to reach adult values at 6–8 months of life.

In contrast, intestinal transit times in neonates and infants are shorter when compared with adults. This will affect the contact time of the drug with the intestinal mucosa and may affect drug specific bioavailability.

The lower bile acid synthesis and pool may affect both micelle formation and enterohepatic recirculation in infants.

Pancreatic lipase is low at birth and reaches an adult level from 9 to 12 months of life onwards. However, this transient deficiency is – at least in part – compensated by exogenous lipase in the mother's milk and gastric lipase.

The main driver of absorption, but also metabolism, for most drugs is the intestinal mucosa. Besides the intestinal surface area, developmental maturation in the activity of drug metabolising enzymes (e.g. CYP3A)

Table 1 Examples of the impact of maturational changes on oral and non-oral absorption of formulations

Oral	
Swallowing	Liquids or mini-tablets are preferred formulations in the first years of life.
Gastric pH	Higher bioavailability following oral penicillin administration in newborns compared with infants or children.
Gastric emptying	The peak concentration of a given compound, e.g. paracetamol, is delayed and lower in infants compared with children.
Intestinal enzymatic activity	First-pass effect is lower and bioavailability higher following oral midazolam in (pre)term neonates, because of lower intestinal (CYP3A) drug metabolism.
Pancreas activity and bile	Reduced uptake of lipophilic drugs, fat-soluble vitamins or enteral-hepatic recirculation.
Microbiome	The need for vitamin K supplementation in the first months of life to avoid vitamin K deficiency subsequently disappears, because vitamin K is generated by the intestinal microflora once this flora is established.
Co-morbidity	Bioavailability after oral administration may be different in the setting of diarrhoea or critical illness. Another, more reliable, route (e.g. intravenous) should be considered.
Non-oral	
Transcutaneous	The higher surface area and the higher permeability results in extensive absorption of iodine or corticosteroids following cutaneous application, and subsequent endocrine disorders. Patches are specific formulations developed for a continuous, stable release. Manipulations (e.g. cutting) or cutaneous lesions (e.g. eczema, burned skin) may alter this disposition.
Rectal	Compared with oral administration, rectal administration of paracetamol results in lower, and less predictable, absorption.
Intravitreal	Intravitreal injection of bevacizumab for retinopathy of prematurity results in appearance in the systemic circulation.
Inhalational	Non-bronchial disposition of steroids may result in tongue hypertrophy, oral candidiasis or systemic corticoid effects.
Buccal	The first 'PUMA' formulation is a buccal midazolam (Buccolam®) formulation, to be used in children with seizures.

and efflux transporters (e.g. efflux transporter P-glycoprotein (P-gp)) is an important covariate of the bioavailability and – related to this – the first-pass process. This also includes the appearance of polymorphism (e.g. P-gp) and environmental (e.g. grapefruit juice, type of feeding – breast milk or formula – and co-medication) related effects. There is also increasing interest, from the developmental pharmacology perspective, in the metabolic activity of the intestinal tract through either gut metabolising enzymes, the gut microflora or their interaction. These interactions are not limited to drug metabolism, but may also affect drug transporter activity as well as bioactivation, biotransformation or biodegradation. It has also been reported that the type of feeding, either mother's milk or formula, affects both the intestinal bacterial flora as well as drug metabolism. It is interesting to speculate that the ontogeny of the intestinal microbiome tailors the ontogeny of drug absorption and metabolism.

Non-oral

Developmental changes can also alter the absorption of drugs administered by non-oral routes, and this may be up to the level of clinical relevance, resulting in either effects or side-effects (Table 1). This relates to changes in either size or composition of the relevant absorptive surfaces (e.g. skin, pulmonary tree) and to formulation specific (e.g. rectal) aspects.

To further illustrate this, the more extensive percutaneous absorption of drugs in infants compared with children is in part explained by the thinner stratum corneum, but also by the difference in the ratio between body surface area and weight (proportionally higher in young children) and by differences in regional perfusion. This may result in unanticipated events like methemoglobinaemia following topical EMLA application.

For inhalational drugs, the formulation (aerosol, spacer, nebuliser, dry power) applied is a very important contributor to the effectiveness of disposition in the bronchial tree. In contrast, the absorption of inhalational agents (e.g. sevoflurane) relates to the alveolar surface area and functional residual capacity (FRC). Since neonates have a proportionally higher alveolar capacity and lower FRC, absorption is more rapid in neonates and infants.

Absorption of drugs following rectal administration in general is less predictable and delayed, but in part also depends on the formulation used (e.g. paracetamol, capsular or triglyceride suppository).

Improving knowledge on absorption in children

To learn more on the ontogeny of absorption processes, various research strategies have been suggested. The final aim is to estimate more precisely the impact of age, but also disease characteristics, environmental factors and genetic polymorphisms, on absorption throughout childhood. The available research strategies are multiple and relate to, e.g., *in vitro* drug dissolution and solubility models.[4] This model tests drug dissolving aspects, combining differences in formulations with different food patterns in an 'out-of-patient' setting. Similar mechanism-based or physiologically based pharmacokinetic models (Simcyp, PKSim, GastroPlus) are also used. The backbone of such models is the availability of data on the ontogeny of intestinal physiology, while validation with *in vivo* data is obviously needed to confirm the model predictions. A recent example on sotalol exposure throughout paediatric life had a good predictability of observed data in adults and children, but not yet in neonates and young infants. *In vitro* drug metabolism and transporter studies in intestinal, cutaneous or other samples can be considered. Finally, the first studies on microdosing (stable labelled or radioactive labelled microdose) to study oral bioavailability are ongoing.

Conclusions

Absorption reflects and quantifies the ability of a specific formulation to overcome or cross barriers (e.g. chemical, physical, mechanical, biological) to appear in the systemic circulation. Following oral administration of a given formulation, absorption displays extensive maturation because the gastrointestinal anatomy and function evolve throughout childhood. The ontogeny of absorption is further driven by environmental, disease related or polymorphism related factors. Developmental changes can also alter the absorption through non-oral routes. This relates to changes in either size or composition of the relevant absorptive surfaces (e.g. skin, pulmonary tree) and to formulation specific (e.g. rectal) aspects.

To learn more about the ontogeny of absorption processes, research strategies have been suggested. These research models include *in vitro* drug dissolution and solubility models, mechanistic or physiologically based PK modelling, *in vitro* drug metabolism and transporter studies, and microdosing.

References

1   Kearns GL *et al*. Developmental pharmacology – drug disposition, action, and therapy in infants and children. *N Engl J Med* 2003; 349(12): 1157–1167.
2   Batchelor HK, Marriott JF. Paediatric pharmacokinetics: key considerations. *Br J Clin Pharmacol* 2015; 79(3): 395–404.
3   Mooij MG *et al*. Ontogeny of oral drug absorption processes in children. *Expert Opin Drug Metab Toxicol* 2012; 8(10): 1293–1303.
4   Arahamse E *et al*. Development of the digestive system – experimental challenges and approaches of infant lipid digestion. *Food Dig* 2012; 3(1–3): 63–77.

4

Drug distribution: from birth to adolescence

K Allegaert and JN van den Anker

Introduction

As mentioned earlier (chapter 2), pharmacokinetics aims to describe the relationship between a given drug dosage and a drug concentration–time profile. This mathematical description is, in essence, based on the volume of distribution (V_d) and subsequent total body clearance (either metabolism or primary elimination). The combination of both is reflected in the still commonly used serum elimination half-life ($t_{1/2}$). V_d can be defined as a proportionality constant that links the amount of a given drug to the measured plasma or serum concentration. This volume does not necessarily represent a real physiological volume, but an apparent volume into which the drug would have been distributed (if it were uniformly distributed) to achieve the measured concentration [(V_d, litres) = amount (mg) of the drug/concentration (mg/L)] of the drug. Since V_d determines in part the concentration, this means that drug distribution can alter the desired effects, side-effects and duration of action of a given drug. The most obvious application is to determine the loading dose required (LD), which is the dose needed to attain the target concentration (Ct) [Ct = dose (mg/kg)/V_d (L/kg)]. A drug with a high V_d will need a large loading dose.

When reaching the systemic circulation, a specific compound will distribute in different tissues or organs. This distribution pattern will, in part, depend on physical (e.g. only extracellular or also intracellular, lipophilic or water soluble compound, molecular size, ionisation) and physiological (e.g. protein binding, permeation to deep compartments, tissue uptake) processes. Consequently, distribution is driven by the extent of protein binding, systemic and regional blood flow, permeability of physiological barriers (e.g. meningeal, placental barrier; in part related to drug transporters) and body composition. Obviously, these covariates will display interpatient and intrapatient variability, also in part explained by or reflecting maturational changes or disease related differences.

The learning objectives of this chapter are:

➤ to understand that changes during growth and development in childhood can affect a drug's apparent V_d
➤ to recognise the key developmental factors determining V_d, namely body composition, protein binding capacity and membrane permeability
➤ to be aware that disease related changes (i.e. pathophysiology) can also alter V_d.

Maturational changes throughout childhood

Although the V_d reflects an apparent volume, the estimates are affected by maturational, age-dependent, changes, including but not limited to body composition, protein binding capacity and membrane permeability to reach deep compartments.[1]

The impact of body composition

Age dependent changes in body composition alter the physiological spaces into which a drug will distribute. Neonates and infants have a proportionally higher amount of body water per kilogram of body weight when compared with children and adults, and preterm neonates have an even higher value when compared with term neonates.[2] For the total body water content, this is about 80% in preterm and 70% in term neonates, with a progressive decrease to about 60% at the end of infancy and subsequent stabilisation throughout childhood, as demonstrated in Figure 1. This pattern is similar for the extracellular water content, starting at 40% and decreasing to about 25–30% at the end of infancy. For the lipid compartment, the trends are somewhat more complex, with an initial increase from 10–15% at birth to 20–25% at the end of infancy, and a subsequent decrease back to 10–15% until adolescence.

Larger extracellular and total body water spaces in neonates and infants result in lower plasma concentrations for drugs that distribute into these respective compartments when administered in a weight-based fashion.[3] For lipophilic compounds, the reverse is true. To illustrate this, the V_d of aminoglycosides (water soluble) displays a progressive decrease within neonates (extreme preterm, 0.7 L/kg, to term neonates, 0.5 L/kg) and throughout childhood (0.5 L/kg in neonates, to 0.3 L/kg in young adults). A similar pattern has been described for paracetamol. In contrast, diazepam, a lipophilic compound, has a proportionally lower V_d in the newborn (1.6 L/kg) when compared with children or adults (2.4 L/kg). A similar pattern has been estimated for propofol – another lipophilic

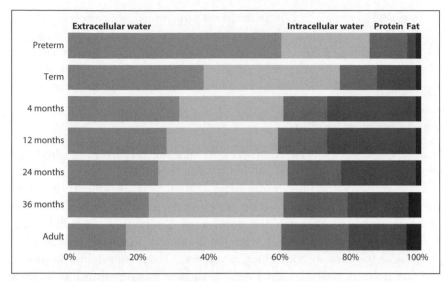

Figure 1 Distribution of body composition

compound – (2.8–5.6 L/kg in the newborn, up to 5.6–8.6 L/kg in toddlers) throughout early childhood.

Protein binding

Protein binding also influences drug distribution. Compared with adults, infants and children have lower concentrations of the principal plasma binding proteins like albumin, alpha-1 acid glycoprotein and plasma globulins. As protein levels reach adult values in infancy, this effect is likely to be most pronounced in newborns and infants. Besides the absolute values or concentrations, competitive binding with endogenous compounds (e.g. bilirubin, free fatty acids) may further affect the binding capacity. In the newborn, there is a simultaneous lower concentration of the plasma proteins, in combination with raised bilirubin and/or raised free fatty acids.

A recent example for illustration is the protein binding of cefazolin to albumin: the free fraction is related to the total concentration and albuminaemia, but – even after considering these covariates – it remains higher in the newborn. Similar patterns have been described for other antibiotics (ampicillin, flucloxacillin), antiepileptics (e.g. phenytoin) and chemotherapeutics (e.g. etoposide). Reduced protein binding increases the free concentration and the free fraction of drugs, thereby influencing the availability of the active drug to diffuse more easily to other compartments, to interact more with receptors and/or to be cleared more rapidly (higher clearance). Similarly, when higher free fractions of a given compound are circulating in the plasma compartment, these fractions are able to penetrate to deeper tissue compartments, resulting in a higher V_d.

In general terms, it can be assumed that the influence of protein binding on free plasma drug concentrations is limited to drugs that have a high degree of protein binding ($>90\%$) and a narrow therapeutic index (e.g. phenytoin, etoposide). This is because only a minor difference in protein binding will result in a significant difference in the free concentration of the given drug.

Membrane permeability

Drug distribution to deep compartments like the cerebrospinal fluid and brain compartment is delayed and limited due to endothelial 'tight junctions' in combination with efflux transporters. This is why intrathecal injections are performed to bypass this barrier for children with, e.g., acute leukaemia or brain tumours. Although the number of observations is still limited, it seems that there are also maturational changes in this barrier, with a progressive increase in both efflux transporter (P-glycoprotein) expression and function, as well as tight junction (higher passive diffusion in early infancy) capacity.

Disease related differences

The phenotypic V_d estimates throughout childhood are, to a large extent, driven by maturational changes. However, these estimates may be further affected by disease related changes in body composition, protein binding capacity or membrane permeability.

Both obesity and malnutrition are of importance in children. At present, a single size descriptor to estimate the V_d values of all drugs in both lean and obese children does not exist, but it is reasonable to anticipate that a higher fat mass mainly alters the distribution of lipophilic drugs and has more limited impact on water soluble compounds. Based on the currently available evidence, protein malnutrition does not extensively affect V_d for most compounds, but does affect absorption, and clearance to a larger extent. Similarly, the presence of a patent ductus arteriosus or sepsis has been associated with a further increase in the V_d in (pre)term neonates, most pronounced for water soluble compounds. Also, the use of extracorporeal membrane oxygenation will affect drug disposition, because of the additional external volume (membrane and tubing), as well as the lower plasma protein and associated fluid retention commonly observed.

Protein binding is obviously affected in the setting of hypo-albuminaemia (e.g. nephrotic syndrome, syndrome of inappropriate ADH secretion (SIADH)), but also environmental aspects (pH, free fatty acids, competitive binding) may affect protein binding characteristics. Competitive binding is a major issue in neonates with hyperbilirubinaemia, since displacement of initially bound bilirubin may result in kernicterus. This is why ceftriaxone should not be given to neonates with hyperbilirubinaemia. Binding characteristics may also relate to disease states, as, e.g., alpha-1 acid glycoprotein will increase after surgery, resulting in a somewhat higher binding capacity for local anaesthetics. Finally, besides maturational changes, membrane permeability may also be affected by disease states. In the setting of meningitis, the associated inflammation will result in less effective tight junctions, and a similar pattern can be anticipated in the setting of severe intracranial trauma.

Conclusions

The V_d is an apparent volume into which the drug has been distributed (if it were uniformly distributed) to achieve the measured concentration [$(V_d$, litres) = amount (mg)/concentration (mg/L)]. V_d depends on physical (e.g. only extracellular, or also intracellular, lipophilic or water soluble compound, molecular size, ionisation) and physiological (e.g. protein binding, permeation to deep compartments, tissue uptake) processes. Because of this, V_d also depends on maturational, age dependent, changes, including body composition, protein binding capacity, and membrane permeability. Finally, V_d may also depend on disease characteristics like obesity or malnutrition, sepsis, patent ductus arteriosus, regional perfusion/inflammation or treatment modalities (extra-corporeal membrane oxygenation).

References

1 Batchelor HK, Marriott JF. Paediatric pharmacokinetics: key considerations. *Br J Clin Pharmacol* 2015; 79(3): 395–404.
2 Kearns GL *et al*. Developmental pharmacology—drug disposition, action, and therapy in infants and children. *N Engl J Med* 2003; 349(12): 1157–1167.
3 Rakhmanina NY, van den Anker JN. Pharmacological research in pediatrics: from neonates to adolescents. *Adv Drug Deliv Rev* 2006; 58(1): 4–14.

5

Drug metabolism

K Allegaert and JN van den Anker

Introduction

This chapter focuses on drug metabolism in children.

The learning objectives of this chapter are:

> to understand that the biological purpose of drug metabolism is to convert compounds into more polar, water soluble compounds to facilitate subsequent elimination by the bile or urinary route

> to understand that the major drug metabolism pathways are commonly divided into phase I and phase II reactions

> to understand that phase I involves processes including oxidation, reduction, hydration or hydrolysis

> to understand that phase II involves glucuronidation, sulfation, methylation, acetylation or glutathione conjugation

> to understand that throughout childhood, the main factors determining drug metabolism relate to growth and maturation.

Drug metabolism: an overview

As mentioned earlier (chapter 2), pharmacokinetics aim to describe the relationship between a given drug dosage and a drug concentration–time profile. This is in essence based on distribution (chapter 4) and clearance. Clearance is defined as the volume of fluid that, for a given time interval, is completely cleared of a specific compound through either metabolism (chapter 5) or primary elimination (chapter 6). Clearance represents the capacity to eliminate a given drug from the body and thereby reflects the average steady state or median concentration achieved with a maintenance dose.

Metabolic clearance relates to the regional blood flow, the compound specific extraction rate and the intrinsic isoenzyme specific capacity. The biological purpose of drug metabolism – similar to the metabolism of endogenous compounds – is to convert compounds into more polar (e.g. through oxidation, glucuronidation), water soluble compounds to facilitate subsequent elimination via bile or the urinary route. However, some prodrugs first have to undergo metabolism to become active compounds (e.g. codeine to morphine, mycophenolate mofetil to mycophenolic acid, cyclophosphamide to 4-hydroxy cyclophosphamide, ifosfamide to 4-OH-ifosfamide, enalapril to enalaprilat).[1]

It is generally claimed that the major site of drug metabolism is within the liver, although the first-pass effect is also driven by intestinal drug metabolism, while other organs like kidneys, lung, blood cells (e.g. esterase function, red blood cells), placenta or brain may also display relevant drug metabolic capacity. The major pathways involved in drug metabolism are commonly divided into phase I or phase II reactions. Phase I mainly covers 'destructive' processes and results in structural changes of the compound, while phase II reactions are synthetic in their pattern. Phase I involves processes like oxidation, reduction, hydration or hydrolysis. The most relevant group of isoenzymes is the cytochrome P450 (CYP) enzymes, with a major contribution of CYP3A4/5 isoenzymes involved in the metabolism of about 50–60% of all therapeutic drugs currently on the market. Other relevant isoenzymes are CYP1A2, CYP2B6, CYP2C8-10, CYP2C19, CYP2D6 and CYP2E1. Phase II involves glucuronidation, sulfation, methylation, acetylation or glutathione conjugation. The most relevant group of isoenzymes involved is the UDP-glucuronosyltransferases (UGT). Because of substrate specificity, drug–drug interactions mainly relate to phase I processes, while phase II metabolism is important for detoxification (e.g. paracetamol metabolism) of reactive molecules initially produced by phase I metabolism.

The phenotypic drug metabolising capacity observed or estimated in an individual patient is affected by multiple covariates. Throughout childhood, the most obvious covariates relate to growth and maturation, and are reflected or quantified by weight, length, age, body surface area or lean body mass. These maturational differences often result in different disposition patterns throughout childhood when children are compared with adults, and are of clinical relevance to determine doses, or may explain differences in (side) effects. The grey baby syndrome following chloramphenicol exposure relates to impaired glucuronidation; valproate hepatotoxicity in infants and children is likely to relate to differences in capacity of specific isoenzymes (CYP2A6 and different UGTs); while ifosfamide renal tubular toxicity can also be explained by differences in the ontogeny of specific isoenzymes (CYP3A4 vs CYP2B6 ontogeny) in the kidney.[2]

The maturational, i.e. ontogeny related, variability is further affected by interfering disease characteristics (e.g. hepatic failure, renal impairment, haemodynamic changes, sepsis), treatment modalities (e.g. co-medication, extracorporeal membrane oxygenation, whole body cooling) or other specific covariates (e.g. pharmacogenetics, environmental factors, co-treatment with other drugs). All these covariates will affect interpatient as well as intrapatient variability in drug metabolism. In this chapter, we will only focus on adaptations over age; other aspects are covered elsewhere (chapter 8, chapter 10, chapter 11).

Maturational changes throughout childhood

Metabolic clearance relates to regional blood flow, extraction rate and intrinsic isoenzyme specific capacity, and all these aspects may display age related differences. The extraction rate depends on the free concentration or fraction (cf. chapter 4). The ratio of liver weight to body weight is greater in infants and toddlers, and subsequently decreases with age. Related to this, the regional liver blood flow is also higher during infancy and in young children. Finally, the intrinsic clearance capacity relates to the overall microsomal as well as isoenzyme specific activity.

Liver microsomal protein content (20–25 mg/g liver proteins) is low in neonates and subsequently increases with age to reach a maximum level of microsomal protein content (40 mg/g) at about 30 years of age. However, a picture showing that drug metabolism is low in neonates, rising throughout infancy, early childhood and prepuberty to reach adult levels in puberty is too simplistic. Hines *et al.*[3] suggested more recently three different developmental patterns for drug metabolism enzymes: high in fetal life to low or absent postnatally (class 1), stable throughout development (class 2), or low in fetal life to high postnatally (class 3) (Figure 1). Moreover, for a specific isoenzyme, significant inter-individual variation is observed in the timing of these perinatal changes, creating isoenzyme specific windows of hypervariability. This results in age related differences and changes in fractional elimination

Class 1	Class 2	Class 3	
ADH1A		ADH1B	EPHX2
CYP3A7	CYP3A5	ADH1C	FMO3
FMO1	GSTA1	AOX	GSTM
GSTP	GSTA2	CYP1A2	SULT2A1
SULT1E1	SULT1A1	CYP2C9	UGT1A1
SULT1A3		CYP2D6	UGT1A6
		CYP2E1	UGT2B7
		CYP3A4	PON1
		EPHX1	

Figure 1 Human hepatic drug metabolism ontogeny

pathways for specific drugs, and may affect, for example, the magnitude and extent of drug–drug interactions or age related (side) effects. Genetics, comorbidity or environmental issues interact significantly with these developmental changes; ontogeny is only one of the relevant covariates. Finally, it seems that the age dependent isoenzyme specific activity may also be organ specific: CYP3A7 decreases after birth and almost disappears after infancy, but remains relevant in the bronchial tree.

Maturational changes in phase I enzymes

Phase I covers both non-CYP and CYP mediated reactions. Non-CYP mediated isoenzymes relate to flavin-containing mono-oxygenases (FMOs), alcohol, and aldehyde dehydrogenases (ADHs) and esterases. It seems that the FMO-1 activity is high at birth, with a subsequent decrease over the first two years of life (class 1), while FMO-3 ontogeny is the opposite, being low at birth with an age dependent increase (class 3). Overall alcohol dehydrogenase capacity in the newborn liver is about 10% of the adult capacity; however, there are different patterns of ontogeny for different isoenzymes, with a high fetal activity and a subsequent decreasing activity for ADH1 (class 1), and the reverse for ADH2 and ADH3 (class 3). Based on *in vivo* observations (e.g. N1-methylnicotinamide to pyridine conversion), it has been suggested that aldehyde oxidase is lower throughout infancy. Esterase function already matures from at least 28 weeks of gestational age onwards, as reflected in, for example, effective remifentanil or propacetamol degradation in neonatal blood samples (class 2).

CYP1A2 hepatic protein concentrations and *in vitro* activity are very low, with a slow developmental pattern after birth, starting with 5% at birth, to 25% at the end of infancy, and up to only 50% at the age of six years. This is in line with the available *in vivo* observations on, for example, caffeine metabolism and clearance. CYP2B6 expression and activity increases significantly (twofold) in the first month of life, with subsequent conflicting information either suggesting that there are no additional changes between 1 month and 18 years, or a sevenfold increase between 1 year and adulthood. *In vivo* observations relate to ifosfamide, efavirenz or methadone disposition. The CYP2C subfamily covers CYP2C8, 2C9, 2C18 and 2C19. CYP2C9 ontogeny is faster and earlier (from birth onwards) when compared with CYP2C19 ontogeny (only slowly rising in the first 6 months of life). Related *in vivo* observations from the CYP2C subfamily include ibuprofen and warfarin (both 2C9) and pantoprazole (2C19). CYP2D6 is already present in fetal liver tissue, with a subsequent increase in neonatal life and early infancy, with more uncertainty on how the maturational pattern subsequently evolves. Similar patterns have been described for *in vitro* observations on dextromethorphan or tramadol disposition. The CYP3A subfamily covers CYP3A4, CYP3A5 and CYP3A7, with completely different age related activity patterns. CYP3A7 has a high activity during fetal life and early infancy, with a subsequent decrease for hepatic but not for bronchial mucosal tissue. In contrast, CYP3A4/5 matures slowly and only reaches an adult level of activity at the end of infancy. The most extensively evaluated *in vitro* CYP3A4 model compound is midazolam.

Maturational changes in phase II enzymes

Phase II enzymes catalyse different conjugation reactions, including sulfation (SULT), acetylation (N-acetyl transferases; NAT), glutathione conjugation mediated by glutathione transferases (GST), and, most importantly, glucuronidation (UGT). Compared with glucuronidation, sulfation activity is already higher in early infancy, but still limited because of an overall lower capacity. Sulfation is the second major phase II metabolic pathway (catechol or phenol sulfotransferases). Compared with the CYP patterns, drugs are quite commonly metabolised by different UGT isoforms and/or sulfotransferases. Consequently, the isoenzyme specific ontogenic pattern is more difficult to describe based on *in vivo* observations. Moreover, the ratio of glucuronidation to sulfation may also differ throughout development, as illustrated for, for example, paracetamol metabolism. In contrast, this seems not to be the case for, for example, chloramphenicol or propofol. Glutathione conjugation is already at a relevant level of activity at birth (65–70% of the adult level) and is of relevance for, for example, paracetamol detoxification. Based on isoniazid *in vivo* observations, relevant phenotypic acetylation activity and the impact of the different polymorphisms ('slow', 'intermediate' and 'rapid' acetylators) have been described in infants.

The UGTs are responsible for the glucuronidation of hundreds of hydrophobic endogenous compounds and drugs, including morphine or chloramphenicol (both UGT2B7), propofol (UGT1A9) and paracetamol (UGT1A6/1A9). *In vitro* ontogeny data are limited. In fetal liver samples, activity towards substrates was low (1–10% of adult levels) for UGT1A1, UGT1A3, UGT2B6, UGT2B15 and UGT2B17. After birth, UGT1A9 and UGT2B4 activities remain significantly lower in infants (0.5–2 years) than in older children and adults.

How this knowledge can be used to improve pharmacotherapy

The information above on maturation of drug metabolism can be used to predict compound specific or isoenzyme specific patterns. For compound specific patterns, drug metabolising enzymes are important determinants of drug disposition. The fact that their activities are not stable throughout childhood commonly results in different pharmacokinetics and different disposition of drugs metabolised by these enzymes.[3] The consequence of this isoenzyme specific ontogeny is not just maturational related lower total clearance, but it also leads to age related variation of the contribution by different pathways, as has been illustrated for, for example, dextromethorphan metabolism. The urine ratio of the different metabolites evolves through infancy because of the initially faster CYP2D6 activity, subsequently taken over by the increasing CYP3A4 capacity. This is also of relevance to predicting or anticipating drug–drug interactions (chapter 11).

Isoenzyme specific patterns can also be used to estimate or predict drug disposition. The impact of developmental changes in drug metabolism on drug efficacy and safety throughout paediatric life has been studied increasingly, and more and more compound specific observations have been reported. Translation of existing knowledge to dosing guidelines and clinical trial design is needed urgently. It should be noted that extrapolation can avoid some pharmacokinetic studies by reducing the need to study the compound in each subpopulation if the drug's pharmacokinetics can be predicted reliably. Such extrapolations can be performed between populations or between drugs that undergo elimination through the same route.

Conclusions

The phenotypic drug metabolising capacity observed or estimated is affected by multiple covariates. Throughout childhood, the most obvious covariates relate to growth and maturation. Thinking of drug metabolism as low in neonates, rising throughout infancy, early childhood and prepuberty to reach adult levels in puberty is too simplistic. Genetics, comorbidity or environmental issues further interact with these developmental changes; ontogeny is only one of the relevant covariates. Translation of the existing knowledge on ontogeny into age adjusted dosing guidelines and clinical trial design is a powerful tool to improve pharmacotherapy, clinical study design and to predict effects/side-effects throughout childhood.

References

1   Kearns GL *et al*. Developmental pharmacology—drug disposition, action, and therapy in infants and children. *N Engl J Med* 2003; 349(12): 1157–1167.
2   de Wildt SN. Profound changes in drug metabolism enzymes and possible effects on drug therapy in neonates and children. *Expert Opin Drug Metab Toxicol* 2011; 7(8): 935–948.
3   Hines RN. Developmental expression of drug metabolizing enzymes: impact on disposition in neonates and young children. *Int J Pharm* 2013; 452(1–2): 3–7.

6

Drug elimination

D Mekahli and K Allegaert

Introduction

Drugs can be eliminated either unaltered (as the mother compound) or in the form of metabolites. The objectives for this chapter are to learn that:

➤ generally the most important route of elimination is renal
➤ renal elimination covers glomerular filtration rate (GFR) and renal tubular transport
➤ these renal processes do not necessarily mature simultaneously
➤ assessment of renal function by a single plasma creatinine measurement has serious limitations
➤ the rate of maturation of different elimination routes (either hepatic or renal) also varies.

Background

Drug clearance represents the capacity to excrete a given drug from the body and thereby reflects the average steady state or median concentration achieved with a maintenance dose. Clearance is defined as the volume of fluid that, for a given time interval, is completely cleared of a specific compound through either metabolism (chapter 5) or elimination. As mentioned above, the most important route of elimination is renal, except for specific compounds or situations where non-renal routes predominate, such as exhalation (e.g. inhalational anaesthetics), transcutaneous elimination (e.g. transcutaneous water losses in preterm neonates), or where hepato-biliary elimination (e.g. micafungin) may be of relevance. This elimination covers the mother compound and also the drug metabolites (both active and inactive).

Maturational changes in renal elimination capacity

The final destiny of the majority of drugs and their metabolites is elimination by the renal route. Consequently, it is important to understand the maturation of renal elimination capacity. Maturation of renal elimination capacity is a continuous process, which starts during fetal organogenesis and only completes at the end of childhood. Renal elimination covers both GFR and renal tubular transport activity (both excretion and absorption). Intriguingly, these processes do not mature simultaneously.[1] This is because the developmental increase in glomerular filtration relies on the extent of glomerulogenesis (completed at about 34 weeks' gestational age), but also depends on the perinatal changes in renal and intrarenal blood flow.[2] Maturational patterns of tubular functions are much less explored.

Given these two driving forces, GFR maturation depends on aspects of maturation at birth (e.g. birth weight, gestational age) as well as postnatal changes (e.g. postnatal age). To further put this into some perspective, the GFR is $20-45$ mL/min/1.73 m^2 in the term neonate, with a subsequent progressive increase of $5-10$ mL/min/1.73 m^2/week. When corrected for body surface area, GFR values reach adult values in the second half of infancy (at 8 months). When expressed in a weight corrected approach (/kg), GFR relative to age is several-fold higher in toddlers than adults. Similarly, renal tubular functions (secretion, absorption) also display maturation, but with a somewhat later onset and rate, to reach adult capacity at the end of the first year of life. Tubular secretion of organic anions at birth is about 20–30% of adult values, but the ontogeny of individual transporters in the renal tubular cells is largely unknown.

How to assess the renal elimination capacity

GFR estimates based on single plasma creatinine measurement are commonly used. However, before creatinaemia can be used to estimate renal drug elimination capacity, there are some analytical issues that need to be considered. Creatinaemia *at birth* does not yet reflect neonatal renal function, but instead reflects maternal renal clearance. In early postnatal life and because of passive leakage into the tubules, creatinine clearance does not yet fully reflect GFR. The postnatal pattern in creatinine trends is based on an initial increase in creatinine. This increase is most pronounced and delayed in the most immature neonates. This is followed by a subsequent decrease, most delayed in the most immature neonates. Finally, absolute creatinine values also depend on the technique used to quantify them. It is generally accepted that the Jaffe colorimetric quantification method overestimates the creatinine concentration when compared with an isotope dilution mass spectroscopy (IDMS) traceable enzymatic technique. The extent of the absolute differences between both techniques and reference values for neonates are provided in Table 1.

In a regular, non-complicated medical setting (no critical illness, no renal impairment), the clinician will very likely rely on the general trends in renal maturation or single creatinine values. In contrast, in cases with altered

Table 1 Postnatal trends (consecutive days) in median serum creatinine values for different birth weight categories. Serum creatinine was quantified by either enzymatic analysis or the Jaffe quantification method. Differences in median values are between 0.1 and 0.245 mg/dL.

<1 kg	D1	D2	D3	D4	D5	D6	D7	D8	D14	D21	D28	D42
Enzyme	0.58	0.85	0.91	0.88	0.825	0.82	0.75	0.73	0.695	0.58	0.465	0.42
Jaffe	0.75	1	1.09	1.09	0.98	0.93	0.88	0.84	0.765	0.68	0.61	0.54
Diff	0.17	0.15	0.18	0.21	0.155	0.11	0.13	0.11	0.07	0.1	0.145	0.12
1–2 kg												
Enzyme	0.61	0.82	0.77	0.68	0.63	0.64	0.59	0.585	0.59	0.51	0.43	0.375
Jaffe	0.78	0.97	0.95	0.88	0.85	0.81	0.77	0.775	0.72	0.63	0.58	0.52
Diff	0.17	0.15	0.18	0.2	0.22	0.17	0.18	0.19	0.13	0.12	0.15	0.145
2–3 kg												
Enzyme	0.64	0.79	0.68	0.56	0.49	0.46	0.48	0.45	0.47	0.37	0.34	0.29
Jaffe	0.8	0.95	0.88	0.78	0.74	0.705	0.65	0.66	0.62	0.6	0.535	0.46
Diff	0.16	0.16	0.2	0.22	0.25	0.245	0.17	0.21	0.15	0.23	0.195	0.17
>3 kg												
Enzyme	0.65	0.71	0.63	0.5	0.45	0.41	0.4	0.4	0.375	0.35	0.3	0.27
Jaffe	0.88	0.935	0.81	0.71	0.66	0.67	0.65	0.63	0.59	0.55	0.505	0.51
Diff	0.23	0.225	0.18	0.21	0.21	0.26	0.25	0.23	0.215	0.2	0.205	0.24

renal function (congenital, acquired, drug induced) and in the setting of pharmacotherapy with narrow safety margins (e.g. chemotherapy), GFR estimates through repeated creatinine measurements, cystatin C or technetium-99 m diethylene-triamine-pentacetate (DTPA) may be more appropriate. Creatinine clearance can be calculated based on serum and urine creatinine measurements [$CL_{crea} = Crea_{ur}$ (mg/dL) × urine volume (mL/min)/$Crea_{ser}$], preferably based on 24 hour urine collections. Indirect calculations based on only serum creatinine values are also commonly used. When these conversion formulae are applied, it is also of relevance to know whether or not an IDMS traceable creatinine measurement technique has been used. Box 1 provides an overview of the two different formulae and how to apply these formulae throughout childhood.

Box 1 Schwartz Formulae

How to estimate creatinine clearance (CL_{crea}) from serum creatinine ($crea_{ser}$) values based on Schwartz estimates (IDMS = isotope dilution mass spectroscopy).

Original Schwartz estimate: Serum creatinine ($crea_{ser}$) is measured based on a non-IDMS traceable assay, most likely Jaffe colorimetric technique.

$$CL_{crea} = [K \times height/crea_{ser}]$$

K = age related factor 0.33, in low birth weight
infant, < 1 year
0.45, in term infant, < 1 year
0.55, child or adolescent girl
0.70, adolescent boy

Revised Schwartz estimate: Serum creatinine ($crea_{ser}$) is measured based on an IDMS traceable assay, most likely an enzymatic technique.

$$CL_{crea} = [0.413 \times height/crea_{ser}]$$

How does this relate to renal drug clearance?

Developmental changes in renal elimination capacity can dramatically affect drug clearance of compounds with extensive or exclusive renal elimination. Consequently, for drugs that are primarily eliminated by the renal route, clinicians must tailor dosing regimens to both maturational as well as other covariates [factors such as congenital or acquired renal impairment, co-treatment with ibuprofen, perinatal asphyxia, or patients post chemotherapy with renal toxicity (cisplatinum, ifosfamide, methotrexate)].

A commonly used example to illustrate this is the correlation between maturation of aminoglycoside clearance reflecting GFR ontogeny (Figure 1). Similar patterns are reflected in the age-dependent trends in the clearance of vancomycin or penicillins. These patterns are accounted for in dosage recommendations by several sources.

Compound specific maturation may also be affected by renal tubular transport processes (passive/active) or plasma protein binding aspects (e.g. cefazolin, vancomycin, flucloxacillin). Furthermore, concomitant administration of medications (prenatal lung maturation with betamethasone,

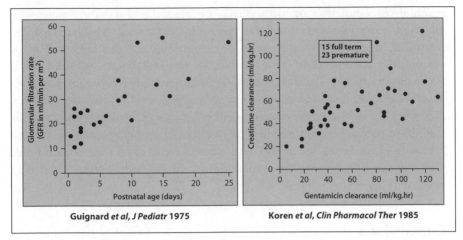

Figure 1 Correlation between the ontogeny of glomerular filtration and gentamicin clearance[3,4]

ibuprofen/indomethacin in neonates or young infants, cisplatinum nephro-toxicity) or disease characteristics (e.g. peripartum asphyxia) may result in extensive intrapatient variability in renal function, resulting in the suggestion to consider monitoring renal function more regularly in these circumstances.

When trying to improve individualised pharmacotherapy and patient safety, it is important to stress two additional emerging concepts: critical illness related hyperfiltration (also known as augmented renal clearance – ARC) and, secondly, the complex interaction between maturational trends in metabolic and renal elimination clearance throughout childhood. These phenomena should prompt increased vigilance for adverse events or failed therapy, and may require therapeutic drug monitoring in some situations. Drug dosing in renal replacement therapy is another important area of research but is outside the scope of this chapter.[4]

We still commonly anticipate that a critically ill patient is more likely to display reduced renal clearance capacity, and assessment tools, e.g. creatinine serum values, have been developed to quantify the reduction in clearance, not augmented clearance. For compounds where the link between dose and effect cannot be observed directly (e.g. antibiotics) and that undergo clearance through renal elimination, this may be of clinical relevance. Augmented renal clearance has been observed in about 25% of adult intensive care patients. This may also be the case in infants and children, but the integration of these concepts into developmental pharmacology is partly hampered by the interfering maturational covariates.

Similarly, we have to take into account that the maturation of differ-ent elimination routes (either hepatic or renal) may be different. This may result in accumulation of metabolites, because the elimination pathways are even more immature than the metabolic pathways. As illustrated for tramadol, and more recently also for morphine, midazolam and cefotaxime, the concentration–time profiles of the metabolites (O-desmethyl-tramadol, morphine-3 and morphine-6 glucuronide, 1-hydroxy-midazolam-glucuronide, desacetyl-cefotaxime) not only depend on the formation of these metabolites, but also on their subsequent clearance via renal elimination. For the above-mentioned compounds, this results in higher metabolite plasma concentrations. Given the pharmacodynamic effects of all these metabolites, this may be of relevance to predict or anticipate (side) effects following routine doses of these drugs.

Conclusions

The most relevant route of drug elimination is the renal route, and this relates to both the mother compound and the metabolites. Renal elimination covers GFR and renal tubular transport (excretion, absorption – active/passive). These processes do not necessarily mature simultaneously. When corrected for body surface area ($/m^2$), GFR values reach adult values in the second half of infancy. When expressed in a weight corrected approach (/kg), GFR relative to age is several-fold higher in toddlers.

Although commonly used, assessment of renal function by a single measurement of plasma creatinine has serious limitations. These limitations include differences in analytical methods applied, intrapatient variability, and the difficulty in detecting augmented renal clearance. The maturational slope of distinct elimination routes (either hepatic or renal) is different. This may result in accumulation of metabolites not due to enhanced metabolite formation (via hepatic metabolism), but due to immature elimination capacity.

References

1 Kearns GL *et al.* Developmental pharmacology—drug disposition, action, and therapy in infants and children. *N Engl J Med* 2003; 349(12): 1157–1167.
2 Schreuder MF *et al.* The interplay between drugs and the kidney in premature neonates. *Pediatr Nephrol* 2014; 29(11): 2083–2091.
3 Guignard JP *et al.* Glomerular filtration rate in the first three weeks of life. *J Pediatr* 1975; 87(2): 268–272.
4 Koren G *et al.* A simple method for the estimation of glomerular filtration rate by gentamicin pharmacokinetics during routine drug monitoring in the newborn. *Clin Pharmacol Ther* 1985; 38(6): 680–685.
5 Zuppa AF. Understanding renal replacement therapy and dosing of drugs in pediatric patients with kidney disease. *J Clin Pharmacol* 2012; 52(Suppl 1): 134S–140S.

7

Pharmacodynamics: practical examples

JN van den Anker and K Allegaert

Introduction

Drug therapy is a very powerful tool to improve the medical outcome of children. Yet caregivers still commonly prescribe drug formulations and dosing regimens that initially were developed for adults, extrapolating from indications validated in adult medicine and based on the pathophysiology proper to the adult patient. Pharmacokinetics (PK; absorption, distribution and elimination, through either metabolism or primary renal elimination, **ADME**) estimates the relationship between a drug concentration at a specific site (e.g. plasma, cerebrospinal fluid) and time (i.e. what the body does to the drug). Pharmacodynamics (PD) estimates the relationship between a drug concentration and (side) effects (i.e. what the drug does to the body). Drugs will interact at a specific site, usually a receptor or an enzyme, with a subsequent alteration of their function.

The learning objectives of this chapter are:

> to recognise that age dependent differences in drug action may have a PK and/or a PD basis
> to understand that differences in developmental pharmacology result in differences in drug potency, efficacy and/or toxicity
> to be aware that age related developmental changes in the expression and functionality of receptors and differences in disease status may alter PD, i.e. the pharmacological response or side-effect to a given concentration of a given compound.

Most of the variability observed in pharmacological effects relates to differences in PK, and maturational PD can only be considered once the PK aspects have been taken into account. We aim to illustrate both differences in effects and side-effects, based on available observations in neonates.

Inotropic agents in the neonatal myocardium act in a more limited fashion than inotropic agents in the myocardium of children or adults. This is due to a lower ratio of active myofilaments to non-contractile elements, higher cardiac output per unit surface area, greater stiffness of the ventricles and less developed cardiac sympathetic nerves. Related to differences in side-effects, neonates appear to be less susceptible to renal toxicity induced by aminoglycosides as compared with children and adults. A reduced capacity for intracellular accumulation of aminoglycosides in the tubular epithelial cells of the renal cortex (e.g. differences in megalin and tubulin expression) seems to be the underlying mechanism of this characteristic.

Although developmental PD remains neglected, we have to be aware that both developmental PK and PD will be considered by the authorities and will affect to a large extent the design of a specific paediatric drug development programme (paediatric study decision tree). If it is reasonable to assume that there is a similar concentration–response relationship in children (similar disease progression, similar response to intervention), only PK and safety studies are needed in the different subpopulations. If there is not such a similar concentration–response relationship, PK efficacy and safety trials are needed. In the latter scenario, the availability of a PD measurement ('biomarker', B 1.7.3.) to predict efficacy will determine the final study design (e.g. conduct PK/PD studies to get a concentration–response relationship for the PD measurement).[1]

Practical examples of developmental PD

Age dependent differences in wanted and unwanted (side) effects of drugs may have a PK basis, a PD basis, or both. Besides the earlier mentioned illustrations in neonates (cardiac, aminoglycoside toxicity), other examples are provided to stress the relevance of developmental PD.[2] We hereby some-what arbitrarily link these examples to specific paediatric subpopulations, although overlap between the different subpopulations is possible.

Neonates and infants

- Dexamethasone and the associated risk for impaired neurodevelopmental outcome and cerebral palsy; the reason for administering dexamethasone was to wean neonates as quickly as possible off the ventilator to prevent further damage to the lungs in an attempt to mitigate the development of chronic lung disease. The unwanted side-effect of this treatment has been a significant decrease in brain volume in these vulnerable patients.
- Oxygenation saturation levels and the subsequent differences in mortality and morbidity (bronchopulmonary dysplasia, retinopathy of prematur-ity) in preterm neonates; the reason for administering a low amount of oxygen was a successful attempt to prevent retinopathy of prematurity.

The unwanted side-effect of this treatment was a significant increase in mortality due to pulmonary disease.

- Impact of ibuprofen or indomethacin on renal function; the reason for administering ibuprofen or indomethacin was to close a patent ductus arteriosus. The unwanted side-effect of this treatment was impaired renal function, because neonatal renal function largely depends on the prostaglandin driven dilatation of the afferent renal arterioli.
- Exposure to antibiotics and its impact on weight gain and body composition through its effects on the intestinal microflora.
- Neonatal hypoglycaemia and hyperglycaemia, or hypothyroidism and neurocognitive outcome because of the higher sensitivity of the central nervous system to glucose and thyroid hormone in early infancy.
- Developmental toxicology for, e.g., valproate (hepatic failure) or ifosfamide (renal tubular cell dysfunction, Fanconi) due to age related differences in drug metabolism.
- The lymphocyte proliferation response with the same ciclosporin concentration is twofold lower in infants compared with other paediatric populations.
- Paradoxical seizures due to proportional excitatory gamma-aminobutyric acid (GABA) receptor overexpression results in a higher incidence of seizures in infancy.

Children and adolescents

- Impact of steroid exposure on growth.
- Impact of both disease and treatment on normal pubertal development.
- Impact of ethanol, nicotine or other illicit drugs on brain development and maturation and subsequent neurodevelopmental and behavioural outcome.
- Limited to absent effects of tricyclic antidepressants because of a neurodevelopmental delay in the expression and activation of the norepinephrine system.
- Differences in oncological disease patterns in children compared with adolescents and young adults, with significant higher morbidity and mortality in adolescents and young adults; likely to be multifactorial.
- The anticoagulant response to warfarin is higher in prepubertal children, independent from plasma S-warfarin concentrations or vitamin K levels. This suggests a higher sensitivity to warfarin in children, likely due to differences in concentrations of several coagulation factors.

Biomarkers to address the PD gap in children

Related to the above mentioned paediatric study decision tree there is an obvious need to address the 'PD gap' in paediatric drug development.[3] The US National Institutes of Health (NIH) definition of a biomarker is 'any characteristic that is objectively measured and evaluated as an indicator of normal biologic processes, pathogenic processes, but also to quantify the response to a therapeutic (pharmacologic) intervention'. Consequently, biomarkers can be used to quantify disease response or progression (e.g. liver enzymes for hepatitis, creatinine for renal dysfunction, exhaled nitric oxide for bronchial inflammation) or predict a given drug exposure or effect (e.g. polymorphisms of drug metabolising enzymes or receptors), or can be PD (neuro-imaging techniques, neurocognitive outcome assessment, blood pressure, histamine response, pupillary diameter) biomarkers. Biomarkers can also be used as surrogate endpoints, linking pathophysiological processes to clinical endpoints. In some instances, biomarkers are even substitutes for clinical endpoints, and may facilitate the drug approval process.

While the concept of biomarkers can be applied to children as well as to adults, it is obvious that issues like disease incidence, severity, progression and the subsequent response to a specific pharmacological intervention are likely to be different between children and adults, and even within the paediatric population (preterm neonates to adolescents). There is an obvious opportunity to develop or tailor biomarkers to paediatric drug development as a proven method to address the PD gap in paediatrics. Preferably, such biomarkers should be non-invasive, with limited discomfort (if any), and feasible to use within the routine setting of clinical patient care.

To further illustrate this, we refer to the following examples: (1) pupillary measurement to assess the impact of analgesics; (2) the assessment of microcirculation based on laser Doppler flowmetry (cutaneous), capillary glycocalyx and density (mucosal), or retinal imaging (systemic); (3) different breath tests to assess intestinal drug metabolism, gastric emptying or intestinal transit time; (4) exhaled nitric oxide or advanced lung function testing to assess pulmonary diseases; (5) documentation of age dependent reference values for electrocardiograms (ECGs; e.g. maturational and activity related differences in the corrected QT interval (abbreviated QTc, the QT interval being defined from the beginning of the QRS complex to the end of the T wave), to subsequently assess the impact of drugs on QT_c times) or (6) electroencephalograms (EEGs; maturational patterns to subsequently assess the impact of drugs, therapeutic inventions such as whole body cooling, or diseases); (7) prediction of long term neurocognitive outcome based on validated Bayley assessment tools at 18–24 months of life; or (8) the validation of the 6-minutes walking test in children with neuromuscular diseases.

Although all these examples remain somewhat disease specific and anecdotal, they do illustrate the feasibility, the relevance and the urgent need to further develop and validate such 'surrogate' endpoints, thereby linking pathophysiological processes to clinical endpoints in children, similar to the efforts made for diseases that are much more common in adults.

Conclusions

PD estimates the relationship between a drug concentration and (side) effects (i.e. what the drug does to the body). Similar to PK, developmental changes in PD should be considered.

Developmental PD is still neglected. However, we must be aware that both developmental PK and PD are considered by the authorities and will affect to a large extent the design of a specific paediatric drug development programme (paediatric study decision tree).

Although all the examples provided in the PD and the biomarker section remain somewhat anecdotal, they do illustrate the relevance and the urgent need to further develop biomarkers as 'surrogate' endpoints, linking pathophysiological processes to clinical endpoints in children.

References

1 Manolis E, Pons G. Proposals for model-based paediatric medicinal development within the current European Union regulatory framework. *Br J Clin Pharmacol* 2009; 68(4): 493–501.

2 Kearns GL *et al*. Developmental pharmacology—drug disposition, action, and therapy in infants and children. *N Engl J Med* 2003; 349(12): 1157–1167.

3 Kearns GL. Beyond biomarkers: an opportunity to address the 'pharmacodynamic gap' in pediatric drug development. *Biomarkers Med* 2010; 4(6): 783–786.

8

Pharmacogenetics and pharmacogenomics

T de Beaumais and E Jacqz-Aigrain

Introduction

Genomics refers to the identification of genetically determined variations associated with a functional impairment or disease predisposition. Postgenomics refers to the regulation of gene expression and aims to study how genes are transcribed into mRNA (transcriptomics) and produce proteins (proteomics), to quantify metabolites and determine how they influence cellular/tissue biochemistry and metabolism (metabolomics).

Pharmacogenetics is defined as the study of genetic variations, primarily single nucleotide polymorphisms (SNPs) associated with inter-individual differences in drug response, and aims to individualise drug therapy in order to optimise efficacy and reduce toxicity.

The terms pharmacogenetics and pharmacogenomics are frequently used interchangeably in the absence of a consensus definition of these two terms, although in addition to pharmacogenetics, pharmacogenomics aims to develop genomic technologies to discover targets for new drugs.

In contrast to the adult situation, in children a limited number of pharmacogenetic polymorphisms have been studied. Indeed, diseases are different in children, the impact of maturation on gene expression results in genotype–phenotype correlations changing with age, and epigenetic factors may play a major role in the regulation of gene expression over the different age groups, starting during fetal life.

The learning objectives of this chapter are to understand that:

➤ genotype refers to the genetic make-up characterising each individual
➤ phenotype is the observable constitution of each individual, resulting from interactions between genotype and environmental factors
➤ genetic polymorphisms affect key players of drug disposition and effects, including adverse drug reactions

➤ genotype/phenotype correlation changes with age as maturation progresses, and therefore differs between adults and children

➤ in developed healthcare systems, pharmacogenetics and pharmacogenomics are anticipated to play an increasing role in routine paediatric healthcare in the near future.

Pharmacogenetic and epigenetic mechanisms

Pharmacogenetics

Most pharmacogenetic polymorphisms are variations of gene coding regions (exons), including DNA point mutations (SNPs), deletions, rearrangements and amplifications, although alleles' intronic mutations, polymorphisms affecting gene regulation and mRNA processing, are also reported. Pharmacogenetics results in individual variability in gene expression. However, it should be kept in mind that pharmacogenetic markers, i.e. the genotype, only explain part of inter-individual variability, and that phenotype is dependent also on postgenomic events and physiological, pathological and environmental factors (Figure 1).

Epigenetics

Epigenetics is the study of inherited changes in gene expression and phenotype caused by mechanisms other than changes in the underlying DNA sequence. The key epigenetic modifications include three mechanisms: histone and chromatin modifications, changes in DNA methylation, and gene silencing through RNAi.

Gene expression, i.e. individual epigenetic status, changes with age, nutrition and environmental factors. Epigenetics is also a possible link between early life events, such as diet during early development, and adult chronic diseases. It is also modified by maternal factors, as animal experiments have demonstrated that the mother's diet during pregnancy shapes the epigenome of her offspring.

Pharmacogenetic polymorphisms in children

Many pharmacogenetic polymorphisms affecting drug disposition (drug metabolising enzymes and transporters) or drug effect (drug targets) have been characterised in adults. Selected examples include the VKORC1/ CYP2C9 – warfarin, the CYP2D6 – tamoxifen, and the CYP2C19 – clopidogrel.[1]

In children, it has been clear for many years that developmental changes in drug exposure and effects result from interactions between ontogeny and pharmacogenetics, requiring validation of age specific dosage schedules.[2,3]

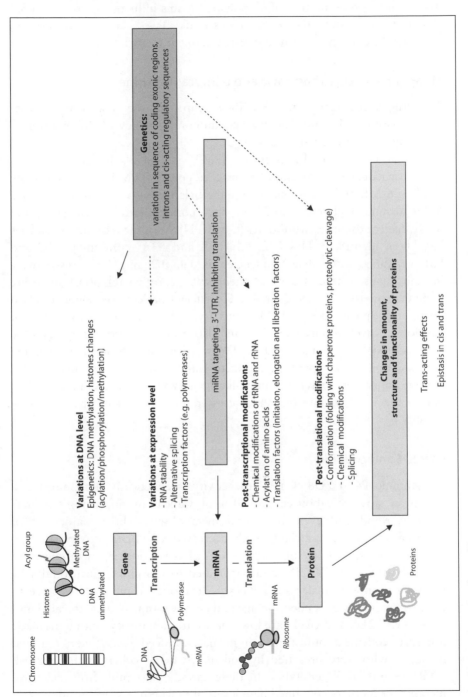

Figure 1 Pharmacogenetic polymorphism

Key examples in children

An exhaustive presentation of all polymorphisms influencing drug response in children is beyond the remit of this book. Two examples are used to illustrate the concept of adapting drug treatment to variability.

Thiopurine methyltransferase and 6-mercaptopurine

The drug 6-mercaptopurine (6-MP) is central to the treatment of acute lymphoblastic leukaemia, the most common malignancy of childhood, representing 80% of paediatric leukaemia.

Thiopurine S-methyltransferase (TPMT) is one of the best examples of pharmacogenetic variation in drug response. TPMT metabolises the prodrug 6-MP and is responsible for the balance with formation of active 6-thioguanine nucleotides (6-TGN), incorporated into nucleic acids and methylmercaptopurine metabolites (6-MMPN). Major loss of function alleles have been identified: TPMT*2, *3C/*3B and *3A (combining *3C and *3B variants), with allele frequencies of 0.4, 0.2 and 4.4% respectively in Caucasians. There is a close phenotype–genotype relationship: severe bone marrow toxicity occurs in TPMT deficient patients receiving standard doses of thiopurine drugs; TPMT heterozygotes are at an increased risk of developing myelosuppression, but are also prone to better early response as measured by minimal residual disease after mercaptopurine including consolidation.[4] Additional genetic factors are currently being investigated. Dosage adjustment based on individual genotype is now recommended as one of the ways to improve the success rate of treatment and to reduce toxicity.[5]

CYP2D6 and codeine

Cytochrome P450 2D6 (CYP2D6) activity is genetically determined and results in slow metabolisers (5–10% of Caucasian populations), intermediate, rapid and even ultra-rapid metabolisers. Three major loss of function alleles are associated with decreased CYP2D6 activity. In paediatrics, one important substrate of CYP2D6 is codeine, metabolised to morphine through CYP2D6 and conjugated to morphine glucuronides by UDP-glucuronosyltransferases (UGTs). Metabolic profile and response to codeine are highly dependent on age and genetics. In neonates, the activities of both CYP2D6 and UGTs are low, related to immaturity, with a dramatic impact of codeine administration in neonates. Indeed, deaths were reported in babies who were breastfed by codeine treated mothers with high risk CYP2D6 and UGT genotypes. In these cases, breast milk from extensive metaboliser mothers contained high levels of morphine, which accumulated, reaching high toxic levels in the newborn, as morphine was not eliminated, because of low activity in neonates. Taken together, these data opened a pro–con debate regarding whether or not to use codeine in children.[6] The CYP2D6 polymorphism is also involved in the variability of response to psychotropic drugs and antidepressants, and genotyping may identify patients who will not respond to treatment or who will develop toxic effects.

Conclusions

Few biomarkers, pharmacogenetic or otherwise, are currently validated or used in paediatrics. Some key pharmacogenetic biomarkers are already important for drug evaluation and development, but also for effective drug treatment in adults and children.[1,7] As research evolves, pharmacogenetics will likely begin to play a more mainstream role in paediatric care, as the relevant laboratory methods become more affordable for developed healthcare systems.

References

1   Becquemont L *et al*. Practical recommendations for pharmacogenomics-based prescription. 2010 ESF-UB Conference on Pharmacogenetics and Pharmacogenomics. *Pharmacogenomics* 2010; 12: 113–124.
2   Kearns GL *et al*. Developmental pharmacology–drug disposition, action, and therapy in infants and children. *N Engl J Med* 2003; 349: 1157–1167.
3   Leeder JS *et al*. Understanding the relative roles of pharmacogenetics and ontogeny in pediatric drug development and regulatory science. *J Clin Pharmacol* 2010; 50: 1377–1387.
4   Adam de Beaumais T *et al*. Determinants of mercaptopurine toxicity in paediatric acute lymphoblastic leukemia maintenance therapy. *Br J Clin Pharmacol* 2011; 71: 575–584.
5   Lennard L. Implementation of TPMT testing. *Br J Clin Pharmacol* 2014; 77: 704–714.
6   Tremlett M *et al*. Pro–con debate: is codeine a drug that still has a useful role in pediatric practice? *Paediatr Anaest* 2010; 20: 183–194.
7   Elie V *et al*. Pharmacogenetics and individualized therapy in children: immunosuppressants, antidepressants and anti-inflammatory drugs. *Pharmacogenomics* 2011; 12: 827–843.

9

Modelling and simulation: pharmacometrics

W Zhao

Introduction

Pharmacological research in children is an important component of drug development programmes. The overall goal is the determination of safe and effective dosing regimens for children. The introduction of the Paediatric Regulation by the European Union (EU), together with the renewal of the Pediatric Rule by the Food and Drug Administration (FDA) on the requirements for paediatric labelling made it mandatory for sponsors to develop drugs for the paediatric population. The development of paediatric dosing regimens is, in general, more complex because of the diversity in this population, ranging from preterm neonates weighing 500 grams to adolescents weighing 100 kilograms. To effectively optimise drug therapy in children, a thorough understanding of developmental pharmacokinetics (PK) (chapter 2) and pharmacodynamics (PD) (chapter 7) is essential.[1]

There has been a growing interest in exploring innovative methodology to optimise drug evaluation and establish evidence-based pharmacotherapy in paediatric clinical practice. In this context, pharmacometrics presents a promising and valuable approach.[2,3] Pharmacometrics is the science of quantitative pharmacology. In its application to paediatrics, it involves primarily developmental PK and PD modelling and simulation (M&S), which can combine information from many diverse sources, such as about drug characteristics, developmental physiology and pharmacology, paediatric disease progression, and statistics.[4]

In this chapter, the principles and methods of PK–PD modelling and simulation are explained. The illustrated examples should be helpful to demonstrate and explain the key elements of M&S application in personalised therapy in children.

The learning objectives of this chapter are:

> to understand the principles of PK–PD M&S in children
> to describe the processes of development and validation of a population PK–PD model
> to provide an example illustrating how to apply M&S to personalised therapy.

PK–PD M&S in children

PK has been defined as 'how the body handles the drug' and describes the relationship between drug dosing and the drug concentration–time profile in the body. PD has been defined as 'how the drug affects the body' and describes the relationship between concentration and effects; an effect can be either efficacy or an adverse event. Two methods are available to analyse concentration–time and concentration–effect datasets obtained in children: the standard two-stage approach and the model-based population approach using non-linear mixed effect models.

Standard two-stage approach, or classical approach

The standard two-stage approach, or classical approach, consists of a first step of estimation of each child's individual PK parameters (i.e. clearance, volume of distribution, area under concentration–time curve) based on individual concentration–time profiles, followed by a second step of description of individual data by summary statistics such as means and standard deviations of PK parameters, and difference in clinical outcome between baseline and end of trial. Such an empirical approach can provide an adequate description of the data but does not allow for making subsequent predictions or understanding the underlying parameters that drive the data. In addition, this methodology requires a relatively high number of samples from each individual patient, which presents a major barrier to performing clinical research in children.

Population approach

The population approach is based on simultaneous analysis of all data of the entire population using a non-linear mixed-effects model, while still taking into account that different observations come from different patients. Such data could be drug concentrations, blood sampling time and dosing regimen in the case of PK data, or physiological data, disease or effect parameters and adverse events in the case of PD data. 'Non-linear' refers to the fact that the dependent variable (i.e. concentration) is non-linearly related to the model parameters and independent variables. 'Mixed effects' refers to the model parameterisation; parameters that do no vary across individuals are referred to as fixed effects; parameters that vary across individuals are referred to as random effects.

The population approach allows not only for the analysis of dense data, but also for sparse and unbalanced data. This feature makes population approaches perfectly suitable in paediatric research, as usually only a limited number of observations can be obtained in paediatric subjects due to ethical and practical constraints discussed in other chapters. Consequently, when designing a paediatric population PK or PK–PD study, blood samples can be collected at different times or set to alternating sampling schemes in subgroups of patients. Samples collected during routine clinical practice (e.g. biochemical tests) that are left over can also be used for data analysis. As a result of this methodology, the burden for the paediatric patient is reduced and the statistical power to develop a population PK or PK–PD model is not affected or can even be improved.

In recent years, PK–PD M&S has become a mainstay for optimising drug therapy in paediatric patients. Drug therapy is optimised primarily through the estimation of population PK and PD parameters and understanding different levels of covariate influence on PK–PD, and thus dosing regimen. The PK parameters that are important for dosing are well known. Clearance is the most important, as it determines the maintenance dose. Volume of distribution is important for the loading dose. The impact of covariates on PK and PD are more important in children than in adults, because of the large range and developmental change of influential covariates such as body weight and age. Paediatric dosing regimens are most often based on patients' developmental factors (correlating with body size) such as body weight, body surface area, or age. The goal of these dosing regimens is to generate similar drug exposure across the whole paediatric population adjusted for developmental PD. It is important to recognise that changes in physiology that characterise development may not correspond to predefined age groups (neonates, infants, children and adolescents) and are also not linearly related to weight. Children are in a continuously and dynamically changing state of growth and development.

Although other model-based approaches have also been used in paediatric clinical pharmacology, in addition to population PK–PD, such as physiologically based PK modelling and non-parametric approaches, these topics are beyond the scope of this chapter.

Development of PK–PD model

The first phase of a population PK–PD analysis usually involves determining the most appropriate structural model to describe the observations. The choice of structural model (e.g. one-, two- or three-compartment model;

linear; non-linear) is based upon the best prior information about the drug. Published adult population PK models or the results of non-compartment studies may provide the starting estimates of the parameters and likely models. The statistical submodel, which accounts for the inter-individual, intra-individual and residual variability, is then tested and evaluated.

After the preliminary analyses are complete and the structural model and statistical submodel have been identified, the next stage is to try to explain inter-individual variability by examining the influence of covariates. The influence of developmental changes in the paediatric population can be explored primarily by using size (weight) and/or age as covariates. Weight is a critical element when applying population approaches to children. It can range more than 200-fold between preterm neonates and adolescents, and closely correlates with other developmental factors. Allometric scaling,[5] based on sound biological principles, is often used to account for the impact of weight on PK parameters in children, using equations 1 and 2.

$$CL_{child} = CL_{standard} \times (WT_{child}/WT_{standard})^{PWR} \tag{1}$$

$$V_{child} = V_{standard} \times (WT_{child}/WT_{standard})^{PWR} \tag{2}$$

where CL is clearance ($CL_{standard}$ represents clearance in a typical patient weighing $WT_{standard}$, usually a 70 kg adult, whereas CL_{child} is clearance in a typical child), V is volume of distribution and WT is body weight.

The exponents (denoted as 'PWR' above) can either be fixed – 0.75 for clearance and 1 for volume of distribution – or estimated with the dataset. It is of practical importance to report PK parameters in terms of a standard weight, allowing direct comparison between different studies and better understanding of developmental changes. The allometric predictions are not changed by the choice of the standard weight. Of note, allometric scaling is insufficient to describe clearance in neonates and infants.[6] The maturation and organ function must also be taken into account (equation 3).

$$CL_{neonate} = CL_{adult} \times (WT_{neonate}/WT_{adult})^{PWR} \times MA \times OF \tag{3}$$

where MA is maturation and OF is organ function.

The impact of age should be evaluated separately from the side-effects. It can have a non-linear relationship to the model parameters, and therefore graphics are useful to determine the relationship between age and the parameters of the interest. When attempting to evaluate age as an influential covariate for neonates, postmenstrual age should be tested first. Postmenstrual age is considered to be an adequate marker of many aspects of ontogeny. The impact of postnatal age and gestational age at birth should also be evaluated as separate covariates, thus recognising that maturation occurs at different rates *in utero* versus in the postnatal environment.

Other covariates that have been identified as important in paediatric PK analysis include renal function, hepatic function, nutrition, pharmacogenetics, ethnicity, drug–drug interactions, extracorporeal membrane oxygenation, hypothermia and disease characteristics. The diversity of the paediatric population and numerous covariates emphasise the importance of performing PK studies in special paediatric patients in order to optimise dosing regimens.

Validation of the model

A proper validation of the model includes an internal evaluation followed by an external evaluation and a prospective clinical study to evaluate the model-based dosing regimen.

Various techniques are available for the internal and external evaluation of the model, including goodness-of-fits plots (individual predicted versus observed concentrations; population predicted versus observed concentrations; conditional weighted residual error versus time; conditional weighted residual error versus population predicted concentrations), bootstrapping, visual predictive checks, normalised prediction distribution errors, etc. The technical aspects and advantages or disadvantages of each validation method can be found in tutorial papers.[7,8] It should be emphasised that in order to define whether a model is useful and valid for dosing optimisation, a thorough evaluation based on a combination of these evaluation methods is necessary.

M&S applications in personalised therapy

The dramatic physiological and maturational processes during the first month of life produce dynamic alterations in drug PK. To effectively optimise drug therapy in neonates, a thorough understanding of developmental PK and the impacts of covariates on neonatal PK are essential. We present a population PK model of vancomycin to illustrate how to use M&S techniques to enable personalised therapy in neonates.

Vancomycin is a glycopeptide antibiotic used for more than 50 years in neonates. It is primarily effective against Gram positive cocci. *Staphylococcus aureus* and *Staphylococcus epidermidis*, including both methicillin-susceptible (MSSA and MSSE respectively, for *S. aureus* and *S. epidermidis*) or methicillin-resistant (MRSA and MRSE respectively, for *S. aureus* and *S. epidermidis*) species, are usually sensitive to vancomycin.[9] Vancomycin PK has shown large inter-individual variability. As vancomycin is primarily eliminated by glomerular filtration, renal maturation, renal function and body weight should be the most important factors influencing PK. 'Classical' weight-based (mg/kg) dosing regimens integrated these factors as categorical variables, and the corresponding dose was calculated for the different neonatal age groups (i.e. neonates less than 29 weeks' postmenstrual age, 15 mg/kg every 24 hours; neonates 29–35 weeks' postmenstrual age, 15 mg/kg every 12 hours; neonates over 35 weeks' postmenstrual age, 15 mg/kg every 8 hours) in order to obtain similar drug exposure to that achieved in adults.

This approach obviously simplifies the major impacts of developmental factors on PK parameters. It assumes an 'average neonate' with an 'average weight', and a simple linear maturation relationship between weight and drug clearance in each age group. Our recent study of vancomycin continuous infusion in neonates highlighted this problem.[10] Standard weight-based dosing regimens of vancomycin were used in three intensive care units and provided the expected 'average' concentration in the neonatal population; however, variability was extremely large. Only 41% of neonates had concentrations in the target range of 15–25 mg/L.

In order to personalise vancomycin therapy in neonates, we conducted a population PK study based on samples collected in neonatal clinical practice. Applying modelling techniques, a one-compartment model with first-order elimination was developed. Covariate analysis identified that current weight significantly influenced clearance and volume of distribution, with power functions of 0.513 for clearance and 0.898 for volume of distribution. Vancomycin clearance also significantly increased with increases in birth weight, postnatal age and renal function (see the following equations for CL and Vd). The model was then validated internally using the methods described above.

After the model was built and validated, an optimised dosing regimen, taking into account birth weight, current weight, postnatal age and serum creatinine, was developed based on the model.

$$\text{Loading dose (mg)} = \text{Target concentrations} * V$$

$$\text{Maintenance dose (mg) per 24 hours}$$

$$= \text{Target concentration} * CL * 24 \text{ hours}$$

$$Vd = 0.791 * \left(\frac{WT}{1416}\right)^{0.898}$$

$$CL = 0.0571 * \left(\frac{WT}{1416}\right)^{0.513} * \left(\frac{bWT}{1010}\right)^{0.599}$$

$$* \left(1 + 0.282 * \left(\frac{PNA}{17}\right)\right) * \left(\frac{1}{\left(\frac{CR}{42}\right)^{0.525}}\right)$$

Where CL is clearance in L/h, Vd volume of distribution in L, WT current weight in g, bWT birth weight in g, PNA postnatal age in days, and CR serum creatinine concentration in μmol/L.

Clinical trial simulation showed that the optimised dosing regimen could result a higher percentage of neonates reaching the therapeutic range and early dosage adaptation (6–12 h post dose). A prospective validation study in 58 neonates confirmed the results of the clinical trial simulation. The percentage of patients reaching the recommended target levels increased from 41% in the original population to 71% in the model guided optimised dosing population. After taking into account the first TDM measurement, this level increased to nearly 100%. A major improvement in individual vancomycin therapy was thereby achieved by using modelling and simulation techniques. Consequently, the corresponding software has been set up in neonatal intensive care units to individualise vancomycin dose, and undoubtedly optimisation of prescriptions will be applicable to other antibiotics prescribed for neonates and children.

Conclusions

Population PK–PD analysis is indispensable in paediatrics to understand developmental pharmacology. Investigating PK–PD variability in children and identification of relevant covariates can be used to improve drug dosing and develop personalised drug therapy. Successful integration of model-based dosage individualisation into paediatric clinical practice needs close collaboration between paediatric clinical pharmacologists, pharmacists and paediatricians.

References

1   Kearns GL *et al*. Developmental pharmacology--drug disposition, action, and therapy in infants and children. *N Engl J Med* 2003; 349: 1157–1167.
2   Manolis E, Pons G. Proposals for model-based paediatric medicinal development within the current European Union regulatory framework. *Br J Clin Pharmacol* 2009; 68: 493–501.
3   Barrett JS *et al*. Pharmacometrics: A multidisciplinary field to facilitate critical thinking in drug development and translational research settings. *J Clin Pharmacol* 2008 48: 632–649.
4   Zhao W *et al*. Dosage individualization in children: integration of pharmacometrics in clinical practice. *World J Pediatr* 2014; 10: 197–203
5   Anderson BJ, Holford NH. Mechanism-based concepts of size and maturity in pharmacokinetics. *Annu Rev Pharmacol Toxicol* 2008; 48: 303–332.
6   Tod M *et al*. Facilitation of drug evaluation in children by population methods and modelling. *Clin Pharmacokinet* 2008; 47(4): 231–243.
7   De Cock RF *et al*. The role of population PK–PD modelling in paediatric clinical research. *Eur J Clin Pharmacol* 2011; 67 Suppl 1: 5–16.
8   Keizer RJ *et al*. Modelling and simulation workbench for NONMEM: tutorial on Pirana, PsN, and Xpose. *CPT Pharmacometrics Syst Pharmacol* 2013; 2: e50.
9   Jacqz-Aigrain E *et al*. Use of antibacterial agents in the neonate: 50 years of experience with vancomycin administration. *Semin Fetal Neonatal Med* 2013; 18: 28–34.
10 Zhao W *et al*. Vancomycin continuous infusion in neonates: dosing optimisation and therapeutic drug monitoring. *Arch Dis Child* 2013; 98: 449–453.

Further recommended reading

Tatarinova T *et al*. Two general methods for population pharmacokinetic modeling: non-parametric adaptive grid and non-parametric Bayesian. *J Pharmacokinet Pharmacodyn* 2013; 40(2): 189–199.

Upton RN *et al*. An introduction to physiologically-based pharmacokinetic models. *Paediatr Anaesth* 2016; 26(11): 1036–1046.

Villiger A *et al*. Using physiologically based pharmacokinetic (PBPK) modelling to gain insights into the effect of physiological factors on oral absorption in paediatric populations. *AAPS J* 2016; 18(4): 933–947.

10

Adverse drug reactions

MJ Rieder

Introduction

While drug therapy has unquestionably improved care for children, this has not been without cost or risk. One of the most important problems associated with drug therapy is the risk of adverse drug events. Given the common use of drugs for therapy of children and the increasing complexity of care – especially for the growing number of children with chronic diseases – it is imperative that child healthcare workers have an approach to possible adverse drug events in children.

The learning objectives of this chapter are:

➤ to understand the burden of adverse drug reactions (ADRs) in children
➤ to develop awareness of risk factors for ADRs
➤ to recognise the role of classification systems for ADRs
➤ to describe the clinical approach to a suspected adverse drug event in a child.

ADRs and adverse drug events

An adverse drug event is when an undesired effect is associated with the use of a drug. This is a broad term including medication errors that occur when a drug is given in the wrong dose or to the wrong patient, or the wrong drug is given. In the context of therapy for children, it should be noted that medication errors appear to occur at a higher frequency among children than among adults, and indeed have been associated with several significant events in the history of drug regulation. ADRs are typically defined as noxious or undesired events that occur when a drug is administered via the usual route in the usual dose for therapy or prevention of disease.[1]

Burden of adverse drug reactions in children

The general rate of ADRs is considered to be 5% at best, with risks rising sharply for certain classes of drugs and certain classes of patients. This is a minimal ADR rate, and for many drugs and patients the rate is much higher; as an example, rates of ADRs to potent drugs such as anticonvulsants or chemotherapy are typically much higher than 5% – in the case of certain chemotherapeutic agents, to rates approaching 100%; for some groups of patients, such as premature infants in the neonatal intensive care unit (NICU), it has been estimated that, if they remain in the NICU long enough, the rate of ADRs also approaches 100%.

The importance of ADRs in the clinical care of children relates not only to their frequency but also to mortality; it has been estimated that, in developed countries, ADRs are among the top four or five causes of death. An example is in oncology: up to half of the deaths in childhood cancer, and up to two-thirds of long-term morbidity, are direct consequences of chemotherapy. In addition to risks of mortality and morbidity, ADRs have a significant economic burden; it has been estimated that ADRs cost the US healthcare system as much as $150 billion per year. Much of this cost is for monitoring for potential adverse events. Finally, ADRs represent an emotional and psychological burden for patients and their families and create many problems for healthcare providers, not the least of which is the selection of drugs for therapy when there is history of a possible ADR. In this context, having an organised approach to the assessment and treatment of a potential adverse drug event is crucially important in ensuring that accurate information and guidance is provided to those caring for the patient in the future.

Risk factors for adverse drug reactions

The risk for ADRs is not uniformly distributed, and there are well described risk factors that increase the risk for ADRs (Table 1). These risk factors are not independent, and indeed several are closely related. As an example, and building on the issues cited above, a premature infant in the NICU has several related risk factors, including polypharmacy, developmental impairment in the organs of excretion and being at the extremes of age, the latter two being clearly related; it is thus not surprising that they are at an increased risk for ADRs. Similarly, a child with cancer receiving chemotherapy also has several risk factors, including polypharmacy and high doses being needed as part of their therapeutic regimen. Again, the increased risk for ADRs in this context is not surprising.

The issue of genetic polymorphisms is a recent and important consideration. It is now clear that polymorphisms of CYP2D6 – notably the ultrarapid metaboliser phenotype – are associated with a higher risk of ADRs to drugs

Table 1 Risk factors for adverse drug reactions
Previous history of an adverse drug reaction
Polypharmacy
Extremes of age
Impairment of the organs of excretion
Female gender
Larger drug doses
Certain genetic polymorphisms

such as codeine. As our appreciation of the importance of genetic and other factors in drug disposition increases, it is likely that other polymorphisms will be identified that are important determinants of drug safety in children.

Classification of adverse drug reactions

A classification system for ADRs that provides both mechanistic insights as well as considerations for management is the modified system of Rawlins and Thompson (Figure 1). Focusing on immediate ADRs, the two most relevant broad categories are type A ('augmented'), or predictable, ADRs and type B ('bizarre'), or unpredictable, ADRs.

Type A, or predictable, ADRs are the most common type of ADRs and are mechanistically linked to the pharmacological activity of the drug. These ADRs include side-effects, which are often mild and self-limited. 'Treating through' may be a useful clinical approach, as many of these ADRs diminish in severity over time. Type B, or unpredictable, ADRs are less common but frequently more severe, and as they are often not immediately predictable from the known pharmacological action of the drug, are difficult to anticipate and plan for. These ADRs typically require discontinuation of the drug; in the case of immune-mediated ADRs, symptoms may continue or even worsen despite discontinuation of the drug.

Other ADR classification systems also exist but are beyond the scope of this chapter.[4,5]

Clinical approach to suspected adverse drug events

An organised approach to the clinical evaluation of suspected adverse drug events is a core competency for child healthcare workers, given the frequency and magnitude of drug use in children. An approach that can be used involves the five As: appreciation, assessment, analysis, assistance and aftermath.

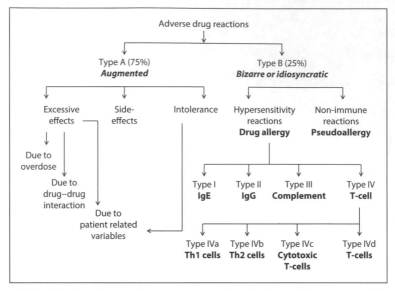

Figure 1 Classification of adverse drug reactions, based on Rawlins and Thompson and the revised Gell and Coombs system for hypersensitivity[2,3]

Appreciation

A diagnosis cannot be made if the clinician is unaware of an ADR's existence. Healthcare workers must appreciate the possibility of an ADR when unexpected or undesired events occur during or shortly after a course of drug therapy. As well, it cannot be assumed that ADR patterns are the same in children as in adults. When the unexpected happens in the presence of a drug, suspect a possible ADR, especially when this is a new drug or at least a new drug to paediatrics.

Assessment

The next step is assessment, in which all of the relevant clinical information is collected in order to inform the differential diagnosis. It is important to have a complete grasp of the patient, the details of therapy and other important variables. This includes a careful history and physical examination, which remains the basis of ADR diagnosis. Care must be taken in this; as an example, having a rash that develops before therapy starts is a fairly good indicator that the drug is not responsible for the rash. The details of physical examination are often neglected in the assessment of a possible adverse drug event, which is unfortunate as, for example, some rashes are much more and some much less likely to be due to drug therapy. As an example, a non-pruritic, non-urticarial diffuse rash – typically called maculopapular – developing after 4 or 5 days of therapy is much less likely to be due to drugs than is an urticarial rash developing shortly after starting therapy. Similarly, Stevens-Johnson syndrome is most commonly due to drugs, while erythema multiforme major is more commonly due to infection. In this context, accurate identification of rashes is very important.[6] In the experience of this author, Stevens-Johnson syndrome is commonly over-diagnosed, given that the mucositis associated with Stevens-Johnson syndrome is classically haemorrhagic and inflammatory rather than the painless mucosal oedema commonly seen with erythema multiforme major.

In addition to having a complete clinical picture of the patient, it is important to consider the disease being treated and the drug used. In this context it may be necessary to consult drug information resources; the average clinician uses between 100 and 200 drugs routinely, while there are more than 3500 drugs available on many national formularies. It is also important to acknowledge that key data on the adverse effects of drugs in children – especially for new drugs – may be unavailable.

Analysis

The next step is crucial, which is the conduct of a careful differential diagnosis. This addresses the key question: is this a drug related event or not? Key considerations in the construction of a differential diagnosis include evaluating the original indication for therapy. Thus, the event under consideration may be due to drug therapy or may be due to the disease being treated. As part of this process, it is important to recognise that patients and families tend to blame undesired effects on drugs, while clinicians tend to blame the disease being treated, with the truth often lying somewhere in between. In order to make this crucial decision, additional information is often necessary. Drug information pharmacists are an invaluable resource for this, given that, frequently, child specific information on ADRs is difficult to find.

Assistance

Once a diagnosis has been reached, the clinician needs to consider two important management points. An important but often neglected part of the management of an ADR is the treatment of the initial disease of interest. If the problem has resolved, as in the case of an infection that has been treated effectively, then no further management may be needed. Conversely, in the event that the initial disorder is not being optimally controlled or if ongoing therapy is needed, then careful consideration must be given to what this should be, including which drugs are likely to be safe. Thus when the diagnosis is made that the event in question is an ADR, an important and immediate consideration is whether the drug should or should not be stopped. This decision varies with different types of ADRs. As an example, treating through (continuing therapy in the expectation that the ADR will abate over time) is an acceptable strategy for many side-effects; for example, the fine hand tremor seen with initial use of inhaled beta agonists such as salbutamol (albuterol) typically diminishes reasonably quickly even in the face of continuing therapy. In contrast, in the face of allergic or serious idiosyncratic ADRs such as drug allergy or Stevens-Johnson syndrome, it is imperative to discontinue therapy as quickly as the diagnosis is made.

For life-threatening ADRs such as anaphylaxis, prompt and aggressive management of airway, breathing and circulation is crucial. However, for most ADRs the management of the ADR is dependent on the nature and severity of symptoms, and is typically supportive care, given that the natural history of most ADRs is resolution once the drug is discontinued. For some severe ADRs such as drug hypersensitivity it may be necessary to use immunomodulatory therapy, but this decision should be made in consultation with an expert in the care of these patients.

Aftermath

The last and one of the most important steps in approaching an ADR is dealing with the aftermath. One obvious area is in the selection of future therapy. Generally, it is prudent to avoid the drug in question and drugs of the same class, notably when the ADR has been serious.

In addition to the obvious impact on future therapy of restricting therapeutic choices, there are other effects. The fact of having had an ADR has clearly been demonstrated to be a determination of the likelihood of compliance with future therapy. Simply put, a patient who has had an ADR is significantly less likely to be compliant with therapy. The fact of an ADR is also likely to impact on the effectiveness of the physician–patient or physician–family relationship. The best way to approach this is straightforward. It is best to be honest with the patient and family, acknowledge the fact of the ADR as a separate problem, and discuss both the immediate concerns and the potential impact on future therapy. This is even more effective when patients and families are advised about the possibility of an ADR prior to starting therapy.

In addition to the impact on the patient, part of dealing with the aftermath is information sharing. Many children, notably those with complex or chronic disease, are cared for by teams of clinicians and other healthcare professionals. All the members of the circle of care should be made aware of any ADRs and the potential risk of ADRs with future therapy. In addition, information about new or serious ADRs should be shared with drug regulatory agencies. During the drug approval process, studies are rarely conducted in children, and consequently essentially all serious ADRs in new drugs used in children have been identified by an astute clinician. Hence the communication of new and serious ADRS is extremely important for the care of other children.

Conclusions

ADRs are common and important problems in the therapy of children; they are more common in certain groups of children, related to predictable risk factors; ADR monitoring should form part of the management planning for therapy for these patients. While some types of ADRs can be predicted, others cannot and thus vigilance for ADRs is important; the experience of the use of the drug in adults may not always be helpful in guiding use of the drug in children. Having an organised clinical approach to a suspected adverse drug event in children – beginning with appreciation, and proceeding through assessment, analysis, assistance and dealing with the aftermath – is a core clinical skill needed to provide effective and safe drug therapy for children.

References

1 Rieder MJ. New ways to detect adverse drug reactions in pediatrics. *Pediatr Clin N Am* 2012; 59: 1071–1092.
2 Rawlins MD, Thompson JW. Pathogenesis of adverse drug reactions. In: Davies DM, ed. Textbook of Adverse Drug Reactions. Oxford: Oxford University Press, 1977: 10.
3 Pichler WJ, ed. Drug Hypersensitivity. Basel: Karger, 2007.
4 Ferner RE, Aronson JK. EIDOS: a mechanistic classification of adverse drug effects. *Drug Saf* 2010; 33(1): 15–23.
5 Aronson JK, Ferner RE. Preventability of drug-related harms – part II: proposed criteria, based on frameworks that classify adverse drug reactions. *Drug Saf* 2010; 33(11): 995–1002.
6 Noguera-Morel L *et al.* Cutaneous drug reactions in the pediatric population. *Pediatr Clin North Am* 2014; 61: 403–426.

11

Drug interactions

MJ Rieder

Introduction

Drug therapy is one of the cornerstones of healthcare for children and has provided healthcare workers with the ability to cure or control diseases that have been associated with significant mortality and morbidity in children. The great benefits that have been obtained via drug therapy have not come without risk, however. One of the most important risks associated with drug therapy is the risk of adverse drug reactions (ADRs). Among ADRs, drug interactions are increasingly recognised as a problem for patients with complex or chronic therapy.

The learning objectives of this chapter are:

➢ to describe different types of drug interactions
➢ to understand the mechanisms of drug interactions
➢ to recognise potential consequences of drug interactions
➢ to develop a therapeutic plan that takes drug interactions into account.

Drug disposition in children

Drug therapy for children is delivered by a variety of routes, including topically, via intravenous or intramuscular injection, or orally. Due to a number of practical issues, the most common route for drug delivery is oral. The disposition of orally administered drugs is determined by processes known collectively as ADME (absorption, distribution, metabolism and excretion).[1] Drug interactions have been described at all stages of drug disposition but are most commonly associated with alterations in drug clearance.

Types of drug interactions

There are different types of possible drug interaction. While the classical consideration is for drug–drug interactions, the biological fate of drugs is influenced by a number of variables, including diet and disease. Further, drug interactions can involve not only the pharmacokinetics of a drug but also the pharmacodynamics – or mechanism of therapeutic effect – of a drug.

The consequences of drug interactions vary with respect to the mechanism of interaction as well as to the magnitude of the interaction.

Drug–drug interactions occur when the co-administration of more than one drug alters the biological fate or biological action of another drug. An example of this is the increase in tacrolimus blood concentrations – and increased risk of tacrolimus toxicity – when amlodipine is given to children receiving tacrolimus for anti-rejection therapy post transplantation. While drug–drug interactions have been well described in adults and to some extent in older children, there is very limited data on the impact of drug–drug interactions in children under the age of 2, and a recent study suggests that adult data should be interpreted with caution when assessing potential risks among children at this young age. When treating patients with HIV, there is a dedicated website that can help clinicians identify potentially significant drug interactions (www.hiv-druginteractions.org/checker), although this is largely based on adult data.

Drug–food interactions occur when the concurrent consumption of food and administration of the drug impacts on drug effects, typically by altering the biological disposition of the drug. The food most commonly associated with drug interactions is grapefruit. Although grapefruit is known to alter the effect of many drugs, this is not frequently a problem for children given that grapefruit and grapefruit juice are not commonly consumed by children. Drug–food interactions that are more common in children are those related to drug administration to children who are being fed via a feeding tube, e.g. the decrease in phenytoin bioavailability seen when the drug is given via a feeding tube.

Drug–disease interactions occur when the biological fate or action of a drug is altered in the presence of disease. An example is the well described increased risk for drug hypersensitivity that is seen in HIV patients with acquired immunodeficiency syndrome. There is some evidence that more common viral infections can alter drug metabolism, but it is unclear as to the overall clinical relevance of these changes. Inflammation is appreciated to significantly impact on drug metabolism, and thus children with critical illness may have impaired drug clearance during the acute phase of their illness.

While all three types of drug interactions have been described in children, interactions of the greatest clinical concern for children are typically drug–drug interactions.

Mechanisms of drug interactions

The mechanisms of drug interactions vary but fall into several general themes. One broad group of drug interactions occur related to impaired drug clearance. There are a number of drugs that are known to inhibit the metabolism of other drugs, often related to metabolism by similar pathways. Typically these interactions involve phase I metabolism, with the iso-enzyme most frequently involved being CYP3A4 (Table 1). In the case of drug–food interactions, inhibition of drug metabolism was the mechanism by which the interaction between grapefruit juice and drugs was first described. Drug interactions can also impact on renal excretion of drugs.

While some drugs inhibit the metabolism of other drugs, other drugs can increase the clearance of concurrently administered drugs, typically by induction of drug metabolism. Again CYP3A4 is often the iso-enzyme of interest in the case of induction of drug metabolism (Table 1).[2]

As noted above, there is a paucity of evidence to guide therapy with respect to drug interactions in children under the age of 2. This is in part due to lack of research but is also an issue related to the well-known ontogeny of drug clearance systems, which is most marked in very young children. As well, related to ontogeny, the route of clearance may be different in very young children than in older children or adults. Thus many of the sophisticated modelling exercises that can be undertaken in adults or older children are difficult to extrapolate to very young children.

Drug interactions can also occur on a pharmacodynamic basis. A classical example of this is long QT interval. Many drugs are known to prolong the QT interval.[3] The clinical significance of this for therapy for children remains unclear, but it does appear that children who have long QT syndrome are at increased risk for adverse events related to the use of drugs that prolong QT interval, notably in the context of anaesthesia. The extent to which this is relevant to drugs such as antipsychotic drugs remains unclear.

Consequences of drug interactions

The consequences of drug interactions are dependent on the mechanism of the drug interaction. As an example, drug interactions that result in impaired drug clearance – e.g. by inhibition of drug metabolism – typically result in an enhanced drug effect or an increased risk of drug toxicity. In contrast, drug interactions that result in increased drug clearance – e.g. when enzyme induction increases drug metabolism – may be associated with reduced drug efficacy. In the case of prodrugs, the converse may apply. As an example, inhibiting the metabolism of warfarin will result in an increased risk of bleeding (drug toxicity) while inhibiting the oxidation of codeine – a prodrug converted to morphine by CYP2D6 – will reduce codeine's analgesic efficacy.

Table 1 Common inducers and inhibitors of CYP3A4	
Inducers	**Inhibitors**
Carbamazepine	Amprenavir
Efavirenz	Azithromycin
Nevirapine	Chloramphenicol
Phenytoin	Clarithromycin
Rifampin	Clotrimazole
Oxcarbazepine	Ciclosporin
Phenobarbital	Erythromycin
	Fluconazole
	Isoniazid
	Ketoconazole
	Metronidazole
	Miconazole
	Ranitidine
	Ritonavir
	Saquinavir
	Sertraline
	Valproic acid

While therapeutic failure is an obviously undesirable consequence of a drug interaction, the most common concern about drug interactions is drug toxicity and the possibility of adverse drug events. The manifestations of adverse events are dependent on the individual drug. When adverse events – or therapeutic efficacy – are related to measurable drug concentrations in readily available biological fluids, then therapeutic drug monitoring offers the potential to monitor – and predict – whether a drug interaction occurs, notably when a new drug is added to the therapeutic regimen. As an example, if a child receiving ciclosporin for anti-rejection therapy post transplantation has clarithromycin added to the therapeutic regimen – e.g. for the therapy of presumptive *Mycoplasma* pneumonia – then there is the possibility of a drug interaction, as ciclosporin is principally metabolised by CYP3A4 and CYP3A5, while clarithromycin inhibits CYP3A4 on a variable basis. As the toxicity of ciclosporin – notably renal toxicity – is known to be concentration dependent, as predicated by plasma ciclosporin concentrations, the potential for adverse consequences of concurrent clarithromycin therapy can be evaluated by more intensive monitoring of serum ciclosporin concentrations, while risk can then be managed by dose adjustment.

A clinical approach to drug interactions in children

The problem of drug interactions is most commonly an issue in the case of children on chronic therapy, notably when this is complex therapy involving several or many drugs. Children for whom this is a consideration include, among others, children with epilepsy, children with cancer and children who have undergone organ transplantation. Healthcare workers caring for these children therefore need to take this into account when developing a therapeutic plan for these children and when monitoring therapy for these children, especially when new drugs are added to the therapeutic regimen or when the child's condition changes.

Initial steps include considering the drugs being used in the light of the known pharmacology of these drugs, especially for the therapy of the disease of interest. Known drug interactions need to be considered, with the caveat that what is known in adults and older children may not apply to children under the age of 2. In the case of children at special risk, the therapeutic plan should take this into account. The potential for drug interactions should be discussed with the child's family and the importance of communication when unexpected events occur should be emphasised.

Ongoing considerations include the need for monitoring, which is of special relevance when there are changes in therapy, especially when these changes involve changes in dosage or the addition of new drugs to the therapeutic regimen or replacement of one drug with another. In these circumstances, enhanced monitoring may be necessary and it may be prudent, for drugs for which this is available, to use therapeutic drug monitoring to assist the clinician in the assessment of potential drug interactions. In the case of a drug interaction, prompt attention to this is important. The first step is to prevent harm, which may involve stopping or altering therapy, e.g. by changing dose while concurrent therapy is being administered. The second step is to ensure that attention is paid to the therapeutic goal for which therapy was initially prescribed. During this process, communication with other members of the child's healthcare team – e.g., consultants in other disciplines who may be involved in the care of the child – is critically important, as is communication with the child and their family. Finally, in the case of very young children or new drugs it is important that new patterns of drug interactions are reported to the respective drug regulatory agency as well as published in the peer reviewed literature to inform fellow paediatricians and pharmacists, so that other children can avoid the risk of drug toxicity or therapeutic failure.

Conclusions

The effects of drugs may be altered by interactions with other drugs, diet or disease. These interactions may increase or decrease drug effect and may or may not be similar to those seen in adults, and this is of special importance for children on chronic and complex therapy. Healthcare workers caring for children with chronic and complex therapy need to be alert to the possibility of drug interactions, notably when new drugs are added to the therapeutic regimen. Communication is a key component of not only managing drug interactions but also in preventing them.

References

1 de Wildt SN *et al*. Drug metabolism for the paediatrician. *Arch Dis Child* 2014; 99:1137–1142.
2 Salem F *et al*. Do children have the same vulnerability to metabolic drug-drug interactions as adults? A critical review of the literature. *J Clin Pharmacol* 2013 May; 53(5):559–566.
3 Trinkley KE *et al*. QT interval prolongation and the risk of torsades de pointes: Essentials for clinicians. *Curr Med Res Opinion* 2013; 29:1719–1726.

12

Pregnancy and lactation

K Allegaert and K Van Calsteren

Introduction

Most drugs are not thoroughly evaluated for use during pregnancy, at delivery or post-partum (e.g. during breastfeeding). This is to a large extent similar to the extensive off-label, unlicensed pharmacotherapy in the paediatric subpopulations. Consequently, labelling includes almost nothing about dosing, efficacy, or maternal, fetal or newborn safety, with the default setting that the drug has not been studied during pregnancy or breastfeeding.[1] Despite this, women often need treatment for a range of conditions during both pregnancy and breastfeeding. Drugs may have harmful effects on the fetus at any time during pregnancy, illustrated by the thalidomide disaster that initiated the legal initiatives on drug evaluation and safety. A decision on drug treatment should always be a balanced decision, comparing outcome to the absence of any treatment. Similarly, breastfeeding is beneficial and the optimal feeding for newborns and infants, but may result in breastfeeding related drug exposure. Consequently, the ultimate goal of using maternal medications during breastfeeding is dual: provide safe and effective pharmacotherapy for the maternal condition(s) and still assure safety of the nursing infant or its tolerance to adverse events related to the maternal pharmacotherapy.

The learning objectives of this chapter are:

➤ to provide introductory information related to maternal–fetal–infant pharmacokinetics
➤ to give guidance on drugs during pregnancy, the initiation and maintenance of breastfeeding, and drugs during breastfeeding
➤ to suggest potential sources of information for individual advice, since knowledge on this topic is evolving.

Perinatal pharmacokinetics

Clinical pharmacology aims to predict drug related effects based on drug- and patient-specific pharmacokinetics (PK, concentration–time), and pharmacodynamics (PD, concentration–effect). Pregnancy (mother, fetus) and early infancy require a specific approach. For aspects of PK/PD in infants, refer to previous chapters (chapters 4–8). Pregnancy also results in extensive alterations in PK with subsequent extensive inter-individual variability in drug response.[2,3] These changes are mainly driven by raised maternal metabolism (e.g. cardiac output, metabolic activity) and hormonal changes (oestrogens, progesterone). In general, renal elimination is higher during pregnancy (i.e. higher glomerular filtration rate, higher active renal tubular transport). Similarly, the basal metabolic activity is also increased. This commonly results in increased drug metabolism (phase I or II processes), although these changes are isoenzyme specific. Although rarely, pregnancy may even result in reduced enzymatic activity. Additionally, changes in body weight or binding capacity (protein changes, pH) may affect the volume of distribution. Finally, duration of pregnancy, comorbidity (e.g. pre-eclampsia) or labour itself may further affect variability in drug disposition and response.

The placenta provides a link between the circulations of two distinct individuals (mother and fetus) but also acts as a barrier to protect the fetus from xenobiotics in the maternal blood. The placenta is described as an organ separating the maternal and fetal circulations. However, the term 'placental barrier' includes a false notion, since the placenta is not a true barrier but instead is active tissue that guides the entry to and from the fetus. As at other barriers, passive diffusion, facilitated diffusion, active transport and drug metabolism have been described at the placental barrier. The same holds true for the fetus. Elimination of drugs from the fetus occurs primarily by diffusion back to the maternal compartment, but this is not the only route of elimination. Significant concentrations of drug metabolites have been found in the fetus, suggesting fetal metabolic clearance. It should be noted that the process of biotransformation usually renders the drug more water-soluble and thus more readily excreted by the (fetal) kidney. This is of concern to the fetus when the drug undergoes metabolism in the fetal compartment, because the greater water-solubility of the metabolite will decrease the ability of the compound to be cleared from the fetus across the placenta. Drugs or metabolites that are 'trapped' in amniotic fluid, meconium, fetal hair or bones also reflect direct fetal clearance.

Maternal–fetal pharmacotherapy

Only rarely, maternal pharmacotherapy has a primary fetal indication (fetal supraventricular tachycardia, prenatal lung maturation, fetal thyroid diseases, antibody-mediated fetal diseases (e.g. allo-immune thrombocytopenia, neonatal haemochromatosis)). These examples further illustrate that the placenta is not a full barrier, nor is the fetus an inactive bystander of maternal drug exposure. Maternal drugs can also have harmful effects on the fetus at any time during pregnancy. This is already the case in the first trimester of pregnancy, with a window of vulnerability between the third and 11th week of pregnancy for structural teratogenic effects, i.e. prenatal toxicity characterised by defects in the developing embryo or fetus. Consequently, this is of relevance to consider when prescribing for a female of childbearing age (e.g. angiotensin-converting enzyme inhibitors, coumarins, antiepileptics, isotretinoin, rubella vaccination). In contrast, drug exposure (e.g. illicit drugs) during the second and third trimesters of pregnancy more generally affects fetal growth or functional development. Finally, perinatal exposure (e.g. opioids, benzodiazepines) may affect neonatal adaptation.

How to handle and assess the available evidence, association or likelihood of fetal harm related to maternal treatment is a difficult balanced decision. This is also reflected by the different approaches applied: strategies vary and evolve. Pregnancy category classifications are one approach, but classifications vary somewhat between different authorities, and these categories do not include risks related to drugs or their metabolites through breast milk. The Food and Drug Administration (FDA) classification uses category A, B, C, D, X and N and requires a relatively large amount of high quality data for a drug to be defined as pregnancy category A. The FDA requests also a narrative description of the evidence available for use of the drug in pregnancy. In contrast to such a classification approach, the *British National Formulary* gives a table of drugs to be avoided or used with caution in pregnancy, and does so using a limited number of key phrases instead of categorisation.

Initiation and maintenance of breastfeeding

A multidisciplinary team of healthcare providers apply general strategies to improve breast feeding initiation and continuation rates, commonly referred to as the Baby Friendly Hospital Initiative (BFHI). The ten steps to successful breastfeeding (Box 1) provide a supportive pathway enabling women to achieve their breastfeeding intentions as well as guidance for training of healthcare workers in breastfeeding support. Non-pharmacological recommendations should be exhausted before adding pharmacological therapy to enhance milk production (galactogogues). Anecdotal evidence suggests the use of metoclopramide, but efficacy and safety data are limited. The same holds for oxytocin and domperidone.

Box 1 10 steps to successfully initiate and maintain breastfeeding

1 Have a written breastfeeding policy that is routinely communicated to all healthcare staff.

2 Train all healthcare staff in skills necessary to implement this policy.

3 Inform all pregnant women about the benefits and management of breastfeeding.

4 Help mothers initiate breastfeeding within a half hour of birth.

5 Show mothers how to breastfeed and how to maintain lactation, even if they are separated from their infants.

6 Give newborn infants no food or drink other than breast milk unless medically indicated.

7 Practise rooming-in – allow mothers and infants to remain together – 24 hours a day.

8 Encourage breastfeeding on demand.

9 Give no artificial teats or pacifiers (also called dummies or soothers) to breastfeeding infants.

10 Foster the establishment of breastfeeding support groups and refer mothers to them on discharge from the hospital or clinic.

Source: Baby Friendly Hospital Initiative, BHFI (www.tensteps.org/breastfeeding-bfhi-training-materials.shtml)

Pharmacotherapy during breastfeeding

Despite the fact that lactating women are regular users of medications and are often advised to discontinue or stop nursing while taking drugs, there are only a limited number of drugs that have been clearly identified as potentially harmful to the newborn.[4] In a cohort of 838 nursing infants with mothers taking medications, the incidence of adverse reactions was 11.2%, and all events were classified as minor reactions associated with antibiotics, analgesics/narcotics, antihistamines, sedatives, antidepressants or antiepileptics. A similar pattern was retrieved in the evaluation of 100 published case reports. None were 'definite', 47% were 'probable', 53% were 'possible'. Central nervous system related drugs accounted for about 50% of the events. These observations suggest that a few simple precautions in drug selection and considering the infant's age are important, and breastfeeding very rarely needs to be discontinued when the mother needs pharmacotherapy.

Maternal exposure to a given dose of drug (D_m) will result in transfer of the drug into the milk (D_i) – albeit very limited. However, concentrations in the human milk usually remain low and the infant's oral bioavailability is

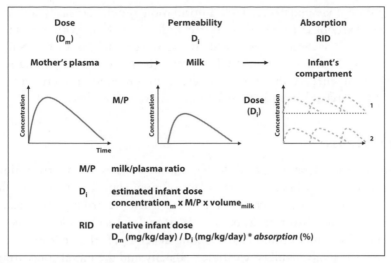

Figure 1 Breastfeeding related drug disposition following maternal drug administration

also a covariate of exposure (RID = relative infant dose, D_m/D_i absorption) (Figure 1). The difference in drug concentration in the infant's compartment (1 vs 2) is explained by either the presence (1) or absence (2) of 'initial concentration due to prenatal exposure', since accumulation relates to dose, duration and the initial concentration in the newborn.

Suggestive indicators of 'likely safe during breastfeeding' are (i) a drug commonly administered to infants (e.g. antibiotics), (ii) a drug that is not absorbed following oral administration (e.g. aminoglycosides, propofol), (iii) a drug not excreted into human milk (e.g. insulin, heparin), and finally (iv) a drug considered safe during pregnancy, since fetal exposure is generally longer and more extensive. In contrast, radioactive labelled diagnostics, lithium, iodine, gold, ergotamine alkaloids and antineoplastics/immune suppressants are high risk drugs, likely not compatible with breastfeeding. Peripartum opioid exposure has also been a focus of interest following a case report of morphine intoxication in a breastfed neonate of a codeine-prescribed mother. Subsequent guidelines (lowest codeine dose possible, maternal exposure <4 days, and switch to non-opioids as soon as possible, monitor maternal and neonatal sedation) resulted in an eightfold reduction (5/238, 2.1%) in the incidence of neonatal sedation and was only associated with prolonged (>4 days) maternal codeine intake.

Sources of information

The knowledge on clinical pharmacology in pregnancy, postpartum and breastfeeding is rapidly evolving and has become a field of active clinical research, albeit sometimes an emotional, opinion driven topic.[5]

This means that updated reliable information should be easily accessible. Besides textbooks, LactMed – a free online database with information on drugs and lactation – is one of the newest additions to the National Library of Medicine's TOXNET system (http://toxnet.nlm.nih.gov/cgi-bin/sis/htmlgen?LACT). The Motherisk programme also provides an updated, searchable website (www.motherisk.org) for advice.

Conclusions

Pregnancy and lactation affect PK/PD, but most drugs are poorly evaluated in this context. During the first trimester of pregnancy, a window of vulnerability already exists, which is of relevance when prescribing for females of childbearing age. Most drugs do appear in the mother's milk, but the final concentration–time profile in the infant depends on the concentration in the milk, the bioavailability, clearance capacity and the initial concentration (fetal and neonatal, or only neonatal exposure). Reliable information sources have become available, reflecting increasing interest in the topic.

References

1 Ramoz LL, Patel-Shori NM. Recent changes in pregnancy and lactation labeling: retirement of risk categories. *Pharmacotherapy* 2014; 34(4): 389–395.
2 Thomas SH, Yates LM. Prescribing without evidence – pregnancy. *Br J Clin Pharmacol* 2012; 74(4): 691–697.
3 Feghali M, Venkataramanan R. Pharmacokinetics of drugs in pregnancy. Semin Perinatol. 2015; 39(7): 512–519.
4 Sachs HC; Committee on drugs. The transfer of drugs and therapeutics into human breast milk: an update on selected topics. *Pediatrics* 2013; 132(3): e796–809.
5 Temming LA *et al*. Clinical management of medications in pregnancy and lactation. *Am J Obstet Gynecol* 2016; 214(6): 698–702.

13

Paediatric clinical pharmacology

I Choonara, K Hoppu, S Ito and GL Kearns

Introduction

The need for improved development, scientific study, regulatory assessment and appropriate use of paediatric medicines has been recognised internationally, especially in the paediatric medicines initiatives of the USA, EU, China and World Health Organization (WHO). Implementation of all the paediatric studies mandated by these initiatives requires well trained investigators and other experts, which in many countries do not yet exist in numbers sufficient to embrace the demands associated with paediatric drug development. Building enhanced capacity and strength in paediatric clinical pharmacology across the world is essential to ensuring the success of these initiatives.

The scientific evidence generated by these initiatives needs to be used to promote the rational use of medicines in children, infants and neonates. Paediatric clinical pharmacologists can play a vital role both in generating the new evidence and also in ensuring its application in enhancing the rational use of paediatric medicines.

The learning objectives of this chapter are:

➤ to know the definition of paediatric clinical pharmacology
➤ to recognise the importance of the discipline in promoting the safe and effective use of medicines in children
➤ to understand the value of paediatric clinical pharmacology in supporting paediatric clinical research and the implementation of evidence-based practice
➤ to gain awareness of examples of current national training programmes.

Definition of paediatric clinical pharmacology

Paediatric clinical pharmacology can be defined as a scientific discipline that involves all aspects of the relationship between drugs and humans during growth, development and maturation.[1] Its breadth includes the continuum between drug discovery, development, regulation and utilisation of medicines (as regards compounds and formulations) intended to benefit the paediatric population. Paediatric clinical pharmacology is also concerned with the adverse effects of medicines, their misuse and the economics of drug therapy as one avenue for restoring and/or promoting child health. As the great majority of scientific research and drug development is, for many reasons, first done in adults, paediatric clinical pharmacology adds the translational element of adopting scientific methods and translating scientific information from adults to paediatric patients.

It is recognised that, by virtue of the comprehensive scope of paediatric clinical pharmacology, it represents a discipline that must be multidisciplinary by design, involving a myriad of skills and relevant individuals with these skills who are involved in one or more scientific and/or clinical facet of the discipline (e.g. physicians, biomedical scientists, non-physician healthcare providers such as nurses and pharmacists). Paediatric clinical pharmacology *per se* is therefore generally not recognised as a profession, but rather as a multifaceted field of endeavour that constitutes a scientifically driven professional discipline dependent on a wide variety of highly skilled professionals who are both educated and trained in a comprehensive and complete fashion.

Scope of practice in the field of paediatric clinical pharmacology

Practice environments for paediatric clinical pharmacology are diverse and can include patient care, research, teaching, drug development and drug regulation. Paediatric clinical pharmacologists may participate directly in the care of paediatric patients as either primary caregivers or consultants, or by working in scientific and/or administrative capacities to improve the quality of medicines use in all healthcare settings and all over the world, irrespective of the wealth of the country. At the country level, paediatric clinical pharmacologists can provide valuable services in the development of a national medicines policy. Linked to the principles of good clinical practice (GCP) that underpin the delivery of clinical research, the paediatric clinical pharmacologist role can in part help to ensure that necessary measures to protect the basic rights of paediatric patients who participate in medicines research are developed and maintained. The role of a paediatric clinical pharmacologist often extends to the regulatory assessment of paediatric medicines, the development of national treatment guidelines, proposing inclusion of paediatric medicines in reimbursement lists, and monitoring the performance of medicines in real life after regulatory approval (e.g. through the application of pharmacoepidemiology, pharmacovigilance and pharmacoeconomic principles) to assess the impact on health outcomes.

It should also be recognised that globally more than a third of the population in developing countries and almost half in the least developed countries are in the paediatric age range (i.e. less than 18 years). Recognising the special needs of children with respect to the development and implementation of safe and effective drug treatment is essential and must be fully embraced. To this end, the enhanced availability of the expertise and services that can be provided by paediatric clinical pharmacologists represents a critical need on a global level.

Training in paediatric clinical pharmacology

Despite the fact that training of paediatric clinical pharmacologists has been going on for decades, training capacity remains small. Consequently, the number of trained paediatric clinical pharmacologists in the world is counted in the hundreds, with the majority of countries having 10 or fewer.[2,3] Paediatric clinical pharmacology is a subdiscipline of clinical pharmacology and paediatrics. At present, it is a recognised paediatric medical subspecialty in the UK, USA, Canada and Australia. Within Europe, several countries either have trainees or an informal training programme.[2,4]

While many of the professionals in the world recognised as paediatric clinical pharmacologists have completed both medical education and formal training programmes in paediatrics and clinical pharmacology, it is important to note that individuals outside the profession of medicine (e.g. professionals with degrees in pharmacy, dentistry and psychology, and biomedical scientists) who have also completed formal training in paediatric clinical pharmacology and received certification through examination by country specific credential-awarding boards have made highly significant and important contributions to the discipline. It is this professional diversity that enriches the discipline and will enable it to embrace the challenges of the future. Thus it is critical that the development of training programmes in paediatric clinical pharmacology be multidimensional in scope and appropriate for the professional skill set of qualified individuals who enter training.

It must be emphasised that the value of training in paediatric clinical pharmacology extends beyond the development of specialist paediatric clinical pharmacologists. It is vital that educational curricula for all healthcare professionals involved in the treatment of infants and children contain instruction in the principles of paediatric clinical pharmacology. Similar educational components should also be included in paediatric medical and surgical subspecialty training programmes. The continued development of programmes and practitioners of paediatric clinical pharmacology is essential for these broad educational goals to be accomplished throughout the world.

Examples of current training programmes

UK

The UK has both a recognised training programme and accreditation,[4] coordinated by the Royal College of Paediatrics and Child Health. Applicants need to be medical graduates on a training programme in paediatrics. A minimum of 2 years' general professional training and 2 years of core training in paediatrics are required before applicants are eligible. The actual training programme in paediatric clinical pharmacology is for 3 years. The training programme in the UK has recently been described.[4]

USA

Paediatric (or adult) clinical pharmacology in the USA is not recognised formally as a subspecialty of medicine. The American Board of Clinical Pharmacology (ABCP) was established with collaboration from the three major organisations representing clinical pharmacology in the USA: the American Society for Clinical Pharmacology and Therapeutics, the American College of Clinical Pharmacology and the American Society for Pharmacology and Experimental Therapeutics. ABCP has two primary functions: 1) the administration of a certification examination in clinical and applied pharmacology for physician and non-physician candidates who are suitably qualified in clinical pharmacology, and 2) the registration and accreditation of clinical pharmacology training programmes. Paediatric clinical pharmacology is recognised by the American Academy of Pediatrics as an area of specialisation within paediatric medicine.

The National Institutes of Health (NIH) through its National Institute of General Medical Sciences (NIGMS) has supported training programmes in adult clinical pharmacology through a training grant (T32) funding mechanism. To facilitate training in paediatric clinical pharmacology, Eunice Kennedy Shriver National Institute of Child Health and Human Development (NICHD) provided each NIGMS-supported T32 programme with one training slot for a paediatrician into the clinical pharmacology fellowship programme, of a minimum of 24 months, for completing specialised training and conducting research. NICHD also supported three fellowship training programmes that focused on paediatric/developmental pharmacology research.

Paediatric clinical pharmacology in the USA is multidisciplinary by design. Most paediatric clinical pharmacology programmes in the USA require that candidates either have completed a paediatric medical residency or, for non-physicians (individuals with PharmD, PhD or PharmD/PhD degrees), are licensed healthcare professionals (e.g. pharmacists, nurse practitioners) who have previously completed clinical training that included experience in paediatric therapeutics. This enables the full integration of both physicians and non-physicians in a single paediatric clinical pharmacology programme, thereby providing a unified fellowship training platform that facilitates cross-discipline education provided not only by programme faculty but also by peers. It also magnifies the importance of complementary expertise to this multifaceted specialty.

Canada

In Canada, the Royal College of Physicians and Surgeons of Canada (RCPSC) governs training of medical specialists at each medical school, which leads to professional recognition after successful completion of the training, including the RCPSC certification examination. The subspecialty in clinical pharmacology and toxicology (CPT) is one of the RCPSC recognised medical disciplines. As of 2014, trainees are eligible to apply to CPT programmes if they are currently in one of the five RCPSC-recognised disciplines: internal medicine, paediatrics, psychiatry, anaesthesia, and emergency medicine. The curriculum and training contents, which are available on the RCPSC website (www.royalcollege.ca/portal/page/portal/rc/about), address not only general clinical pharmacology and toxicology common to all of these primary entry disciplines, but also specifics relevant to the primary specialty of each trainee. Therefore, those who are from paediatrics learn both general and paediatric clinical pharmacology and toxicology. In Canada, core paediatrics training is for 3 years, and the CPT subspecialty training is for an additional 2 years. Training objectives are aligned with the CanMEDS 2015 (Canadian Medical Education Directives for Specialists) framework, which describes the roles of medical specialists in the key domain of medical expert, supported by the other domains of communicator, advocate, manager, collaborator, professional and scholar (www.royalcollege.ca/portal/page/portal/rc/canmeds).

Conclusions

Paediatric clinical pharmacology is a scientific discipline that involves all aspects of the relationship between drugs and humans during growth, development and maturation. Building enhanced capacity and strength in paediatric clinical pharmacology across the world is essential to ensure the success of the paediatric medicines initiatives. Paediatric clinical pharmacology is a subdiscipline of clinical pharmacology and paediatrics. In some countries, individuals outside the profession of medicine can also formally train in paediatric clinical pharmacology and receive certification through examination by country specific credential-awarding boards.

References

1 Hoppu K. Drug therapy in paediatric patients. In: Rägo, L *et al.*, eds. *Clinical Pharmacology in Health Care, Teaching and Research*. Geneva: Council for International Organizations of Medical Sciences (CIOMS), 17–18.

2 Bonati M *et al.* Paediatric clinical pharmacology in Europe. *Paediatr Perinat Drug Ther* 2006; 7(3): 134–137.

3 Koren G, Macleod SM. The state of pediatric clinical pharmacology: an international survey of training programs. *Clin Pharmacol Ther* 1989; 46(5): 489–493.

4 Choonara I, Sammons H. Paediatric clinical pharmacology in the UK. *Arch Dis Child* 2014; 99(12): 1143–1146.

14

Education: training programmes and competencies

K Parker and S Ito

Introduction

One of the main objectives of the Global Research in Paediatrics (GRiP) Network of Excellence (www.grip-network.org) was to develop a high quality, pedagogically sound international training framework for paediatric clinical pharmacology. The work included development of a fellowship programme in paediatric clinical pharmacology (PCP) to address the global need for health professionals to be skilled in the areas of drug development and clinical trials. This chapter details how the fellowship was developed in accordance with best practices in curriculum development so that GRiP quality criteria could be achieved.

The learning objectives of this chapter are:

➤ to define the GRiP quality criteria applied to the fellowship programme
➤ to describe how two pedagogical frameworks (Kern[1] and Bloom[2]) were used in the development of the fellowship
➤ to identify the key components of the fellowship curriculum as defined in Kern's model.[1]

Quality criteria for the fellowship programme

The GRiP community is committed to generating and disseminating educational initiatives of the highest quality. The central tenets of high quality education were defined by members of the GRiP community and are as follows.

1 **GRiP education activities are based on assessment of learning needs.**
   Planning of all GRiP educational activities, including the fellowship programme, is based on an assessment of learning needs. Needs assessment is
   performed at programme level for training programmes, and at the level
   of individual participants for courses (modules).
2 **The content of GRiP education is relevant and of high scientific quality.**
   The relevance of the content is based on needs assessment of the
   participants, thorough up-to-date content expertise of the staff and
   teachers, and high quality learning resources made available for the
   participants. The learning objectives, learning resources and competence
   of the teachers selected are described and justified in the documentation
   of the educational activity.
3 **Educational methods employed are effective and will result in the desired
   learning outcomes.**
   Targeted outcomes cannot be reached by delivering appropriate scientific
   content unless the educational methods employed result in learning by the
   participants. The educational methods used are described and justified in
   the documentation of the educational activity.
4 **Assessment of learning outcomes and their relevance is included in all
   educational interventions.**
   As GRiP educational activities are aimed at postgraduate students
   or professional experts, meaningful learning outcomes are related to
   better attitudes, knowledge and skills in the professional work of the
   learners after the interventions. Assessment of learning outcomes needs
   to consider both the relevance of the outcomes and their relationship to
   the learning objectives. The learning outcomes and the methods used
   to assess these outcomes are described and justified in the documentation
   of the educational activity. Assessment of the opinion of the participants
   on the educational intervention and the process can be included, but
   cannot substitute for assessment of learning outcomes.

Developing the fellowship programme

The first step in the building process was to ground the fellowship programme in an existing competency framework. Programme developers chose
the CanMEDS Framework (2005) from the Royal College of Physicians and
Surgeons of Canada.[3] The framework assumes that the professional practice
of physicians consists of several roles that the physician must play. Key
competencies exist for each role, and it was critical to determine how the
programme mapped onto these competencies. Importantly, this competency
framework, developed originally for physician training, has an obvious surface validity in advanced training of other professionals such as pharmacists
and PhD scientists in the field of clinical pharmacology. The content of

the GRiP PCP fellowship curriculum was also developed based on existing training programmes in general clinical pharmacology in countries such as Australia/New Zealand (Australasia), Canada, the UK and USA. In particular, the Canadian postgraduate medical education governed by the Royal College of Physicians and Surgeons of Canada[3] was used as a template for this GRiP PCP fellowship curriculum document.

In order to ensure that the quality criteria are met, developers of the GRiP PCP fellowship programme adopted two well established and widely used frameworks in the field of pedagogy: Bloom's cognitive learning taxonomy and Kern's six steps in the development of a medical curriculum.[2,3]

Bloom's taxonomy of learning

In 1956, Benjamin Bloom and colleagues published a framework for categorising educational goals: *Taxonomy of Educational Objectives*.[2] Commonly known as Bloom's taxonomy, this framework has been applied by generations of school teachers and college instructors in their teaching.

The framework consists of six major categories: knowledge, comprehension, application, analysis, synthesis and evaluation. The categories after knowledge are presented as skills and abilities, with the understanding that knowledge is the necessary precondition for putting these skills and abilities into practice. Further details on the six levels from the original taxonomy are as follows:[*]

- **Knowledge** involves the recall of specifics and universals, the recall of methods and processes, or the recall of a pattern, structure or setting.
- **Comprehension** refers to a type of understanding or apprehension such that the individual knows what is being communicated and can make use of the material or idea being communicated without necessarily relating it to other material or seeing its fullest implications.
- **Application** refers to the use of abstractions in particular and concrete situations.
- **Analysis** represents the breakdown of a communication into its constituent elements or parts such that the relative hierarchy of ideas is made clear and/or the relations between ideas expressed are made explicit.
- **Synthesis** involves the putting together of elements and parts so as to form a whole.
- **Evaluation** engenders judgements about the value of material and methods for given purposes.

[*] from http://cft.vanderbilt.edu/guides-sub-pages/blooms-taxonomy

All GRiP education programming, including the fellowship programme, uses Bloom's taxonomy as a building block for learning objectives so as to achieve quality criteria 3 and 4.[2] The use of Bloom's taxonomy facilitates alignment between learning objectives, the instructional methods needed to achieve them, and the assessment techniques needed to determine whether the learner has achieved the learning objectives.[2]

Kern's model for curriculum development

In order to meet quality criterion 1 and to provide a framework to guide the development of GRiP education, David Kern's model for curriculum development in medical education is essential.[1] This six-step model is a practical, theoretically sound approach to developing, implementing, evaluating and continually improving educational experiences, particularly in the health science field, such as in medicine. Visually rendered in the diagram below (Figure 1), the development of all GRiP education begins with a rationale or problem statement that argues why the development of the programme is important and what problem the programme is designed to address.

Once the problem has been identified (step 1), a targeted needs assessment is required (step 2 in the model and GRiP quality criterion 1) to assess the learning needs of the targeted group and/or institution.

Once the needs assessment has been conducted, the articulation of the learning goals and objectives is step 3. As stated previously, Bloom's taxonomy was used to articulate the learning objectives. Step 4 is to identify the educational strategies that are appropriate for the learning objectives. Step 5 is to implement the programme, and step 6 is to assess the extent

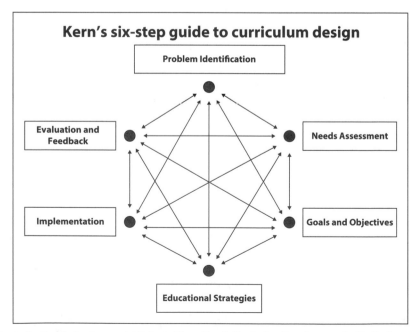

Kern's six-step guide to curriculum design

Problem Identification

Evaluation and Feedback

Needs Assessment

Implementation

Goals and Objectives

Educational Strategies

Figure 1 Kern's six-step model (adapted from Kern's *Curriculum Development for Medical Education: A 6-step Approach*[1])

to which learners achieved the learning objectives and to evaluate the programme more broadly.

Overview of the fellowship curriculum

Rationale/problem identification

Clinical pharmacology encompasses a broad field of therapeutics and its applications in clinical, research and regulatory settings. Because of the discipline's history, patient care provision has formed a key skill set of a clinical pharmacologist, specifically for those in the medical and pharmaceutical profession. Over the years, however, knowledge and skill sets necessary for clinical pharmacology activity have expanded into the area of drug development and clinical drug trials, which are not directly related to clinical care at the patient level. Now it is abundantly clear that such a population-level practice of clinical pharmacology in drug development and clinical trials is possible. This type of practice is not only possible, but also highly sought after due to relative lack of qualified experts, particularly in the field of paediatric clinical pharmacology. A societal need for professional training in paediatric clinical pharmacology with the expanded focus is now clear, aiming for those with a background in medicine, pharmacy or clinical research areas. However, such training opportunities are largely lacking, let alone a standard for the expert education in the field. Recognising the need for such a curriculum with international validity, the GRiP curriculum in paediatric clinical pharmacology has been developed.

Goals and objectives

The aim of the curriculum is to train paediatricians, pharmacists and PhD scientists as experts in paediatric clinical pharmacology for professional competency, knowledge, skills and attitudes. A professional trainee who has successfully completed the fellowship programme will become a Fellow in Paediatric Clinical Pharmacology, competent in drug regulation at local, national and global levels and in the broader area of paediatric drug research. Those training for medicine or pharmacy qualifications will also acquire specialised patient care skills within their respective disciplines. By the end of the training, the Fellow will become a professional expert in paediatric pharmacology who is able to independently function as a consultant with the highest ethical standard. In addition to the research related activity, these professionals will be capable of practising in their clinical domains of patient care settings, and teaching this specialised field to learners at all levels.

Specific learning objectives were written for the topics in Table 1 (educational strategies are described on the GRiP website, www.grip-network.org/index.php/cms/en/training_and_education).

Table 1 Key topics in paediatric clinical pharmacology	
1. Molecular and translational pharmacology	10. Drug interactions
2. Pharmacogenetics/genomics	11. Clinical toxicology
3. Pharmacokinetics (PK)	12. Drug use during pregnancy and lactation
4. Pharmacodynamics (PD)	13. Adverse drug reactions and medication errors
5. Pharmacometrics	14. Substance abuse and drug addiction
6. Pharmacoeconomics and health technology assessment	15. Specific therapeutics areas
7. Drug analyses	16. Pharmaceutical issues
8. Regulatory science of drug development	17. Rational use of medicines in paediatric population
9. Clinical drug research	

Implementation

The following requirements are critical to the successful development of the curriculum and must be in place prior to launch.

A **Organisational requirement**
   1 A clearly defined organisational structure of the curriculum within its institution
   2 A programme director
   3 Administrative staff to support the director
   4 A sufficient number of teaching faculty members
   5 A patient base sufficient for the training
B **Programme support**
   1 Sufficient administrative support from the home institution to the training programme
   2 The programme director, with protected time dedicated for the programme operation
C **Programme committee**
   1 The programme committee supports the programme director for operation of the training programme
   2 The programme committee meets at least every 6 months

Evaluation and assessment

Qualifications for programme completion

The methods used to determine whether the learner has met the learning objectives must be appropriate. For example, a multiple choice test should not be used to assess skill acquisition, nor should performance in a simulator be used to assess basic knowledge of a concept. Furthermore, assessment of students' ability using multiple methods and multiple assessors is strongly recommended in order to accurately determine whether a student has successfully completed the programme. Successful completion of training is based, ideally, on a series of both formative and summative assessments. Specific requirements for programme completion are also largely influenced by the institution in which the programme is based.

Programme evaluation

An evaluation plan for the fellowship curriculum will be co-created with a group of programme stakeholders. The evaluation plan for the curriculum will likely include the collection of the following information for the purposes of programme accountability, ongoing programme development and transportability.

- Feedback from the learners on the quality of their experience in the fellowship
- Feedback from the faculty members on the quality of their experiences delivering the fellowship
- Learner assessment data to determine the extent to which the learners met the learning objectives
- Feedback from members of the four educational institutions to determine best practices in the implementation of the programme across four distinct educational contexts

Conclusions

The GRiP PCP fellowship curriculum was developed according to the guiding principles of the quality criteria, the structures of the existing training programmes in clinical pharmacology in the USA, Canada, UK and Australasia, and the competency framework of the Royal College of Physicians and Surgeons of Canada. Bloom's taxonomy and Kern's model were used to build learning objectives and design the curriculum. Institutions that operate or plan to develop such training programmes may use the fellowship curriculum as a standard template to train those who can eventually lead in various aspects of paediatric drug development, research, regulation, education and clinical care.

References

1 Kern D. *Curriculum Development for Medical Education: A 6-step Approach*. Michigan, USA: Johns Hopkins University Press, 1998.
2 Bloom, BS. *Taxonomy of Educational Objectives*, Handbook I: *The Cognitive Domain*. New York: David McKay Co Inc, 1956.
3 Frank JR *et al*., eds. *CanMEDS 2005 Physician Competency Framework*. Ottawa, Canada: Royal College of Physicians and Surgeons of Canada, 2005. www.royalcollege.ca/canmeds

15

The paediatric drug discovery pipeline

J Lass and I Lutsar

Introduction

Drug discovery and the development pipeline refer to a set of drug candidates that are under development by the pharmaceutical industry. The drug will progress through the research and development (R&D) pipeline if there is proof of concept for efficacy and safety. Before a new medicine is available for use in humans, it will pass through several development phases, such as preclinical and clinical studies. If enough data supporting safety and efficacy are available that is relevant to a particular clinical indication and age group, a manufacturer can apply for a marketing authorisation (MA) for the drug.

The learning objectives of this chapter are:

➤ to understand the key phases in the paediatric drug development pipeline
➤ to recognise the differences in the licensing of medicines for children compared with that for adults
➤ to learn about recent progress in drug development in defined paediatric therapeutic areas and the associated challenges.

Background

The drug development process, demonstrated in Figure 1, can be divided into the following phases:[1]

* Discovery
* Preclinical studies
* Clinical trials (phase I, II and III)
* Post-marketing studies

The development phase including children usually starts with drugs entering phase I and II clinical trials. Phase I studies, which usually commence in older children, typically start during or after phase III studies of that same

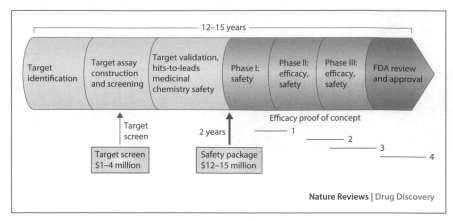

Figure 1 Drug discovery and development pipeline[1]
www.nature.com/nrd/journal/v7/n10/fig_tab/nrd2593_F1.html

agent in adults. When data about the pharmacokinetics, tolerability and safety of the study medicine are available, younger study subjects can then be recruited.

The decade of the 1990s is considered a golden era in the pharmaceutical industry when many blockbuster drugs generating huge annual sales for the developing drug companies came onto the market. After the peak in 1996, the output of new drugs has remained largely static. For example, in 2008, only 21 new medicines were approved for marketing in the USA.[2] This resulted from a reduced output of new medicines from R&D laboratories and has been called a productivity crisis in the pharmaceutical industry.[3] This so-called productivity gap describes the situation when the investments of the pharmaceutical industry do not match the expected product turnover. Also, several backup and 'me too' drug candidates have entered the market instead of the medicines needed for priority therapeutic areas, including paediatrics. At present, there are more than 4300 companies engaged in drug innovation, yet only 6% of these have registered at least one new compound since 1950.[2]

The number of new molecular entities (NMEs) required to achieve one new drug approval is increasing at every stage of development. In 2007–2011, it took an average of 30.4 NMEs in preclinical development to obtain one approval, compared with just 12.4 NMEs in 2003–2007.[4] *De novo* drug discovery is often inefficient. According to a recent analysis, unacceptable safety was the most important reason for drug candidate failure en route to the market, accounting for more than half of all project closures. The majority of preclinical safety closures were related to organ toxicities (cardiovascular toxicity 17%, hepatotoxicity 14%, renal toxicity 8%). The next highest cause of project closure was a lack of efficacy in the chosen disease indication.[3]

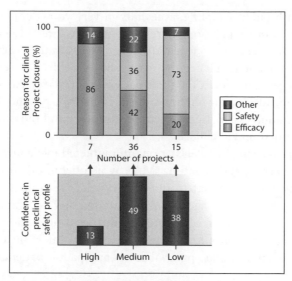

Figure 2 Analysis of project closures due to safety issues[3]

Preclinical and clinical projects that were closed because of safety issues were previously analysed to understand the principal causes of failure.[3] The level of confidence that teams had in their preclinical safety profile (Figure 2 lower graph) was compared with the reasons for project closure in the clinical phase (upper graph). Percentages of projects in each category are shown within bars, and numbers of project closures analysed are shown underneath each bar.

The product pipeline overviews for specific products/therapeutic areas can be seen on the websites of specific pharmaceutical companies.

Licensing of paediatric medicines – adult versus paediatric drug development pipeline

Many diseases occurring in children, particularly acute disorders, can be managed effectively with medicines that are already available. However, many of the medicines used routinely have not undergone formal clinical studies in children, thus often have no paediatric labelling and are used off label.

The early regulatory medicines licensing documents and processes did not automatically include children in the drug development processes. In addition to the ambiguous regulatory situation, there were multiple factors limiting the number of paediatric clinical trials, such as difficulties recruiting patients into studies (due to the small number of children suffering from specific conditions), more complex study design than for adult studies (e.g. age specific drug formulations needed) and technical challenges, e.g. constraints associated with blood sampling, especially in very young children. The first paediatric medicines regulations were established as late as the mid-1990s.

Few diseases occur only in children and necessitate specific medicines not required for adults. Hence the early phases of drug development and clinical trials generally focus on adult patients, and paediatric development has largely depended on the pharmaceutical company's product strategy with respect to the adult population, except for vaccines and those medicines for indications only found in children.

According to current EU legislation, all marketed medicines are required to have a marketing authorisation (MA), which defines their terms of use. If there are enough data on safety and efficacy relevant to a particular clinical indication and a particular age group, a manufacturer can apply for an MA for the drug. A licence is an MA issued by the licensing authority. Approval of new medicinal products for paediatric patients almost invariably occurs after their development and approval for treating adult patients.

Paediatric drug development pipelines of different therapeutic areas

As paediatric drug development usually starts after adult clinical trials, for many therapeutic areas the paediatric pipeline problems are related to the legislative status of a medicinal product or the lack of a child specific drug formulation. Despite the changes in legislation surrounding the approval of medicines for children in Europe and the USA, the paediatric pipeline descriptions do not seem particularly optimistic in any of the therapeutic areas. The bottlenecks of the paediatric drug development pipeline are already well known, e.g. small numbers of patients, limitations of legislation for paediatric medicines and insufficient return on investment.

Here we will provide a robust overview of the following pipelines:

- Child specific therapeutic areas – development of prophylactic vaccines
- The most commonly used drug class in paediatrics: systemic antibacterials
- Drugs for a disease with increasing prevalence in children – type 2 diabetes mellitus
- Medicines for neglected diseases and illnesses mostly affecting children in developing countries where there is a lack of suitable drugs and dosage forms – tuberculosis, HIV and orphan drugs
- Fast developing therapeutic fields in adults, such as oncology

Vaccines

Vaccine development is relatively intensive compared with other therapeutic areas, and the global market for prophylactic vaccines is broader than ever. Today, biopharmaceutical research companies are developing over 200 vaccines for infectious diseases, cancer, neurological disorders, allergies and other diseases. From 1995 to 2008, the number of prophylactic vaccine originators more than doubled.[5] However, the average development time for a vaccine is over 10 years, and each vaccine has a market entry probability of only 6%.[6] The recent analysis shows a continuing decline in vaccine market entry success rates.[7] Also the time for the preclinical development has been found to be significantly longer for prophylactic vaccines compared with other pharmaceuticals (3.7 years vs 2.8 years), and it takes 15–20 years to development a vaccine.[5]

Antibiotics

Systemic antibiotics are the drug class most commonly prescribed to children, and infectious diseases are also the leading cause of death in children younger than 5 years. In older children, pneumonia accounts for 14.1% of all deaths (1.071 million in 2010).[8] The emergence of multidrug-resistant bacteria has challenged clinicians with regard to selection of effective antimicrobial therapy and highlighted the general antibiotic pipeline problem also affecting children. The recent reports by the Infectious Diseases Society of America (IDSA), the European Centre for Disease Prevention and Control, and the European Medicines Agency show that there are few candidate drugs in the pipeline that offer benefits over existing antibacterials. There are only two new antibiotics – telavancin and ceftaroline fosamil – that have been approved since 2009.[9,10] Also it was described that, in 2013, it was mostly small pharmaceutical or biotechnology companies developing antibacterial drugs.[10] As one of the initiatives to improve the situation, IDSA has launched a new collaboration with several societies, titled the 10 × '20 initiative, which aims to support the development of ten new antibiotics by 2020 through the discovery of new drug classes as well as exploring possible new drugs from existing antibiotic classes.[11]

Type 2 diabetes mellitus

Type 2 diabetes mellitus (T2DM) was not a paediatric disease until recently, when the incidence in children and young adolescents began to rise world-wide. The prevalence in the USA increased by 30.5% between 2001 and 2009 in both sexes and all age groups, with a prevalence of 0.46 per 1000.[12] Several new drug groups, such as glucagon-like peptide 1 mimetics (e.g. exenatide) and dipeptidyl peptidase inhibitors (e.g. sitagliptin), are in the pipeline for treatment of T2DM in children. Still, it is not yet comparable with the adult pipeline, where several new drug classes such as incretin-based therapies, sodium glucose cotransporter inhibitors, glucokinase inhibitors, 11β-hydroxysteroid dehydrogenase (HSD)-1 inhibitors, drugs modulating fatty acid metabolism, selective peroxisome proliferator-activated receptor gamma receptor modulators, immunomodulatory drugs and many others are under development. However, at the time of writing, only metformin and insulin are currently licensed for use in the paediatric population.

Tuberculosis

Tuberculosis is among the top causes of death among children, especially in low income countries, with 1 million cases each year occurring in children under 15 years old. The tuberculosis drug pipeline is currently filled with several new drugs that have already reached phase II and III clinical trials. In the past decade, six new compounds specifically developed for tuberculosis have reached the clinical study phase.[13] Nevertheless, the development of novel paediatric medicines for children has lagged behind again – in part for clinical reasons (e.g. difficulties diagnosing pulmonary tuberculosis in children, characterisation of treatment response, and concerns regarding side-effects) and the inherent flaws in paediatric drug development, such as challenges finding optimal trial design or timing the paediatric involvement in development.

HIV infection

The development and pipeline of HIV therapeutics for adults can be considered relatively effective: almost 30 antiretroviral drugs and several additional antiretroviral combinations have been approved since the discovery of HIV. Still, the pipeline for paediatric HIV is narrow. Since HIV is rare in children in high income countries, the development of child friendly formulations suitable for high burden settings is not considered a priority by drug companies.[14] There is also a need to ensure that HIV drugs are appropriate for the conditions of the developing world, where people need simple single fixed-dose regimens for drugs that do not need refrigeration, as over 90% of children with HIV/AIDS live in the developing world.[15]

Orphan drugs

One of the therapeutic areas where drug development is most complicated is developing orphan drugs, since the target population is exceptionally small, again resulting in diminished returns from investment. In 2013, 81 drugs for orphan diseases had marketing authorisations in Europe, but only half of these have become available for children, and 25 potential paediatric products were still off label for children at the time of marketing authorisation.[16]

Oncology

Although many advances have been made in cancer treatments in adults, the development of oncology products for children has lagged behind due to the relatively small market of paediatric oncology, which also does not provide sufficient financial incentive for pharmaceutical companies. New drug development for children with cancer is insufficient also, because most paediatric cancers are divided into several molecularly defined subtypes, meaning once more that fewer patients will be available to participate in clinical trials of relevant biomarker-directed targeted treatments.[17] It has been shown that of 120 oncological medicines approved by the US Food and Drug Administration between 1948 and 2003, only 30 have been used in children.[18]

Neonatology

Another area within which there is limited progress in terms of new and innovative medicines is neonatology. New technologies are needed for treatment of perinatal asphyxia and for promotion of extrauterine lung maturation. Agents with neuroprotective properties are also needed to prevent long term consequences of prematurity.

Means of improvement: drug repurposing

In addition to the *de novo* design of new medicines, a repositioning of 'old' medicines has also been identified as a way forward to help accelerate the process. Repositioning/repurposing is a drug development strategy that consists of finding new therapeutic uses for already known drugs.

A repositioned drug can go directly to preclinical testing and clinical trials. Even if the drug has already been used for a long time, clinical trials are still needed with respect to efficacy (e.g. for the novel indication) and sometimes for safety as well (e.g. when doses higher than the currently approved ones are needed).[19]

Some drug repositioning examples for alternative indications include: thalidomide, which was prescribed as a sedative in the 1960s but has been successfully repositioned for treatment of multiple myeloma; anticonvulsants (carbamazepine, gabapentin, pregabalin) for neuropathic pain; and sildenafil for angina repurposed for persistent pulmonary hypertension.

Conclusion

Despite the production of some remarkable drugs for diseases such as HIV and rheumatoid arthritis during recent decades, paediatric drug development still lags behind. This could be enhanced by improved regulatory requirements, innovative trial designs and better collaboration between pharmaceutical companies, academia and government.

References

1 Roses AD. Pharmacogenetics in drug discovery and development: a translational perspective. *Nat Rev Drug Discov* 2008; 7: 807–817.

2 Munos B. Lessons from 60 years of pharmaceutical innovation. *Nat Rev Drug Discov* 2009; 8: 959–968.

3 Cook D *et al*. Lessons learned from the fate of AstraZeneca's drug pipeline: a five-dimensional framework. *Nat Rev Drug Discov* 2014; 13(6): 419–431.

4 Moors EHM *et al*. Towards a sustainable system of drug development. *Drug Discov Today* 2014; 19(11): 1711–1720.

5 Davis MM *et al*. Failure-to-success ratios, transition probabilities and phase lengths for prophylactic vaccines versus other pharmaceuticals in the development pipeline. *Vaccine* 2011; 29(51): 9414–9416.

6 Pronker ES *et al*. Risk in vaccine research and development quantified. *PloS One* 2013; 8(3): e57755.

7 Stephens P. Vaccine R&D: Past performance is no guide to the future. *Vaccine* 2014; 32(19): 2139–2142.

8 Liu L *et al*. Global, regional, and national causes of child mortality: an updated systematic analysis for 2010 with time trends since 2000. *Lancet* 2012; 379(9832): 2151–2161.

9 Garazzino S *et al*. New antibiotics for paediatric use: A review of a decade of regulatory trials submitted to the European Medicines Agency from 2000 – Why aren't we doing better? *Int J Antimicrob Agents* 2013; 42(2): 99–118.

10 Boucher HW *et al*. 10 × '20 Progress – development of new drugs active against gram-negative bacilli: an update from the Infectious Diseases Society of America. *Clin Infect Dis* 2013; 56(12): 1685–1694.

11 Infectious Diseases Society of America. The 10 x '20 initiative: pursuing a global commitment to develop 10 new antibacterial drugs by 2020. *Clin Infect Dis* 2010; 50(8): 1081–1083.

12 Dabelea D *et al*. Prevalence of type 1 and type 2 diabetes among children and adolescents from 2001 to 2009. *JAMA* 2014; 311(17): 1778–1786.

13 Ma Z, Lienhardt C. Toward an optimized therapy for tuberculosis? Drugs in clinical trials and in preclinical development. *Clin Chest Med* 2009; 30(4): 755–768.

14 Lallemant M *et al*. Pediatric HIV – a neglected disease? *N Engl J Med* 2011; 365(7): 581–583.

15 Ford N *et al*. Treating HIV in the developing world: getting ahead of the drug development curve. *Drug Discov Today* 2007; 12(1): 1–3.

16 Kreeftmeijer-Vegter AR *et al*. The influence of the European paediatric regulation on marketing authorisation of orphan drugs for children. *Orphanet J Rare Dis* 2014; 9(1): 120.

17 Vassal G *et al*. New drugs for children and adolescents with cancer: the need for novel development pathways. *Lancet Oncol* 2013; 14(3): e117–e124.

18 Adamson PC *et al*. Drug discovery in paediatric oncology: roadblocks to progress. *Nat Rev Clin Oncol* 2014; 11(12): 732–739.

19 Oprea TI *et al*. Drug repurposing from an academic perspective. *Drug Discov Today Ther Strateg* 2012; 8(3–4): 61–69.

Further recommended reading

Berti E *et al*. Tuberculosis in childhood: a systematic review of national and international guidelines. *BMC Infect Dis* 2014; 14 Suppl 1: S3.

Blatt J, Seth JC. Drug repurposing in pediatrics and pediatric hematology oncology. *Drug Discov Today* 2013; 18(1): 4–10.

Brodie MJ. Antiepileptic drug therapy the story so far. *Seizure* 2010; 19(10): 650–655.

Davis MM *et al.* The expanding vaccine development pipeline, 1995–2008. *Vaccine* 2010; 28(5): 1353–1356.

Fonseca V. Diabetes mellitus in the next decade: Novel pipeline medications to treat hyperglycemia. *Clin Ther* 2013; 35(5): 714–723.

Jassal MS, Grace MA. 2050: Ending the odyssey of the great white plague. Part of a series on Pediatric Pharmacology, guest edited by Gianvincenzo Zuccotti, Emilio Clementi, and Massimo Molteni. *Pharmacol Res* 2011; 64(3): 176–179.

Jin G, Wong ST. Toward better drug repositioning: prioritizing and integrating existing methods into efficient pipelines. *Drug Discov Today* 2014; 19(5): 637–644.

Lass J *et al.* Off label use of prescription medicines in children in outpatient setting in Estonia is common. *Pharmacoepidemiol Drug Saf* 2011; 20(5): 474–481.

Lass J *et al.* Antibiotic prescription preferences in paediatric outpatient setting in Estonia and Sweden. *SpringerPlus* 2013; 2(1): 1–8.

Rafols I *et al.* Big pharma, little science? A bibliometric perspective on big pharma's R&D decline. *Technol Forecast Social Change* 2014; 81: 22–38.

Stehr M *et al.* Filling the pipeline – new drugs for an old disease. *Curr Top Med Chem* 2014; 14(1): 110–129.

Swaminathan S, Banu R. Pediatric tuberculosis: global overview and challenges. *Clin Infect Dis* 2010; 50 Suppl 3: S184–S194.

Van Gaal L *et al.* Efficacy and safety of the glucagon-like peptide-1 receptor agonist lixisenatide versus the dipeptidyl peptidase-4 inhibitor sitagliptin in young (<50 years) obese patients with type 2 diabetes mellitus. *J Clin Transl Endocrinol* 2014; 1(2): 31–37.

16

Understanding phase I clinical trials

A Al-Hashimi and DB Hawcutt

Introduction

The transition from preclinical studies to clinical studies is arguably the most exciting stage of drug development. Now the active pharmaceutical ingredient (API) is converted into a drug ready to be administered to patients; only at this stage is the new API finally subjected to the true human physiological and metabolic complexities, after years of preclinical testing. This stage in pharmaceutical drug development is referred to as a phase I clinical trial.

The learning objectives of this chapter are:

➢ to understand the aims of phase I clinical trials in children and the associated challenges
➢ to gain insight into how paediatric phase I studies are designed
➢ to learn strategies to improve study design relating to informed consent and blood sampling
➢ to recognise the benefits of developing specialist centres to deliver phase I studies.

Background

Phase I study classification in paediatrics is significantly different to that in adults. In adults, the majority of phase I studies involve the API being given to healthy volunteers (often staff volunteers from within the pharmaceutical company). The exceptions to this, where phase I studies are conducted on the target patient population, are undertaken in areas like chemotherapy in oncology and some advanced therapies such as biologics and gene and cell therapy. Paediatrics also uses a 'first in patient' approach, so the trial participant(s) are affected by the condition the drug is designed to treat.

The aim of phase I studies is to establish pharmacokinetic (PK) information to guide the dose to be used in the following phases of drug development. It is also the beginning of the collection of drug safety data. Prior to paediatric phase I studies, adult phase I studies are normally undertaken to provide additional PK and safety data, and the design of paediatric studies often captures pharmacodynamics (PD) and efficacy information as well. The study design most commonly used in children is therefore termed a phase Ib/IIa, indicating that the study is starting with some prior knowledge and crossing over to what is commonly seen in phase II studies.

Study design

A phase I study is usually designed as a single dose study, investigating safety and PK with multiple PK samples at varying time points, followed by a multiple dose PK study with serial PK collections. An alternative design is a combined multiple dose study with serial and sparse PK samples after the first dose and at steady state to establish PK, safety and some efficacy data for the subsequent phases of development. For studies with significant prior data from adult studies, particularly those with predictable PK and a suitable model to select a single appropriate dose, then one single dose PK study may be sufficient, with serial PK collection followed by efficacy/safety studies with sparse PK samples collected to evaluate multiple dose PK data.

The level and quality of data available prior to the initiation of phase I studies will influence the study design and dose selection. Extending the use of information and conclusions available from adult studies is referred to as extrapolation.[1] Before deciding whether extrapolation is feasible, the following must be assessed: PK/PD data from adults; bioavailability, palatability and excipient content of the paediatric formulation; age of the target population, and therefore the physiological developmental level of each subgroup (hepatic, renal, CYP450 and transporter systems).

A European Medicines Agency (EMA) based, cross-committee working group has established a framework for a systematic approach to extrapolation through setting out when, where and how to apply extrapolation.[1]

Usually in adult phase I clinical trials, the number of patients in each arm is between 10 and 40; however, this is more difficult to predict in paediatrics. In recent guidance, the US Food and Drug Administration (FDA) endorsed work and recommended an approach to prospectively target a 95% confidence interval within 60% and 140% of the geometric mean estimates of clearance and volume of distribution for the drug in each paediatric subgroup with at least 80% power.[2] Using this method with assumptions, it is possible to estimate the sample size for phase I studies.

In paediatric phase I studies investigating conditions also seen in adults, the API would have been tested previously in adult patients. Most commercial studies in paediatrics start later in the product development cycle and as part of a paediatric investigation plan (PIP) agreed with the EMA and/or FDA.[3] The information gained from studies in adults is utilised and modelled to guide the PIP, which then is agreed with the regulatory bodies.

For studies investigating conditions specific to the paediatric population, such as respiratory distress syndrome and congenital heart disease, previous data from adult studies will not be available. A phase I study in healthy adults may be required, if possible, while studies investigating chemotherapy or some advanced biologic therapies will be conducted in the target patient population, as in adults.

Clinical trials in paediatrics: formulation considerations

In phase I studies, the excitement of a new API becoming a medicine must not lead to a rushed transition to clinical studies. To turn an API into a medicine, it must be formulated into a suitable vehicle for the target age group.[4] This will usually include a formulation that is more complicated than simple tablets or capsules. Unfortunately the work required to arrive at a suitable formulation is usually underestimated. The differences between the paediatric subgroups may require more than one formulation to be used to suit enteral or parenteral administrations. Oral solution is the most common form of paediatric formulation for enteral administration, due to its ease of administration and flexibility with doses. Formulating a suitable oral solution that is stable, palatable and delivers safe, accurate dosing is difficult. Development of such a formulation may not be finalised at the phase I stage; however, data generated from preclinical work must be sufficient to confidently allow for such a formulation to be made. The formulation must take into account stability, volume to be administered, palatability and excipient content. Switching formulation is not advisable but might not be avoidable between the age groups or studies as the development plan progresses. Using different formulations with different excipients may lead to unexpected PK/PD data and unsuitable stability both physically and chemically. Problems with formulations may also be found if they specify that they cannot be taken with food, as children often eat smaller meals at more regular intervals. Also, arranging a study that involves fasting is difficult, especially in younger children.

Blood tests in paediatric trials

Invasive procedures such as repeat tissue and blood samples are generally not favoured by children, parents, investigators or ethical committees. Parents and children rightly deserve a protocol that minimises the pain experienced – especially for phase I clinical trials, where there is very little likelihood of the drug producing health benefits in the participating children. For example, the use of local anaesthetic cream prior to insertion of intravenous cannulae is routine. Reduction in the number of these procedures can be achieved by exploring alternative endpoints such as biomarkers, and by the use of non-invasive validated sampling methods such as salivary samples or urinalysis.

The study design must not be rigid and restrictive, and should take into account that blood sampling from children is not as simple as it is in adults. Designers of early phase clinical trials in children should make every effort to customise the study's schedule of procedures to ensure pain and discomfort is reduced. Children require more time for blood samples to be taken, with higher incidences of failed attempts, and have reduced fasting ability and varied sleeping patterns; therefore, a rigid PK sampling schedule could hinder study success. It is worth considering in advance whether, for example, finger prick blood tests are a suitable method for the study design, because if a cannula inserted for blood sampling stops bleeding back, the time taken to use anaesthetic cream and site the new one will mean the sample time point will be missed. Invasive procedures should be reduced to a minimum and should ideally only be used when clinically necessary.

Recommendations about the volumes of blood to be taken from children and neonates have been produced by a number of different bodies in Europe and the USA. The European Commission has included some guidance in the document *Ethical Considerations for Clinical Trials on Medicinal Products Conducted with the Paediatric Population*. This states that 'the following blood volume limits for sampling are recommended (although they are not evidence-based). If an investigator decides to deviate from these, this should be justified (in the protocol and application for ethical review). Per individual, the trial related blood loss (including any losses in the manoeuvre) should not exceed 3% of the total blood volume during a period of 4 weeks and should not exceed 1% at any single time. In the rare case of simultaneous trials, the recommendation of 3% remains the maximum.' The key point is that a very limited amount of blood is available for testing in small children, and the values presented here are the maximums, not targets. When writing protocols for studies in children, investigators must consider as many ways as possible to minimise the volume of blood required.[5]

The protocol must allow and encourage opportunistic blood sampling. Taking extra blood during routine blood sampling for clinical need is better from the patient's perspective than introducing extra episodes of blood sampling specifically for research purposes. If routine blood sampling can be adapted to the optimal timings needed for the study design, this is particularly beneficial.

Consent

Conducting phase I studies does not usually result in a direct benefit to participants. Obtaining consent from parents in these situations is difficult; both parent(s) and child must be engaged in the consenting process with an appropriate level of information provided to the target reader. Ethics committees (institutional review boards; IRBs) will scrutinise the content of the consent, assent and patient information leaflets to ensure they are written in a clear, simple, jargon-free manner that is neither biased nor coercive. It is not the intention of these documents to be exhaustive with detailed information that will overwhelm the parent and the child. The document should include enough information to allow the reader to make an informed decision with a clear understating of what it will entail to be part of the study. The use of question and answer style leaflets is common and desirable, as it breaks the information into smaller segments. It is important to have age appropriate literature for younger participants (chapter 26).

Many factors influence the difficulty of consenting in phase I studies. While some cannot be altered, such as the severity of the disease and availability of alternative treatments, others can be mitigated, such as: complexity and demands of study design on patients and parents; competencies and training of staff; design of patient information leaflets, consent and assent forms; use of scans or biopsies requiring general anaesthesia; insensitivity of requirements for birth control and pregnancy tests; and, finally, the suitability of the research centre to conduct the study.

Phase I accredited centres

Phase I studies in adults usually run in centres dedicated to first-in-human (FIH) studies. Those centres are designed and resourced to meet the inherent elevated risk associated with phase I studies. Most phase I studies in paediatrics are conducted on patients; therefore, they run alongside normal clinics in hospitals which are only required to meet the minimum good clinical practice (GCP) guidelines. This is not sufficient, and was recognised as such by the Medicines and Healthcare products Regulatory Agency (MHRA) following the TGN1412 incident in March 2006. A voluntary accreditation scheme for all units conducting phase I studies was introduced to benchmark the minimum level of setup in phase I units. This accreditation requires the units to provide evidence of appropriate trial design, detailed risk assessment, evidence that facilities and staff are equipped and able to manage medical emergencies, and evidence that all activities are controlled by a robust quality system with written standard operating procedures (SOPs) for every aspect of the unit's activities.[6]

The unit must also consider patient and parental comfort and wellbeing, as the protocol may stipulate a lengthy hospital stay. The unit must provide a welcoming, safe and controlled environment.

Due to the ethical responsibilities of investigators and the vulnerability of children, the highest level of monitoring and safety assurance must be in place for any paediatric study.[7] This is even more acute in phase I studies, with limited or no prior knowledge and experience about the new agent under study. The need for an independent data and safety monitoring committee (DSMC) should be reviewed for phase I and II trials, especially those that include blinding. In phase I and II studies without a DSMC, a robust data monitoring plan must be in place in case any unforeseen risks become apparent throughout the course of the study.

Conclusions

The many differences between children and adults all need to be considered in the design of a phase I clinical trial involving children, and failure to consider each of them in turn can halt the progress of the study. Phase I studies in adults are usually conducted on healthy volunteers who may be driven by compensation. In paediatrics, study design must take into account the preference and convenience of both the children and their parents. For example, the protocol must carefully consider many factors, such as the time required off school and off work, feeding/fasting time and study dietary requirements, sleeping and nap times, distance to research centres, the number and route of blood samples, and so on.

First-in-child studies are complex, and simply repeating the adult study protocol in the paediatric population will seldom result in a successful study and will often require substantial amendments, additional cost and delays to recruitment if it is not rejected (correctly) by the ethics committee. Early investment of efforts in consulting with teams at local sites where the study will run (including paediatricians experienced in delivering these types of study, research pharmacists and research nurses) will greatly reduce the need for further amendments and enhance the possibility of a fruitful outcome.

References

1 European Medicines Agency. *Draft reflection paper on extrapolation of efficacy and safety in paediatric medicine development*, 2016. www.ema.europa.eu/docs/en_GB/document_library/Regulatory_and_procedural_guideline/2016/04/WC500204187.pdf
2 Wang Y *et al.* Clarification on precision criteria to derive sample size when designing pediatric pharmacokinetic studies. *J Clin Pharmacol* 2012; 52(10): 1601–1606.

3 European Medicines Agency. *ICH Topic E 11 Clinical Investigation of Medicinal Products in the Paediatric Population*, 2001. [cited 2015 17th March] www.ema.europa .eu/docs/en_GB/document_library/Scientific_guideline/2009/09/WC500002926.pdf

4 Nunn T, Williams J. Formulation of medicines for children. *Br J Clin Pharmacol* 2005; 59(6): 674–676.

5 Hawcutt D *et al*. Points to consider when planning the collection of blood or tissue samples in clinical trials of investigational medicinal products in children, infants and neonates. In: Rose K, van den Anker JN, eds. *Guide to Paediatric Drug Development and Clinical Research*, Basel: Karger, 2010: 97.

6 Medicines and Healthcare products Regulatory Agency. *Phase I Accreditation Scheme Requirements*. 2015. www.gov.uk/government/uploads/system/uploads/attachment_data/ file/262606/Phase_I_Accreditation_Scheme_requirements.pdf

7 Shaddy RE *et al*. Guidelines for the ethical conduct of studies to evaluate drugs in pediatric populations. *Pediatrics* 2010; 125(4): 850–860.

17

Early phase clinical trials: adaptive designs

S Zohar

Introduction

Phase I dose-finding represents the first translation of basic laboratory work into the clinical setting. Usually, these trials are performed in healthy subjects, except when the drug is cytotoxic and is intended for the treatment of malignancies or for the vaccination of HIV-infected patients. Phase I trials are designed to obtain reliable information on a drug's safety, tolerability and pharmacokinetics (PK). More specifically, in a healthy volunteer study, the objective is to determine the maximum safe dose under a certain PK, pharmacodynamic (PD) and/or safety limit. Following phase I clinical trials, phase II trials aim to explore or obtain evidence of the efficacy of a new drug, combination or procedure, to be confirmed further in phase III randomised clinical trials.

The learning objectives of this chapter are:

- ➤ to understand that early phase clinical trials in paediatrics (excluding those in oncology) focus primarily on efficacy
- ➤ to know that in some paediatric cases, such as in neonates, the endpoints differ from those used in adults, and therefore the statistical methods developed for adults cannot be applied directly to children
- ➤ to recognise that paediatric patients are more heterogeneous than adults with regard to age and metabolic maturity, thus statistical methods should be proposed accordingly
- ➤ to know that, when possible, extrapolation and bridging methods should be used when planning and conducting paediatric clinical trials.

Background

As introduced in the previous section, in paediatrics, classical phase I trials are not often conducted, for ethical reasons. As a consequence, drugs are directly evaluated for efficacy in children with the relevant disease/condition, and the focus is primarily on efficacy, while tolerance is mainly used as a rule for terminating the trial. Furthermore, in some cases such as in neonates, endpoints or administration modes differ from those used in adults, and therefore statistical and simulation methods developed for adults cannot be applied directly to children.

Recently, international guideline committees have recognised the need for modelling and simulation in association with multidisciplinary collaboration to support the choice of doses and design adopted for paediatric clinical research studies; the related need to use existing knowledge by employing extrapolation and bridging techniques has also been acknolwedged.[1]

Standard designs for the early phase are algorithmic dose–escalation schemes, in which the dose of a new drug is gradually increased, starting with a dose level that is not expected to cause any significant toxicity. These types of algorithms are based on standard or modified 3+3 designs used in cancer's early phase research.[2] Such designs can be referred to as 'memory less', since allocation to the next dose level for an incoming group of three patients only depends upon what has happened to the total of three to six patients previously treated at the current dose level. All other information concerning dose levels and probability distribution of toxicities is ignored. Moreover, previous information from preclinical trials and other studies is not taken into account for the design and conduct of such a study. This is a serious shortcoming that has been pointed out by several authors.[2,3]

However, the paradigm of dose selection based on toxicity does not apply for non-life-threatening diseases. In these settings, the specific objective of dose-finding trials is to identify the minimum dose that exhibits adequate drug activity – the minimum effective dose (MED). The MED, 'the smallest dose with a discernible useful effect', defines the targeted dose of phase II trials and could be considered as a dose to which some prespecified proportion of a sample population responds.

The usefulness of clinical trials in children has been debated widely over the last few decades.[4] Some authors have argued that data from adults should be better exploited, both quantitatively and qualitatively, before administering a new drug in children or deciding on a dosage regimen. However, children are not small adults, mostly because of the immaturity of children's renal and metabolic systems, and growth is not a linear variable, which makes it difficult to extrapolate data from adults to children. In children, phase II studies are designed to assess efficacy and safety, using a small sample size based on the optimal dose determined in adults (if applicable). As a result, the dose-finding process has been largely ignored, and trials have focused on one or two dose levels at most. This practice raises concerns about information collected in paediatric studies regarding dose–response curves. Recently, several papers in the *Journal of the American Academy for Pediatrics* have agreed on this topic.[5] With reference to this issue, several authors and specialists have reported a critical need for improvement, starting with increasing the number of clinical trials in children. Arising with this problem is the need for adequate methodology for these trials.

In the following section, two adaptive designs will be presented, introducing dose-finding phase I/II clinical trials. The first design uses binary endpoints for both efficacy and safety; the second design was specifically developed for neonates using other types of endpoints.

Adaptive designs for phase I/II dose-finding trials

The following design was first developed in the oncology setting for binary endpoints and was modified in the setting of this paediatric clinical trial.[6]

Statistical design

The modified bivariate adaptive method, which aims to estimate the safe most successful dose (sMSD), is a Bayesian model-based approach. The objective of this method is to find a dose level that maximises the probability of success at a given dose level under safety restrictions. The design attempts to allocate the maximum number of patients to the estimated sMSD over the whole trial. At the end of the trial, or earlier if the trial stops for safety or efficacy reasons, the estimated sMSD can be calculated with 95% credibility intervals (precision intervals).

The trial consists of the sequential allocation of doses to cohorts of patients (c = 1, 2, 3 or more) until a total number of at least 24 patients has been reached. The first cohort is usually treated with the first dose level, whereas dose levels for the subsequent groups are determined according to the model estimates of the dose–efficacy and dose–safety relationships. The dose allocation procedure is given in Figure 1. If all the dose levels have an efficacy lower than the defined target, and/or if all the dose levels have toxicity higher than the target, the trial is planned to end before the fixed maximal number of patients. An underlying mathematical model expresses the probabilities of response and tolerance as independent functions of dose. (For further statistical details, please see references[6–8].)

The recommended dose level for future experimentation is the one satisfying both efficacy criteria and toxicity restriction. Fixed standards of the minimum probability of response (minimum efficacy target) and the maximum probability of non-tolerance (maximal toxicity target) need to be specified by the trial investigators.

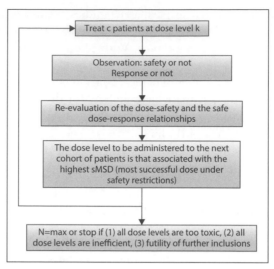

Figure 1 Dose-finding design aiming at estimating the sMSD

Extrapolation and bridging

When possible, it is pertinent and useful to use data from adults, preclinical trials or other sources of external information, to better plan and design the paediatric clinical trials. In a recent methodological paper, Petit *et al.* proposed an extrapolation and bridging method for planning dose-finding studies in children, accounting for metabolic and physiological differences according to age subgroups.[9] In that paper, they presented a unified approach in which: (1) the dose range is calibrated using PK from adults, and allometric and maturation methods; (2) the dose–response model prior parameters, under Bayesian inference, are calibrated using toxicity and efficacy data extrapolated from adults; and (3) in case this parameterisation is far from the data observed in the paediatric study, an adaptive prior approach is recommended for switching to less informative priors.

Adaptive designs in action: an illustrative example

The NEMO (NEonatal seizures with Medication Off-patent) clinical trial was an EU FP7 funded project (www.nemo-europe.com). The aim of this study was to estimate the optimal dose of bumetanide required for the treatment of neonatal seizures not responding to phenobarbitone.[10,11] This optimum dose was defined as the dose that achieves the maximum seizure reduction with an acceptable safety profile out of four dose levels of bumetanide (0.05, 0.1, 0.2 and 0.3 mg/kg). Fixed standards of the minimum probability of response (minimum efficacy target of 50% in this trial) and of the maximum probability of non-tolerance (maximal toxicity target of 10% in this trial) were specified by the investigators before the trial began.

The efficacy primary endpoint was defined as the reduction of electrographic seizure burden by $\geq 80\%$ within hours 3 and 4 after the first bumetanide administration compared with the baseline. The safety endpoints (defined within 48 hours after the first dose) included: (1) the absence of suspected unexpected serious adverse reactions (SUSARs) or absence of serious adverse reactions (SARs) that are at least probably related in $<10\%$; (2) absence of severe hypokalaemia (<2.8 mmol/L) and/or electrocardiogram changes in $<10\%$; and (3) absence of severe dehydration (dehydration with hypotension (mean BP <35 mmHg persistent >1 hour) that requires inotropic support in $<10\%$).

Fourteen evaluable neonates were included in the trial. Four neonates were included at the dose 0.05 mg/kg, three neonates at the dose 0.1 mg/kg, six neonates at the dose 0.2 mg/kg, and one neonate at the dose 0.3 mg/kg.

No toxicities were observed during the trial, according to the definition in the clinical trial protocol. Five efficacy responses were observed: one at the dose 0.05 mg/kg, one at the dose 0.1 mg/kg, and three at the dose 0.2 mg/kg. Figure 2(A) gives the posterior estimated dose–response without toxicity and dose–toxicity relationships at the end of the trial (after the inclusion of 14 neonates). Following completion of the tolerance and efficacy protocol, as defined, there were two dose levels that were estimated to be efficient and safe:

- 0.2 mg/kg, associated with an estimated posterior mean percentage of response without toxicity of 54.3% (95% credibility interval: 33.7–78.4%) and an estimated posterior mean percentage of toxicity of 0.4% (95% credibility interval: 0–15.1%)
- 0.3 mg/kg, associated with an estimated posterior mean percentage of response without toxicity of 78.7% (95% credibility interval: 65.4–89.5%) and an estimated posterior mean percentage of toxicity of 1.3% (95% credibility interval: 0–23.1%)

The sMSD was estimated to be 0.3 mg/kg even if 0.2 mg/kg fulfilled the minimal efficacy threshold. During the trial there were delayed toxicities; hearing loss was observed in three neonates at the following dose levels: 0.05, 0.20 and 0.30 mg/kg. After taking into account the delayed toxicities, the posterior estimated dose–response relationships at the end of the trial, including delayed toxicity, indicate that all doses are estimated to be toxic (Figure 2(B)). The trial was stopped after the inclusion of 14 neonates, as no dose level fulfilled the efficacy criteria under toxicity restrictions.

Adaptive designs dedicated to neonates

In some circumstances, the usual design cannot be just modified and applied to paediatrics, but instead dedicated statistical designs need to be developed.

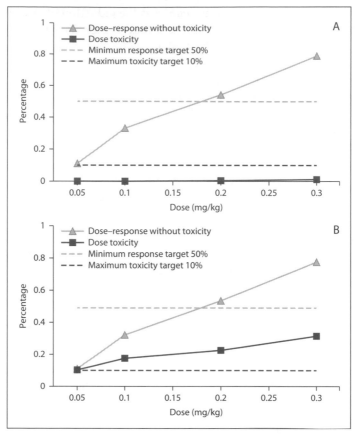

Figure 2 (A) Posterior estimated dose–response without toxicity and dose-toxicity relationships at the end of the trial according to protocol. (B) Posterior estimated dose–response without toxicity and dose-toxicity relationships at the end of the trial adding delayed toxicity

This can be the case when endpoints are not binary, and can even be a combination of several criteria.

This dedicated statistical design was motivated by the need to evaluate a clinical procedure for preterm infants suffering from respiratory distress syndrome. The study used a specific procedure called intubation–surfactant–extubation (INSURE). In this procedure, a surfactant is administered to improve the infant's ability to breathe, but the infant must first be sedated. However, little is known about what the optimal dose of any given sedative may be for the INSURE procedure. Indeed, there is no broad agreement regarding the dosing of any sedatives in neonatology. A common agent for sedation is propofol; however, some doses have been associated with serious adverse events in neonatal or pediatric populations.[12]

To be able to evaluate this procedure and to estimate the optimal dose of propofol, trial investigators have proposed using the Neonatal

Table 1 Neonatal Pain, Agitation and Sedation Scale (N-PASS)[13]				
Assessment	**Sedation**		**Sedation/pain**	**Pain/agitation**
Criteria	−2	−1	0/0	1	2
Crying, irritability	No cry with painful stimuli	Moans or cries minimally with painful stimuli	No sedation/no pain signs	Irritable or crying at intervals Consolable	High-pitched or silent-continuous cry Inconsolable
Behaviour state	No arousal to any stimuli No spontaneous movement	Arouses minimally to stimuli Little spontaneous movement	No sedation/no pain signs	Restless, squirming Awakens frequently	Arching, kicking Constantly awake or Arouses minimally/ no movement (not sedated)
Facial expression	Mouth is lax No expression	Minimal expression with stimuli	No sedation/no pain signs	Any pain expression intermittent	Any pain expression continual
Extremities' tone	No grasp reflex Flaccid tone	Weak grasp reflex – muscle tone	No sedation/no pain signs	Intermittent clenched toes, fists or finger splay Body is not tense	Continual clenched toes, fists, or finger splay Body is tense
Vital signs HR, RR, BP, SaO$_2$	No variability with stimuli Hypoventilation or apnoea	<10% variability from baseline with stimuli	No sedation/no pain signs	↑ 10–20% from baseline SaO$_2$ 76–85% with stimulation – quick recovery	↑ 20% from baseline SaO$_2$ ≤ 75% with stimulation – slow recovery Out of sync with vent

Pain, Agitation and Sedation Scale (N-PASS; www.n-pass.com) (Table 1).[13] The scale ranges from −10 to 10 and includes several criteria.

Investigators wanted the infant to be sedated in good condition but not for too long. This led them to propose a triple outcomes dose-finding design based on two outcomes indicating desirable events (including the N-PASS scale and the patient extubation within 30 minutes), with a third outcome indicating an adverse event as follows:

- good sedation score (GSS) = [−7 < sedation score < −3]
- EXT30 = [complete the INSURE procedure and extubate the infant within 30 minutes]
- HEM (adverse haemodynamic event) = [HR <80 bpm, or SaO$_2$ <60%, or BP drops by >5 mm Hg, at any time during the procedure]

Table 2 Consensus elicited utilities proposed by the trial investigator				
	GSS achieved		GSS not achieved	
	No HEM	HEM	No HEM	HEM
EXT30	100	60	90	40
No EXT30	80	20	70	0

Success was defined by investigators as a GSS and the ability to extubate the infant within 30 minutes from the sedation product injection time (EXT30). Investigators also defined that an acceptable dose level should be associated with at least 60% success and less than 10% experiencing adverse haemodynamic events. The proposed design for this dose-finding trial took into account these specifications and was developed in close coordination with trial investigators. An important aspect was that investigators were asked to assign utilities to clinical outcomes. Indeed, they specified the 'desirability' of each outcome (GSS, EXT30, HEM) that was quantified by a utility, from 100 = best to 0 = worst (Table 2).

A complex underlying statistical model was developed in order to estimate the optimal dose level.[14] At the end of the trial, the dose with the highest posterior mean utility will be recommended for further investigations. At the time of writing the trial has not yet started, but this illustration points out how close collaboration between physicians and statisticians can bring the use of more innovative and ethical methods to paediatrics.

Conclusions

In conclusion, early phase paediatric clinical trials would benefit from improved, modernised and more ethical designs. This is feasible if there is a close collaboration between physicians and statisticians. Dose-finding designs proposed for other indications cannot be directly used in paediatrics and need to be modified accordingly. Paediatric dose-finding studies should base their dose allocation decision rule jointly on efficacy and safety.

Acknowledgement

The NEMO consortium was funded by the European Union Seventh Framework Programme (FP7-HEALTH-2009-4.2-1, grant agreement 241479, NEMO Project): Adapting off-patent medicines to the specific needs of paediatric populations.

References

1   International Conference on Harmonisation of Technical Requirements for Registration of Pharmaceuticals for Human Use (ICH). *Addendum to ich e11: clinical investigation of medicinal products in the pediatric population - e11(r1)*. 2016. www.ich.org/products/guidelines/efficacy/efficacy-single/article/addendum-clinical-investigation-of-medicinal-products-in-the-pediatric-population.html

2   Le Tourneau C *et al*. Dose escalation methods in phase I cancer clinical trials. *J Natl Cancer Inst* 2009; 101(10): 708–720.

3   O'Quigley J, Zohar S. Experimental designs for phase I and phase I/II dose-finding studies. *Br J Cancer* 2006; 94(5): 609–613.

4   Sammons HM. Avoiding clinical trials in children. *Arch Dis Child* 2011; 96(3): 291–292.

5   Denne SC. Pediatric clinical trial registration and trial results: an urgent need for improvement. *Pediatrics* 2012; 129: e1320–1321.

6   Zohar S, O'Quigley J. Identifying the most successful dose (MSD) in dose-finding studies in cancer. *Pharm Stat* 2006; 5(3): 187–199.

7   O'Quigley J *et al*. Dose-finding designs for HIV studies. *Biometrics* 2001; 57: 1018–1029.

8   Zohar S *et al*. Using the continual reassessment method to estimate the minimum effective dose in phase II dose-finding studies: a case study. *Clin Trials* 2013; 10(3): 414–421.

9   Petit C *et al*. Unified approach for extrapolation and bridging of adult information in early-phase dose-finding paediatric studies. *Stat Methods Med Res* 2018; 27(6): 1860–1877.

10 Pressler RM *et al*. NEMO consortium (NEonatal seizure treatment with Medication Off-patent). Bumetanide for neonatal seizures-back from the cotside. *Nat Rev Neurol* 2015; 11(12): 724.

11 Pressler RM *et al*. NEonatalseizure treatment with Medication Off-patent (NEMO) consortium. Bumetanide for the treatment of seizures in newborn babies with hypoxic ischaemic encephalopathy (NEMO): an open-label, dose finding, and feasibility phase 1/2 trial. *Lancet Neurol* 2015; 14(5): 469–477.

12 Sammartino M *et al*. Propofol overdose in a preterm baby: may propofol infusion syndrome arise in two hours? *Paediatr Anaesth* 2010; 20: 973–974.

13 Hummel P *et al*. Validity and reliability of the N-PASS assessment tool with acute pain. *J Perinatol* 2010; 30: 474–478.

14 Thall PF *et al*. Optimizing sedative dose in preterm infants undergoing treatment for respiratory distress syndrome. *J Am Stat Assoc* 2014; 109(507): 931–943.

Further recommended reading

Anderson B, Holford N. Mechanistic basis of using body size and maturation to predict clearance in humans. *Drug Metab Pharmacokinet* 2009; 24: 25–36.

Brasseur D. Paediatric research and the regulation 'better medicines for the children in Europe'. *Eur J Clin Pharmacol* 2011; 67 Suppl 1: 1–3.

Gill D. Ethics Working Group of the Confederation of European Specialists in Paediatrics. Ethical principles and operational guidelines for good clinical practice in paediatric research. Recommendations of the Ethics Working Group of the Confederation of European Specialists in Paediatrics (CESP). *Eur J Pediatr* 2004; 163(2): 53–57.

Taylor RE *et al*. Promoting collaboration between adult and paediatric clinical trial groups. *Clin Oncol* (R Coll Radiol) 2008; 20(9): 714–716.

18

Phase IV studies and pharmacovigilance

I Choonara and HM Sammons

Introduction

All medicines unfortunately have the potential to cause harm. The choice of which drug is best for a particular patient is likely to depend as much on its safety/toxicity as its effectiveness in managing disease. The scientific study of drug toxicity is very different to studying the effectiveness of a drug (phase III studies).

The learning objectives of this chapter are:

➢ to understand the different methods of looking for adverse drug reactions
➢ to recognise that different adverse drug reactions may occur in different paediatric age groups
➢ to know the importance of transparency in the reporting of drug toxicity.

Clinical trials

Clinical trials are essential for determining whether a medicine is effective or not. They are also useful for comparing different medicines in relation to effectiveness. In general, clinical trials, however, are not adequately powered to study drug safety in great detail (especially rare adverse drug reactions), because phase I, II and III studies have limited numbers of patients and are powered to compare the efficacy with current treatment or a placebo. Numerous studies have also shown that the reporting of adverse drug reactions in clinical trials is poor.[1,2] Many clinical trials do not state sufficiently clearly whether adverse drug events occurred and the specific nature of these reactions in children. A systematic review of clinical trials of antiepileptic drugs identified that many trials recruited both adults and children, but that very few analysed paediatric data separately.[1] Two-thirds of the clinical trials of antiepileptic drugs did not even report the number of children recruited. Further, the methods used to identify adverse drug reactions (ADRs) (chapter 10) are rarely reported in detail in publications. Additionally, clinical trials are inadequately powered to compare toxicity between different drugs. It is therefore necessary to perform different studies to look at toxicity.

Prospective cohort studies

Phase IV studies usually consist of a prospective cohort study. These studies are beneficial in terms of both determining the incidence of ADRs and also detecting uncommon ADRs. Prospective cohort studies are usually performed in outpatient settings but can, however, enrol inpatients. The period of observation depends upon the nature of the adverse effect that is under surveillance. Studies of abnormal behaviour following the use of midazolam as a sedative in critically ill children have involved watching the patient for several days only. In contrast, studies looking at the behavioural effect of antiepileptic drugs are longer term studies. Prospective cohort studies can be specific to one drug, a group of drugs or a group of patients with a specific condition.

National pharmacovigilance

Most countries have national systems in place for the detection and reporting of ADRs. It is important to recognise that most ADRs are both unrecognised and unreported. Several systematic reviews have shown that approximately one in ten children in hospital will experience an ADR.[3] Cuba has the most successful national paediatric pharmacovigilance programme. Studies in Cuba have shown that at least 1 in 500 children in the community will experience an ADR each year. It is only by educating health professionals, patients and parents about the importance of recognising and reporting all suspected ADRs that an accurate picture is gained of the side-effect profile of a drug. Recent extension of the yellow card reporting scheme to the Medicines and Healthcare products Regulatory Agency in the UK to include public reporting should help this; however, awareness of this remains low. Information from national pharmacovigilance schemes is frequently shared with the Uppsala Monitoring Centre in Sweden (part of the WHO; World Health Organization), which coordinates pharmacovigilance at a global level.

Evaluating and classifying ADRs

It is important to recognise that most reported ADRs describe adverse events that are likely to be drug related. The collection of details of adverse events within clinical studies is usually conducted using one or a mixture of four methods, namely direct observation, general enquiry, specific enquiry and spontaneous reporting. Which of these is used often dictates the number of events documented, as those methods using specific enquiry scales of known reactions are more likely to give higher numbers than spontaneous reporting.

There are numerous algorithms that enable evaluation of whether a suspected ADR was actually drug related or not (e.g. Naranjo algorithm).[4] Other methods rely on clinical evaluation of each suspected ADR, which can be time-consuming. Unfortunately there is little scientific evidence as to which algorithm or method of evaluation is likely to be most objective. During clinical trials, adverse events are reported and subsequently evaluated in terms of whether they are drug related or not. Unfortunately, many people use the term 'adverse event' rather than 'adverse drug reaction' outside clinical trials. This is confusing, especially as the term 'adverse drug event' is also used to describe medication errors.

ADRs are classified in relation to severity. We have found the most useful classification to be one that classifies ADRs as severe, moderate or mild, as listed below:

- Severe: fatal or potentially life-threatening or causing permanent disability
- Moderate: requiring treatment or prolonging stay in hospital or causing interference with normal daily activities
- Mild: minor reactions that do not require treatment and do not prolong stay in hospital

Age and drug toxicity

Neonates and infants may be more prone to specific ADRs than older children. Valproate induced hepatotoxicity is more likely to occur in children under the age of 3 years than in any other age group. Precipitation of calcium following the co-administration of ceftriaxone and calcium containing solutions has only been reported in young infants. Kernicterus following the displacement of bilirubin from albumin by highly protein bound drugs such as sulfonamides is only a problem in the neonatal period. Apnoea following the use of antihistamines is a problem that has been reported in infancy only. In contrast, dystonic reactions in relation to metoclopramide are more likely to occur in adolescence. Therefore it is important that the age ranges within phase IV studies and pharmacovigilance studies contain sufficient numbers of all paediatric age groups, including neonates if appropriate.

Pharmaceutical industry and academic trials

Paediatricians and investigators need to be aware that information contained in publications of trials, from the pharmaceutical industry or from academia, tends to focus on the primary research question (relating to evidence of efficacy) and often will contain only limited, summary, information about drug toxicity. Unfortunately there were instances in the past of some companies supressing important safety information in order to ensure their medicinal products were authorised and widely prescribed. Importantly, more detailed information is often available in the clinical study report and regulatory documents, which are not often accessible to members of the public or researchers. However, there are now organised initiatives to make sure that information from clinical trials becomes more widely available – to promote data sharing and meta-analysis – and this may help to improve pharmacovigilance efforts.

Conclusions

Drug toxicity is poorly reported in clinical trials. Prospective cohort studies are essential for improving the understanding of drug toxicity. Most ADRs are either unrecognised or unreported. It is the responsibility of all clinicians and pharmacists to look out for ADRs in their patients and to report them when appropriate.

References

1   Anderson M, Choonara I. A systematic review of safety monitoring and drug toxicity in published randomised controlled trials of antiepileptic drugs in children over a 10-year period. *Arch Dis Child* 2010; 95: 731–738.
2   Nor Aripin KNB *et al*. Systematic review of safety in paediatric drug trials published in 2007. *Eur J Clin Pharmacol* 2012; 68: 189–194.
3   Choonara I. Aspects of clinical pharmacology in children – pharmacovigilance and safety. *Eur J Pediatr* 2013; 172: 577–580.
4   Avner M *et al*. Establishing causality in pediatric adverse drug reactions: use of the Naranjo probability scale. *Paediatr Drugs* 2007; 9: 267–270.

19

Non-interventional studies

R Lundin and J Bielicki

Introduction

This chapter aims to introduce non-interventional studies in the context of paediatric drug development, distinguishing them from randomised control trials (RCTs) and other interventional studies. Implications of non-interventional research participation for physicians, pharmacists and patients will be discussed, as well as how to interpret results from such research and incorporate non-interventional findings into everyday clinical practice.

The learning objectives of this chapter are:

➤ to distinguish interventional and non-interventional studies based on study design characteristics
➤ to describe the most commonly applied non-interventional study designs
➤ to understand what participation in non-interventional studies entails for both healthcare providers and patients
➤ to interpret and apply proper significance to strengths and limitations of non-interventional study results
➤ to incorporate non-interventional study results into clinical practice.

Defining non-interventional studies

Implicit in the phrase non-interventional study is the absence of intervention. In the context of paediatric drug development, these are studies where medicinal products are prescribed and administered, and patients are monitored as per regular standards of care. In theory, no additional diagnostic or monitoring procedures are conducted, and drug prescription and administration is not impacted in any way by study participation. This depends upon the definition of additional diagnostic or monitoring procedures, as described later in this chapter, but in general non-interventional research is minimally invasive.

Utility of non-interventional studies

At the other end of the spectrum, RCTs exemplify interventional research. Investigators control who enters an RCT, who receives which treatment, and how patient outcomes will be assessed, as well as controlling external factors like concomitant medications.

While the controlled environment of an RCT is the gold standard for establishing drug efficacy, these studies can be costly and time-consuming and may not be broadly applicable to real-world clinical settings.[1] They are also not well adapted to detect rare adverse events or assess long term treatment outcomes. Non-interventional studies can address these shortcomings and complement RCTs, as they:

- allow inclusion of patients with various comorbidities and concomitant therapies
- provide treatment efficacy data in real-world, day-to-day clinical practice
- allow use of existing and/or routinely collected data.

Types of non-interventional studies

Observational studies

Observational studies can rely on existing data or involve primary data collection. The distinguishing feature is that no intervention is involved on the part of the researcher, either in determining the course of therapy or in evaluation of the outcomes for any patient.[2] It is important to note that regulatory agencies do allow some diagnostic and monitoring procedures in the non-interventional context, a point we elaborate upon later in the section on patient implications.

- **Cohort studies** – These involve primary data collection from patients exposed to a particular therapy or therapies and followed over time to observe efficacy and safety outcomes. Risk ratios describing the relative risk in one exposure group compared with another and incidence rates of the outcomes of interest can be calculated, as well as the time to event for these outcomes. Such studies are ideal for assessing the relationship between drug exposure and multiple outcomes.
- **Cross-sectional studies** – These can involve primary or secondary data collection from patients with a particular disease status or therapeutic exposure, capturing a single point or defined period in time. Data can be used to assess prevalence of a disease or outcome, or in ecologic analysis of the crude relationship between exposure and outcome. Limited by a lack of a temporal link between exposure and outcome, such studies are best suited to exploratory initial research.
- **Case-control studies** – These involve retrospective secondary data collection from patients with an outcome of interest and a group of matched

controls from the exposed population who do not experience that outcome. Odds ratios (analogous to risk ratios) can be calculated comparing the odds of experiencing an outcome among exposed and unexposed patients and, if the cases and controls represent all or a known proportion of the underlying population of interest, incidence rates of outcomes of interest can also be calculated. This design is ideal for rare outcomes of interest and for assessing factors that may mediate the relationship between drug exposure and the outcome of interest.

- **Studies where cases serve as own controls** – In case-crossover studies, cases serve as their own controls, crossing over from exposed and unexposed status throughout a prospective study. In case-time-control studies and self-controlled case series, cases provide their own control data from past periods where they were not exposed to the treatment of interest. All three designs allow for perfect control of all personal characteristics of patients, except characteristics that may change over time.

Post-marketing surveillance studies

Pharmaceutical companies are often required to conduct non-interventional studies after a drug is approved for use, to evaluate its efficacy and safety outside the controlled conditions of an RCT and in a larger, more diverse patient population. The two most common types of post-marketing surveillance studies are:

- Post-authorisation safety studies – These non-interventional studies are conducted after a drug is marketed to assess its safety profile as it is actually used in the real world, including among patients who are not typically included in RCTs, such as pregnant women and neonates. All adverse events can be monitored or a particular safety risk of interest can be the focus of the study. These studies are often used to assess the effects of risk minimisation measures for a particular medicine.
- Post-authorisation efficacy studies (PAES) – These studies are conducted after a drug is marketed, to assess its efficacy as it is actually used in the real world and among patients who are not typically included in RCTs. While efficacy must be established before a drug is approved for marketing, sometimes surrogate efficacy endpoints are used, such as biomarkers of tumour shrinkage for oncology drugs. In these cases, a PAES can be conducted after marketing to assess the actual endpoints such as tumour shrinkage.

Registries

Rather than focusing on populations treated with a particular drug, registries collect observational data on patients with a particular disease or condition. They need not be designed with a particular research question in mind. Standardised data from a registry can provide cases for case-control studies or contribute data to simple cohort studies assessing incidence of a particular outcome. Some registries are structured to collect data on both cases and controls, and on patients exposed and unexposed to various therapies, in which case cohort studies comparing exposed and unexposed populations and case-control studies can be carried out within the registry data.

Drug utilisation studies

These non-interventional studies collect data on how a particular medicine is prescribed and used, and by whom, in real-world settings. Drug utilisation studies facilitate the assessment of how factors like policy changes or media attention can modify the prescription and use of a drug. Data can also be used to compare recommended with actual use and to characterise the population that actually receives a drug.[3]

Participating in non-interventional studies

Implications for healthcare providers

For physicians and other healthcare providers, non-interventional study participation is less involved than interventional study participation. If the study is prospective, healthcare providers should carry on with normal standard of care for all patients, potentially adding only blood draws, questionnaires or surveys. It is important for healthcare providers to remember that simply being observed can lead healthcare providers to inadvertently change their behaviour, and to try to recognise and mitigate this effect as much as possible when participating in any study.

In the case of retrospective or cross-sectional observational research, healthcare providers' participation may entail review of patient records and data entry. In these cases, it is important to obtain ethics committee approval and patient permission to extract these data, and to prevent the transmission of identifiable patient data.

Implications for paediatric patients

By definition, non-interventional studies do not modify patient treatment or assessment in any way. Additional blood draws, surveys or questionnaires of patients or care-givers are not considered interventions by regulatory agencies, and as such may be asked of participants in prospective observational research. Even such minor additional monitoring may be difficult to implement in some populations, such as extremely premature neonates. In many settings it is therefore necessary to obtain informed consent from a child's guardian before participation in non-interventional studies. Patients may also have to be asked for permission to access their medical records for retrospective and cross-sectional non-interventional studies.

Limitations of RCTs

Although RCTs are generally accepted to provide the strongest evidence for drug efficacy, they may not capture the complexity of clinical decision-making and patient behaviour that impacts on observed efficacy in the real world. For instance, concomitant medication use and treatment compliance vary far more in clinical practice than in the controlled setting of an RCT, and can strongly influence the impact of a particular treatment. Additionally, narrow inclusion criteria and small populations in trials often exclude important subgroups and limit identification of rare adverse events, while short treatment and follow-up periods do not provide information on long term efficacy. As such, when the potential benefit of a drug for a particular patient is being evaluating, efficacy data from randomised trials are only directly applicable to patients who match trial participants in terms of physical and clinical characteristics, concomitant therapies, and treatment compliance and tolerance. The external validity, or generalisability, of RCTs is often very low.

Using non-interventional study results to inform prescribing practices

For patients who do not fit the profile of RCT participants, or when more long term or real-world data are needed, non-interventional studies can provide valuable information on drug efficacy and safety. In applying these data to everyday clinical practice, it is important to keep in mind the limitations of non-interventional research and pay close attention to how investigators deal with potential bias and confounding that stems from a lack of randomisation. Several strategies can be applied to the design and analysis of non-interventional studies, including matching, restriction to drug-naive patients, stratification, and statistical modelling. Assessing these factors can help investigators to assign the correct weight to non-interventional data on efficacy and safety when deciding on the appropriate treatment strategy for a particular patient.

It is also important to remember that non-interventional research assumes that treatment allocation is not related to patient outcomes. Some topics are more adapted to this assumption than others; studies of adverse events, for example, are well suited to non-interventional study designs, as adverse effects are not intended and their risk is not known when prescribing patient therapy. Non-interventional studies assessing predicted therapeutic outcomes may need to be interpreted with more care, as blinding and randomisation are the only methods which ensure that patient or prescriber expectations of treatment outcomes do not influence treatment allocation.

Strengths of non-interventional research

- Provide safety and efficacy information, as drug is actually used in clinical practice
- Can involve large, heterogeneous groups of patients or focus on specific vulnerable populations
- Generally better external validity (generalisability) than RCTs
- Allow characterisation of population actually receiving a drug in clinical practice
- Less invasive for patients than interventional research; no need to change standard of care
- Can compare several different treatment alternatives simultaneously
- Can follow patients for longer periods of time and better identify rare adverse events
- Can be conducted quickly, especially if retrospective or cross-sectional, and at less cost than RCTs

Limitations of non-interventional research

- Bias, including selection and information bias, is more common in non-interventional research and more difficult to address than in interventional research
- Confounding caused by underlying differences between patients on different treatments is also a bigger issue in non-interventional versus interventional research, as statistical control is limited to measurable confounders
- May not be suitable for topics where expectations of treatment outcomes are likely to influence treatment allocation
- Non-interventional studies relying on extraction of existing data are limited by completeness and correctness of data available in medical records
- Cross-sectional studies do not allow assessment of causality, because they lack temporal precedence of drug exposure to outcomes of interest
- Difficult to identify selective or misleading reporting of results from non-interventional studies

Conclusions

Non-interventional studies complement and supplement interventional study findings. Participation in such non-interventional studies may present a more appealing benefit–risk profile for patients when compared with interventional studies. Care must be taken to properly interpret results from non-interventional research.

References

1   Avorn J. In defense of pharmacoepidemiology – embracing the yin and yang of drug research. *NEJM* 2007; 357(22): 2219–2221.
2   Rosenbaum PR. *Design of Observational Studies*. New York: Springer, 2010.
3   Strom BL *et al. Textbook of Pharmacoepidemiology*, 2nd edn. West Sussex: John Wiley & Sons Ltd, 2013.

20

Pharmacoepidemiology

A Neubert and R Lundin

Introduction

In this chapter we introduce the research field of pharmacoepidemiology and its relevance to clinical practice in paediatrics.

The learning objectives of this chapter are:

➤ to explain the definition of pharmacoepidemiology
➤ to discuss issues particular to pharmacoepidemiological research in children
➤ to introduce important considerations when searching for appropriate data
➤ to convey the growing need for pharmacoepidemiological research and to describe relevant methodological challenges.

What is pharmacoepidemiology?

Pharmacoepidemiology can be defined as the study of the use of and the effects of drugs in large groups of people. It applies epidemiologic principles and methods to the management of drug safety risk. Key activities in the field of pharmacoepidemiology include: 1) planned surveillance of drug use, efficacy and safety at the population level; 2) estimation of acceptable risk levels based on the natural history of various diseases and the efficacy and safety of comparable treatments for these conditions; 3) development and implementation of measures to mitigate drug safety risk; and 4) evaluation of risk minimisation activity effectiveness.

Why is pharmacoepidemiology needed?

In clinical trials, drug safety and efficacy are studied in a highly controlled environment with a narrowly defined patient population. While this maintains high internal validity for study results, external validity, or generalisability, inevitably suffers. As small samples of homogeneous patients are observed over only a short period of time, clinical trials are consequently not able to detect all potential effects of a therapy. Severe adverse drug events are often rare and therefore need large study populations to be detected. Some adverse effects only occur after long term use or are unique to special populations. In addition, clinical trials are expensive and patient recruitment is often problematic.

Observational pharmacoepidemiological studies may address those questions regarding drug safety and effectiveness that remain unanswered following clinical studies. Although observational studies are more prone to bias and confounding, they are often less costly and easier to conduct and provide data from large, representative population samples over longer periods of time.

Methodological aspects of pharmacoepidemiology

Case reports (sometimes called individual case safety reports; ICSRs) are reports of individual patients who experience some kind of adverse event while taking a drug. Case reports or case series are an important data source for detecting potential drug adverse events as part of routine pharmacovigilance.

Analytical pharmacoepidemiological studies can then evaluate a potential association between drug use and outcomes (beneficial or adverse effects). Various types of non-interventional study designs, such as cohort studies, cross-sectional studies or case-control studies, can be applied,[1] as described in chapter 19.

Identifying acceptable levels of risk associated with a particular therapy involves drug utilisation studies, which aim to describe how drugs are being used in real practice. Simple descriptions of drug use by age, gender and time require information on the source population and drug prescription or dispensing data. More detailed information is necessary to perform qualitative drug utilisation studies that include the concept of appropriateness and are based upon parameters such as indications for use, daily dose and duration of therapy.

Databases for pharmacoepidemiological research

Pharmacoepidemiological studies require valid and complete longitudinal assessment of the population under observation, including information on patient characteristics, patient drug exposure, and outcomes and confounders over time. A large population should be followed for a prolonged period, and it is often useful to have the opportunity to check diagnoses against original records or to go back to the treating physicians if necessary. As prospective cohorts of this type are usually not feasible to construct due to resource constraints, and patient interviews of past prescription drug use and outcomes exhibit relatively low validity, large automated databases are commonly used. Using automated datasets offers additional benefits, including lack of recall bias and selection bias.

The European Medicines Agency (EMA) recommends the use of electronic health records when conducting common pharmacoepidemiological studies such as post-authorisation drug utilisation and safety studies. Healthcare databases comprising patient data, drug exposure, outcomes and confounders are now available in many European countries.[2] The ideal database would include records from inpatient and outpatient care and emergency care, all laboratory and radiological tests, as well as data on prescribed and over-the-counter medication.

Data sources can generally be divided into medical record and administrative databases.[3] Medical record databases contain data collected throughout the process of clinical care. These can include patient demographic information, self-reported medical history, information on relevant behaviours such as diet and exercise, results of clinical and laboratory examinations, diagnoses and any medical treatments including prescription of drugs, referrals to specialists, and inpatient or outpatient procedures. The particular data elements included depend on where the database is housed, who is responsible for data entry and maintenance, and the connectivity between different electronic systems (storing, e.g., laboratory data, hospital admissions, drug prescriptions). For pharmacoepidemiological research, it is important to note that prescription data in medical records databases are often not connected to information on actual drug dispensing. In contrast, administrative databases can contain information on drug dispersal, as they collect data from financial transactions related to medical care.[3]

When choosing a database to answer a particular pharmacoepidemiological question, there are several key factors to consider, the first being the source population of interest. Investigators should clearly define who they want to study based on demographic and clinical characteristics and indications or therapies of interest, and ensure their database contains a large proportion of patients fitting this description.

The chosen database should allow investigators to calculate for how much time an individual patient was observed within the database (calculation of person-time) and to capture all information between the start and the end of follow-up of drug exposure. This enables measurement of frequencies such as the incidence or prevalence for which these time periods would act as denominators.

To study the use and effects of a particular therapy, drug exposure data are essential and should contain an indication for drug use, type of drug, timing and duration of use, and the prescribed dose. These data are often captured better in medical record databases than in administrative or claims databases.

It is equally important to ensure the chosen database contains longitudinal data on outcomes of interest, either as text entries or standardised diagnostic codes. Other secondary outcomes of interest should also be captured, such as quality of life measures.

Finally, it is necessary to confirm that the database contains relevant covariates, as these are crucial for multivariate analysis to rule out confounding. Some covariates that are commonly assessed include age, gender, socioeconomic status, health related behaviours, ethnicity and comorbidities.

Pharmacoepidemiological research in children

There is an enhanced need to build paediatric pharmacoepidemiological research capacity in the areas of drug utilisation, safety and effectiveness, in the light of the scarcity of data from children in clinical trials.

Unique aspects of paediatric population

Observational pharmacoepidemiological research in children is different from that in adults, as paediatric prescription drug uses differ from those of adults. Different physiological and lifecycle issues are of importance, such as intrauterine or breastfeeding exposure to maternal therapeutics, the effect of drugs on maturation, and adverse drug reactions specific to children.[4]

Patterns of drug use also differ in paediatrics, partly driven by the lack of trial data on drug efficacy and safety in children (chapter 28). Prescription of off-label or unlicensed medicines remains common. Doses are sometimes chosen or calculated in a non-standardised way, with limited information available to treating physicians on the risks or benefits of these drugs administered at these doses in children or infants. There is some evidence that paediatric off-label or unlicensed drug use is more often related to adverse drug reactions.[4,5]

Sample size considerations

Sample size is one of the major issues when studying drug use in the paediatric population. In the developed world, the paediatric population is small in general and relatively healthy when compared with older populations. Children and adolescents account for less than 25% of the population of 0–80 years of age. Thus, the number of patients needing a treatment or available to provide efficacy and safety data is always going to be smaller.

Furthermore, the paediatric population ranges from birth to the completion of the 18th year of age. With respect to the use of medicines, this cannot be seen as one homogeneous population. Growth and development during these first years of life affect many physiological processes depending on age in different ways. This results in different responses to drugs

Table 1 ICH paediatric age sub-classifications and developmental stages

Age	Sub-classification	Developmental stage
<37 weeks	Preterm neonates	Survival
<28 days	Newborns and neonates	Adoption
1 month to 2 years	Infants	Growth and proliferation
>2 to <11 years	Children	Training, differentiation
>11 years	Adolescents	Gaining reproductive capacity

from the pharmacokinetic and pharmacodynamics perspective, depending on age. To accommodate these differences, the paediatric population has been subclassified by the International Conference on Harmonization (ICH) into different age groups (Table 1). Each age group has its own characteristics and needs to be studied separately, but it is important to balance this with the fact that in order to achieve sufficient statistical power certain numbers of patients are necessary.

Defining drug dosing in children

Among adults, drug utilisation is often summarised using the proportion prescribed or received of the defined daily dose (DDD), which is the approved average maintenance dose per day for a drug used for its main adult indication. DDD is based on average adult age and weight, and as such is not applicable to children. While efforts have been made to estimate paediatric DDD for therapeutics commonly used by children, these standardised measures are difficult to create and validate due to the heterogeneity of the paediatric population and the fact that drugs are generally dosed for children on a mg/kg basis.[6]

Some alternatives commonly used in paediatric drug utilisation studies are days of therapy (DOT) or length of therapy (LOT). DOT is calculated by adding the days of therapy for each individual drug a patient receives in a given period. For instance, if the patient takes drug A for 5 days and drug B for 10 days over the same 10 day period, the DOT would be 15 days. LOT differs slightly in that it only reflects the overall length of therapy, such that in this example the LOT would be 10 days.

Depending on the objectives of the pharmacoepidemiological study and the classes of drugs examined, a drug utilisation measure may also be appropriate for use among children. This measure evaluates the number of drugs that make up a certain percentage of use for a particular indication in a particular population. For example, the drug utilisation measure of 90% of antibiotics used to treat lower urinary tract infections among paediatric outpatients would consist of a list of all antibiotics making up 90% of those prescribed for lower urinary tract infections among children in the community setting.

Conclusions

Observational studies to investigate drug safety and effectiveness are especially important in children compared with adults, as the number of paediatric clinical trials remains low. There have been promising developments encouraging greater inclusion of neonates and children in pharmacoepidemiological research since the Paediatric Regulation came into force in Europe in 2007 and paediatric investigation plans (PIPs) became part of new licensing applications.

While pharmacoepidemiological research in children applies the same principles as research among adults, implementation of these principles does differ. Paediatric research must take into account physiological and developmental differences, differing drug utilisation patterns and measures of drug use, issues with off-label use and sample size challenges.

Many automated databases used for pharmacoepidemiological research among adults are also appropriate for paediatric research if sufficient numbers of children are included; however, there is still a need for prospective cohorts of paediatric patients. To this end, research networks warrant further development to facilitate international or multisource database studies, which would confer the advantage of larger sample sizes and allow for detailed evaluation of drug specific and dose specific risks as well as comparisons between countries.

References

1   Verhamme K, Sturkenboom M. Study designs in paediatric pharmacoepidemiology. *Eur J Clin Pharmacol* 2011; 67 Suppl 1: 67–74.
2   Neubert A *et al*. Databases for pediatric medicine research in Europe – assessment and critical appraisal. *Pharmacoepidemiol Drug Saf* 2008; 17(12): 1155–1167.
3   Hennessy S. Use of health care databases in pharmacoepidemiology. *Basic Clin Pharmacol Toxicol* 2006; 98(3): 311–313.
4   Bellis JR *et al*. Adverse drug reactions and off-label and unlicensed medicines in children: a prospective cohort study of unplanned admissions to a paediatric hospital. *Br J Clin Pharmacol* 2014; 77(3): 545–553.
5   Neubert A *et al*. The impact of unlicensed and off-label drug use on adverse drug reactions in paediatric patients. *Drug Saf* 2004; 27(13): 1059–1067.
6   Gravatt LA, Pakyz AL. Challenges in measuring antibiotic consumption. *Curr Infect Dis Rep* 2013; 15(6): 559–563.

21

Innovative strategies in paediatric drug development

*G Pons, S Zohar, E Bellissant, C Chiron and
A Saint-Raymond*

Introduction

Despite the development of paediatric investigation plans since the European Paediatric Regulation came into force, medicines for children are still limited by insufficient evaluation in each age group, a lack of age appropriate formulations, and widespread off-label prescribing. However, medicines research in children can be facilitated by the use of novel study designs. In this chapter we will focus on innovative methodological approaches that can be used to increase the feasibility and safety of paediatric clinical research, and also specific methodological tools facilitating the measurement of therapeutic effects in young children.

The learning objectives of this chapter are:

➢ to understand that innovative methodologies in paediatric drug development can protect children from the potential harm of poorly designed clinical studies
➢ to recognise that innovative strategies should be used to facilitate the performance of clinical studies in children and improve cost-effectiveness
➢ to understand that the measurement of the effect of drugs in children requires adapted endpoints and methodology, especially in the youngest age groups.

Prevention of the potential harms of clinical research in children

Harmfulness of clinical studies is related to various factors, including pain, stress, blood deprivation and, potentially, exposure to radioactive isotopes. Exposure to clinical trials and investigational new drugs should be limited to the minimum required.

Prevention of pain and stress

To prevent pain and stress related to blood sampling in children, the use of local anaesthesia and of catheters to avoid repeated venepuncture should be advocated. The assessment of efficacy should be performed where possible through non-invasive procedures such as transcutaneous methods, but such non-invasive methods have to be carefully validated to yield appropriate and reliable surrogate markers.

Prevention of blood loss

To restrict blood loss, a small number of small volume blood samples should be drawn per patient and microassays developed with appropriate sensitivity and specificity. To perform pharmacokinetic (PK) and pharmacokinetic–pharmacodynamic (PK–PD) studies, the use of population approaches has to be further developed.[1] While the 'rich data' individual approach requires many blood samples in a few patients, the population approach (pop-PK) requires fewer blood samples per patient in a larger number of patients (chapter 9).

Alternative approaches, such as salivary sampling, may potentially be misleading. Despite evidence of good correlations between saliva and plasma drug concentration for certain drugs, the large scatter of data points around the correlation line may prevent appropriate estimation of a plasma concentration from concomitant saliva concentrations.

Prevention of exposure to radioactive compounds

Stable isotopes
Irradiation by the use of radioactive compounds must be avoided in children, and the use of stable isotopes should be favoured. The use of the labelling of medicinal products by stable isotopes is of great potential interest in children for bioavailability studies, PK studies during repeated dose treatment, for metabolic studies, and for measuring treatment compliance.[2]

Microdosing
Two different microdose approaches have been proposed in humans in early stage drug development.[3] The first approach would involve not more than a total dose of 100 μg that can be administered as a single dose or divided doses in any subject. This could be useful to investigate target receptor binding or tissue distribution in a positron emission tomography (PET) study. A second use could be to assess PK with or without the use of an isotopically labelled agent. The second microdose approach is one that involves fewer than five administrations of a maximum of 100 μg per administration (a total of 500 μg per subject). This can be useful for applications similar

to the first microdose approach described above, but with less active PET ligands. In some situations, it could be appropriate to carry out a clinical microdose study using the intravenous (IV) route on a product intended for oral administration and for which an oral non-clinical toxicology package already exists. In this case, the IV microdose can be qualified by the existing oral toxicity studies where adequate exposure margins have been achieved. It is not recommended to investigate IV local tolerance of the drug substance in this situation, because the administered dose is very low (100 μg maximum). If a novel IV vehicle is being employed, then local tolerance of the vehicle should be assessed.

Microdosing has recently been used in 52 'babies' in the PAMPER study. The PAMPER study showed the feasibility and validity of microdosing accelerator mass spectrometry (AMS) PK studies in children. This methodology may provide a safer and more ethically robust approach for paediatric PK studies in certain drug models than more traditional PK study designs. The parameters and validation methods for microdosing AMS PK studies need to be reflected in regulatory guidance from the European Medicines Agency (EMA), US Food and Drug Administration (FDA) and other authorities.[4]

Paediatric microdosing may be used for elucidating age-related changes in oral absorption to guide dosing of new formulations. Bioavailability of a new oral formulation is traditionally tested in a crossover design. The drug is given on two different occasions, once orally and once intravenously, each followed by multiple blood samples to measure drug concentrations and then determine oral bioavailability. In children, this study design is usually not acceptable for both practical and ethical reasons, including extensive blood sampling and the administration of non-therapeutic doses, respectively. Given these limitations, microdosing presents an interesting alternative method to study oral drug disposition in children and can also delineate developmental changes in (intestinal) drug metabolising enzymes. Microdosing is a relatively novel technique used in adults to estimate PK and bioavailability, with the main advantage of the absence of therapeutic or adverse effects. The technique seems most valid when linearity exists between the microdose and therapeutic dose. The use of microdosing in the drug development process was endorsed by the EMA in 2009.

Prevention of exposure to unnecessary clinical investigations

Restricting exposure to clinical studies and to investigational new drugs whenever possible requires avoiding unnecessary studies. The lowest possible age limit to which adult data can be extrapolated should be determined case by case and extrapolation used accordingly as much as possible. Unnecessary studies can also be avoided by the use of existing data, both published and unpublished. For example, the bioavailability of paediatric formulations measured in healthy adult volunteers can be used as the human model and only confirmatory data required in children. Population PK analysis (chapter 2 and chapter 9) can sometimes be performed on published data, avoiding additional studies on the influence of maturation on paediatric PK. Meta-analysis of previously published data should also be performed whenever possible.

Optimisation of drug development in children

Pilot observational exploratory studies may be of great potential interest in order to optimise drug development in children. Such studies would allow estimation of the order of magnitude of the treatment effect (each patient being its own control) to record the variability of the endpoint(s) of interest – all useful information for the calculation of the required sample size. These types of studies may also be of interest to identify the potential target population, as has been used for infantile epilepsy syndromes.[5]

Clinical studies should be combined whenever possible with PK studies by recording simultaneously PD endpoints along with collecting PK samples and collecting PK samples during efficacy and safety studies as well.

Extrapolation

In order to extrapolate adult data down to the lowest possible age limit in children, data on the maturational profiles relevant to PK should be used, as well as the profiles relating to developmental PK–PD and safety (e.g. level of drug systemic exposure, minimum and peak plasma concentrations, and area under the plasma concentration–time curve). Knowledge of the ontogeny of the processes involved in drug elimination is very useful for planning paediatric PK studies, because this can guide the lowest possible age limit for age down-extrapolation from adults to children. This knowledge facilitates optimisation of the age distribution targets in patient recruitment and quantitative modelling of the influence of maturation, thus facilitating clinical trial simulation.

Recruitment of paediatric patients

Sequential approaches can be used for dose-finding studies during phase II as well as for comparative trials during phase III of drug development.

Adaptive phase II designs

Dose-finding parallel group studies are difficult to perform in children due to the relatively narrow dose range and the small interval between tested doses, the important inter-individual variability and therefore the lack of statistical power. This could in theory be increased by higher participant numbers, but this is very difficult in children. The new continual reassessment method has been proposed and successfully used in children.

The modified bivariate adaptive method that aims to estimate the safe most successful dose (sMSD) is a Bayesian model-based approach. The objective of this method is to find a dose level that maximises the probability of success under safety restrictions. The design attempts to allocate the maximum number of patients to the estimated sMSD over the whole trial. At the end of the trial, or earlier if the trial stops for safety or efficacy reasons, the estimated sMSD can be calculated with 95% credibility intervals (precision intervals).

The continuous reassessment method is an adaptive sequential Bayesian method. This method consists of the sequential allocation of doses to cohorts of patients ($c = 1$, 2, 3 or more) until a total number of at least 24 patients has been reached. The first cohort is usually treated with the first dose level, whereas dose levels for the subsequent groups are determined according to the model estimates of the dose–efficacy and dose–safety relationships. The dose allocation procedure is given in chapter 17. The recommended dose level for future experimentation is the one satisfying both efficacy criteria and toxicity restriction. Fixed standards of the minimum probability of response (minimum efficacy target) and the maximum probability of non-tolerance (maximal toxicity target) need to be specified by the trial investigators.

Intravenous ibuprofen for PDA as an example

Intravenous ibuprofen (IBU) has been found to be as effective as indomethacin for the treatment of patent ductus arteriosus (PDA) in preterm infants and has been associated with fewer adverse effects in comparative phase III studies. The dose regimen used (10 – 5 – 5 mg/kg/day for 3 days) was based on limited PK data, and no phase II study was available to determine the optimal dose of IBU for this indication.

The present study (Table 1) was designed to determine the minimum effective dose regimen (MEDR) of IBU (one course) required to close ductus arteriosus in preterm infants.[6] A double-blind dose-finding study was conducted using the continual reassessment method, a Bayesian sequential design. Two distinct target closure rates were initially chosen according to postmenstrual age (PMA) at birth: 80% in infants with a PMA of 27–29 weeks, and 50% in infants with a PMA < 27 weeks. Forty neonates (20 in each PMA group) with PDA were treated between days 3 and 5 of life. Four different dose regimens were tested: loading doses of 5, 10, 15 or 20 mg/kg, followed by two doses (half loading dose) at 24-h intervals. Efficacy was evaluated by echocardiography 24 h after the third infusion. In infants with a PMA of 27–29 weeks, the estimated MEDR was 10 – 5 – 5 mg/kg, with a final estimated probability of success of 77% (95% credibility interval: 56–92%). The 15 – 7.5 – 7.5 mg/kg dose regimen had a better estimated probability of success (88%; 95% credibility interval:

Table 1 Bayesian sequential analysis of a dose-finding study of curative intravenous ibuprofen in patent ductus arteriosus in neonates[6]

Patients	Dose	Dose (mg/kg)			
		5	10	15	20
		A priori estimated probabilities of success (%)			
		0.6	0.8	0.9	0.95
		A posteriori estimated probabilities of success (%)			
1	10	0.481	0.683	0.812	0.891
2	5	0.370	0.544	0.682	0.787
3	15	0.539	0.744	0.861	0.925
4	10	0.512	0.717	0.840	0.915
5	15	0.467	0.667	0.799	0.882
6	15	0.500	0.703	0.829	0.903
7	10	0.519	0.723	0.845	0.914
8	15	0.553	0.757	0.870	0.931
9	10	0.567	0.771	0.880	0.938

68–97%) but resulted in more minor renal adverse effects. In contrast, in infants with a PMA < 27 weeks, the estimated MEDR was 20 – 10 – 10 mg/kg, with an estimated probability of success of 54.8% (95% credibility interval: 22–84%), whereas the conventional dose regimen resulted in a low estimated probability of success (30.6%; 95% credibility interval: 13–56%). In these infants, compared with those with a PMA of 27–29 weeks, minor renal adverse effects were more frequent from the 10–5–5 mg/kg/day dose regimen and did not appear to be clearly dose related.[6]

This study confirms that the currently recommended dose regimen (10 – 5 – 5 mg/kg) of IBU is associated with a high closure rate (80%) and few adverse effects in premature infants with a PMA of 27–29 weeks. The failure rate was much higher below 27 weeks. A higher dose regimen (20 – 10 – 10 mg/kg) might achieve a higher closure rate. However, tolerability and safety of this dose regimen should be assessed in a larger population before considering the use of these doses for ductus arteriosus closure.

This method has the advantage of not requiring a placebo group, allowing each patient to receive a dose closer to this optimal dose. This method requires only a limited number of patients (15–20). The flaws of the method are that until now it requires the use of a qualitative parameter, a rapid evaluation of the response, and very efficient organisation throughout the duration of the trial.

Sequential phase III designs

Phase III comparative studies tend to take longer than expected due to the difficulty in enrolling children. It has been observed in an adult study of lidocaine versus placebo after myocardial infarction that the treatment may be deleterious and cause more deaths than observed post infarct in the placebo group; a subsequent post-hoc analysis revealed the trial could have been stopped one year earlier, saving many patients from death caused by lidocaine. The sequential phase III study design, such as use of the triangular test, consists of performing sequential statistical comparisons while maintaining type I and II errors. This can enable trials to be stopped as soon as the initial hypothesis can be adequately tested, thus restricting the number of recruited patients to the minimum necessary.

Example of sequential phase III study design

The presented study was performed in infants. In brief, the triangular test uses a sequential plan defined by two perpendicular axes. The horizontal axis corresponds to a first statistic, V, which represents the quantity of information accumulated since the beginning of the trial, and the vertical axis corresponds to a second statistic, Z, which represents the benefit with the experimental treatment compared with the control. Two straight lines, called the boundaries of the test, delineate a continuation region (between these two lines) from the regions of non-rejection of the inefficacy hypothesis (below the bottom line) and of rejection of the inefficacy hypothesis (above the top line).

Because the two boundaries intersect, the continuation region is closed. The equations of the straight line boundaries depend on the values of the benefit to detect, of its standard deviation, and of the type I and II error rates, as well as on the frequency of the analyses, defined in terms of the number of patients included between two analyses. Because this number generally varies at each analysis, the boundaries need to be adjusted concomitantly, thus defining a continuation region with a shape of a Christmas tree. At each analysis, the two statistics V and Z are calculated from all the data collected since the beginning of the study and define a point (V, Z) on the sequential plan. The consecutive points define a sample path from the left to the right of the sequential plan. As long as the sample path stays within the two boundaries, the study is continued and new patients are included. When the sample path crosses one of the boundaries, the study is stopped and the conclusion is obtained: crossing the bottom boundary causes the inefficacy hypothesis not to be rejected, whereas crossing the top boundary causes the inefficacy hypothesis to be rejected. In this study, the monitoring and the sequential analyses were performed on the main endpoint for efficacy with the PEST statistical software R3 (version 3) on an IBM PS/2 microcomputer. Once the trial was stopped, the final analysis on the main endpoint was performed with the same program, allowing us to obtain an unbiased estimate of each treatment efficacy and a significance level taking into account the sequential nature of the analyses.

This placebo controlled, randomised double-blind study was aimed at assessing the efficacy of metoclopramide (0.2 mg/kg three times daily during 14 days) on gastro-oesophageal reflux in infancy.[7] The main endpoint was the relative variation of the percentage of time at $pH < 4$ between inclusion (day 0) and evaluation (day 14) assessed on two 24-hour oesophageal pH recordings. Statistical analysis was performed with the use of a sequential method, the triangular test. The study was stopped after the seventh analysis (39 infants evaluated: 20 placebo and 19 metoclopramide) without showing the expected benefit. Improvement on the main endpoint was $30\% \pm 48\%$ (mean ± standard deviation). Corresponding unbiased median estimates were 22% for placebo and 39% for metoclopramide ($p = 0.28$, sequential analysis). On day 14, the percentage of time at $pH < 4$ was $8.1\% \pm 11.7\%$ for placebo and $6.7\% \pm 9.2\%$ for metoclopramide ($p = 0.68$, t test), and the number of reflux episodes >5 minutes was 3.0 ± 3.5 for placebo and 1.9 ± 3.0 for metoclopramide ($p = 0.33$, t test). If a tendency for a superior improvement with metoclopramide than with the placebo was observed on the main endpoint, it was lower than expected and the difference was not significant. Compared with the corresponding single-stage design, the triangular test, shown in Figure 1, allowed the investigators to stop the study with a 15% reduction in sample size.[7]

These data illustrate the potential of using a sequential method such as the triangular test in clinical trials where difficulties in patient recruitment are anticipated. This approach could be useful to assist in the planning of paediatric clinical trials. Sequential approaches such as the triangular test are of great potential interest in phase III comparative clinical trials in that they allow recruitment of a smaller number of patients, since the study can be stopped as soon as information sufficient to conclude has been collected.

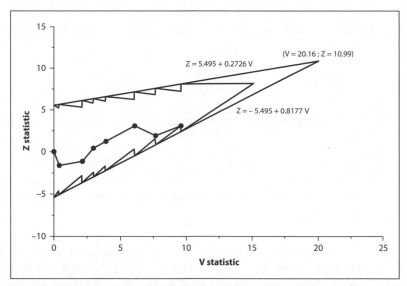

Figure 1 Sequential analysis of a study of the efficacy of metoclopramide (triangular test and sample path) versus placebo in the gastro-oesophageal reflux in infants[7]

Responder population enrichment

Responder population enrichment has been used to decrease the variability of the response and to increase the statistical power in order to facilitate the demonstration of efficacy.

Example

Stiripentol (STP) is a new antiepileptic drug that can potentiate the effect of other antiseizure medications via its inhibition of several cytochrome P450 isoenzymes. Evidence supporting the efficacy of stiripentol in combination with carbamazepine (CBZ) has been reported in an open trial in children with epilepsy. The aim of the trial was to study STP as an add-on therapy to CBZ in refractory partial epilepsy in children.[8] An enrichment and withdrawal design was used (Figure 2). After a 1 month single-blind placebo baseline followed by a 3 month open add-on STP, 32 out of 67 patients were responders. They were double blindly randomised for 2 months either to STP ($n = 17$) or placebo ($n = 15$). If seizures increased by at least 50% after randomisation compared with the baseline, patients dropped out of the study (primary endpoint). During the double blind phase, six patients on STP (35%) and eight on placebo (53%) dropped out (not significant). However, seizure rate (secondary endpoint) decreased significantly more on STP (−75%) than on placebo (−22%). During the double blind phase, the STP dose was

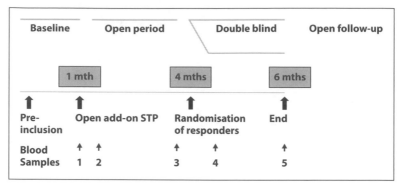

Figure 2 Responder population enrichment withdrawal placebo controlled trial – stiripentol in partial epilepsy in children[8]

81 ± 15 mg/kg/day (minimum plasma concentration (C_{min}): 11.0 ± 5.5 mg/L) and the CBZ dose 12.6 ± 5.6 mg/kg/day (C_{min}: 12.8 ± 2.6 mg/L) in the STP group, while CBZ dose was 17.0 ± 7.0 mg/kg/day (C_{min}: 7.1 ± 1.6 mg/L) in the placebo group. This study design allowed limitation of the number of patients recruited and the risk of worsening seizure control. STP proved to reduce seizure rate as an add-on to CBZ in children with refractory partial epilepsy, although the difference in the primary endpoint was not significant.[8]

Clinical trial simulation

Clinical trial mathematical modelling and *in silico* simulation is a potentially promising avenue to explore, but is beyond the scope of this book. Relevant references are included below.

Use of child-appropriate assessment tools

Appropriate tools have to be developed for the measurement of drug effect, because children cannot cooperate and do not express their distress in the same way as adults. Appropriate scales for measuring the magnitude of response to medicinal products had to be developed for pain and have, for example, to be further developed for the measurement of sedation and of muscular strength. Similarly, new clinical and biological endpoints and surrogate markers have to be validated in children.

Appropriate endpoints for the assessment of pain in children

The use of age appropriate pain scales is discussed in chapter 60. The scales for pain and appropriate tools for the measurement of analgesic efficacy vary not only with age but also with clinical conditions (e.g. postoperative pain), particularly in young children.

Appropriate methodological tools for the assessment of unexpected adverse events specific to children

Adequate methodological tools have to be appropriately chosen for the post-marketing assessment of unpredicted late toxicity of medicinal products on developing organs, and are of particular interest in children for long term or rare adverse events. These tools are mainly observational studies, which are discussed elsewhere in this book. Long-term prospective follow-up studies (including of growth, maturation, intellectual, psychological and reproductive development) can help to identify adverse drug reactions that occur far beyond the period of drug exposure. These are important, given past therapeutic catastrophes such as phocomelia related to thalidomide exposure during pregnancy, adenocarcinoma of the vagina after intrauterine diethylstilboestrol exposure, and delayed ovarian toxicity relating to high dose busulfan before bone marrow transplant. Appropriate methodological approaches should be used to identify rare adverse events; comparative parallel cohort studies and case-studies nested within these cohort studies are of particular potential interest in children (chapter 19).[9]

Observational studies for efficacy

Although such an approach would currently not be accepted by regulatory authorities for marketing authorisation, there are extreme situations where no one could propose a comparative trial in order to demonstrate causality that is universally accepted facing the magnitude of the treatment effect. Who would propose a comparative trial to demonstrate the preventive efficacy of a parachute?[10] The causal relationship between, e.g., tobacco use and lung cancer is accepted on the basis of the strength of the association demonstrated through non-interventional epidemiology studies. As such, tobacco use is considered the leading cause of disease, disability and death in the USA. There are other examples, e.g. asbestos and asbestosis.

For ethical reasons, when the magnitude of a treatment effect is expected to be large, through preliminary observational studies, the search for the demonstration of efficacy should at least plan a sequential comparative trial, e.g. the triangular test, in order to stop the trial as soon as sufficient information has been collected to reach a conclusion, and use withdrawal of individual patients before the end of the individual observation period for lack of efficacy via criteria well defined before the onset of the trial.

Conclusions

Innovative methodologies are potentially useful tools to facilitate drug evaluation in children. They are presently not expected to replace classical approaches. The validity of these approaches and their limitations need to be properly evaluated for appropriate levels of evidence of efficacy and safety. Due to the constraints of drug evaluation in children, paediatric clinical pharmacology represents a challenging area for methodological creativity, which may ultimately also benefit other areas of drug evaluation and development, including in adults.

References

1 Manolis E, Pons G. Proposals for model-based paediatric medicinal development within the current European Union regulatory framework. *Br J Clin Pharmacol* 2009; 68(4): 493–501.
2 Pons G, Rey E. Stable isotopes labeling of drugs in pediatric clinical pharmacology. *Pediatrics* 1999; 104(3 pt 2): 633–639.
3 European Medicines Agency. ICH guideline M3(R2) on non-clinical safety studies for the conduct of human clinical trials and marketing authorisation for pharmaceuticals. EMA/CPMP/ICH/286/1995. 2009. Available at: www.ema.europa.eu/docs/en_GB/document_library/Scientific_guideline/2009/09/WC500002720.pdf [last accessed 2 March 2018].
4 Crawley F *et al*. PS-128 The ethics of microdosing studies in children: the experience of the Era-net Priomedchild Project Pamper. *Arch Dis Child* 2014; 99(suppl 2): A156–A57.
5 Chiron C *et al*. Antiepileptic drug development in children: considerations for a revisited strategy. *Drugs* 2008; 68(1): 17–25.
6 Desfrere L *et al*. Dose-finding study of ibuprofen in patent ductus arteriosus using the continual reassessment method. *J Clin Pharm Ther* 2005; 30(2): 121–132.
7 Bellissant E *et al*. The triangular test to assess the efficacy of metoclopramide in gastroesophageal reflux. *Clin Pharmacol Ther* 1997; 61(3): 377–384.
8 Chiron C *et al*. Stiripentol in childhood partial epilepsy: randomized placebo-controlled trial with enrichment and withdrawal design. *J Child Neurol* 2006; 21(6): 496–502.
9 Mikaeloff Y *et al*. Nonsteroidal anti-inflammatory drug use and the risk of severe skin and soft tissue complications in patients with varicella or zoster disease. *Br J Clin Pharmacol* 2008; 65(2): 203–209.
10 Smith GC, Pell JP. Parachute use to prevent death and major trauma related to gravitational challenge: systematic review of randomised controlled trials. *BMJ (Clinical Research Ed)* 2003; 327(7429): 1459–1461.

Further recommended reading

Bensouda-Grimaldi L *et al*. Pharmaco-epidemiology to evaluate medicines in pediatric patients. *Arch Pediatr* 2008; 15(5): 814–816 [in French].
Gao Y *et al*. Could saliva stand for plasma in theophylline monitoring in asthmatic children? Still a controversial problem. *Fundam Clin Pharmacol* 1992; 6: 191–196.
Leroy S *et al*. Hospitalization for severe bacterial infections in children after exposure to NSAIDs: a prospective adverse drug reaction reporting study. *Clin Drug Investig* 2010; 30(3): 179–185.
Lesko SM, Mitchell AA. An assessment of the safety of pediatric ibuprofen. A practitioner-based randomized clinical trial. *JAMA* 1995; 273(12): 929–933.

22

The role of the pharmaceutical industry in developing medicines for children

SP Tansey

Introduction

This chapter will aim to outline how the pharmaceutical industry contributes to the development of children's medicines.

The learning objectives of this chapter are to understand how industry:

➤ identifies new medicines for children
➤ supports the conduct of clinical trials in children
➤ uses alternative ways to collect evidence
➤ conducts studies after a medicine is licensed.

Deciding which medicines to develop for children

At an early stage of identification of a potential new medicine (either a small molecule or a biologic), the target product profile will be developed. This profile will outline the desirable product specifications, including not only the planned indication(s), but also the target population and the desired safety profile for the medicine. From this target product profile the industry team will start to outline a clinical development plan that will support the use of the medicine in the planned population, which may or may not include children.

An important aspect for companies to consider when deciding whether to move forward with a clinical development plan for a new medicine is whether the cost of the clinical programme will be recouped by the profits made once the product is on the market. This is an important factor taken into account when deciding which medicines to continue to develop.

For large pharmaceutical companies, both top management and shareholders will be involved in decisions about prioritisation of the portfolio. Smaller biotechnology companies will also need to be able to show the potential for profitability and recouping research and development costs when applying for venture capital funding to support their clinical development programmes.

ICH E11 states that data on the use of medicinal products in the paediatric population should be generated unless use of those products in children is inappropriate.[1] In some cases (e.g. a medicine to treat respiratory distress syndrome in neonates), it will not be relevant to obtain data in all age groups of children, and doing so will not be expected; a waiver would be granted from carrying out clinical trials in other age groups. Paediatric clinical trial information should ultimately be included on the product label (e.g. the summary of product characteristics (SmPC) in Europe) in the section relating to paediatric use.

If a disease or condition affects both adults and children, e.g. asthma, the traditional view is that clinical trials in the least vulnerable population (e.g. adults followed by older children) are carried out first before exposing younger children to the investigational medicinal product. In a similar way, clinical trials with an investigational product will usually be carried out in older children before exposing infants and neonates. However, it may be preferable to develop medicines for children and neonates at the same time as for adults if there is a significant therapeutic need in these populations and dosing regimens and safety assessments can be designed rationally.

Categories of potential new paediatric medicines

- New medicine identified for a disease/condition occurring in adults or children
- New medicine identified for use in a disease/condition only occurring in children
- Medicine already licensed for adult use developed for the same indication in children, e.g. medicines licensed prior to 2007 for infection
- Medicine already licensed for adult use and developed for a different indication in children, e.g. propranolol for cavernous haemangioma
- New formulation or route of administration of a medicine that is already licensed for adult use in a different form
- Generics
- Biosimilars

Most of these products will trigger a paediatric investigation plan (PIP) (chapter 28). Generics and biosimilars do not usually require a PIP. New formulations of medicines that are already licensed for adult use in a different form and developed for submission as a paediatric use marketing authorisation (PUMA) may not be required to address all age groups in the PIP application.

Generic products

The World Health Organization (WHO) definition is that a generic drug 'is a pharmaceutical product, usually intended to be interchangeable with an innovator product, that is manufactured without a licence from the innovator company and marketed after the expiry date of the patent or other exclusive rights'.

Further preclinical and clinical data to obtain a marketing authorisation for a generic are not usually required, except to demonstrate that there is pharmaceutical equivalence and bioequivalence. Bioequivalence studies must show that the product behaves in the same way (has the same pharmacokinetic properties) as the innovator drug. Generics generally have a lower price and so may be the only way that less resourced settings can access a medicine.

Biosimilars

The definition given by the European Medicines Agency (EMA) for a similar biological or 'biosimilar' medicine is that it is 'a biological medicine that is similar to another biological medicine that has already been authorised for use'. Biological medicines are complex because of secondary and tertiary structures of protein and patterns of glycosylation. This means that equivalence is not required or possible in the same way that it is for small molecules/generics.

Multiple biosimilar products have now been approved and launched in Europe, resulting in increased patient access to these products. The number of biosimilar products approved in the USA is much smaller to date. Additionally, there are likely to be more developed as the patents for biologicals developed in the last decade start to expire. Unlike for generics, for biological products, because of the complex structure and manufacturing processes, several clinical trials will be required in order to submit for a licence.

Clinical trials are required to show that the biosimilar:

- is similar to the reference medicine
- does not have any meaningful differences from the reference medicine in terms of quality, safety or efficacy.

As with generics, there are significant economic drivers for the development of the biosimilar market. It remains to be seen whether those drivers are sufficient to overcome the obstacles to biosimilar development.

What industry brings to the conduct of clinical trials in children

Paediatric clinical trials are conducted by industry in order to support safety and efficacy claims made on the product label or summary of product characteristics. In other words, clinical trials are planned to show that when the medicine is administered as per the recommended dosage schedule, it has been demonstrated to be efficacious and safe under clinical trial conditions. This information is an important component of the benefit–risk ratio when physicians decide whether to prescribe a medicine for one of their paediatric patients.

Regulators (e.g. the EMA and/or US Food and Drug Administration (FDA)) will generally have agreed the design of the proposed paediatric clinical trial(s) with the sponsoring company in advance of submission.

Reasons why industry carries out clinical trials in children

- To obtain evidence on safety and efficacy to support an application for a marketing authorisation application (MAA) or investigational new drug (IND)
- To obtain evidence for a health technology assessment, i.e. quality of life/health outcomes/ health economics data
- To investigate a safety signal after a medicine is licensed
- To support new claims or a new indication in a marketed product

Industry's role in support of paediatric clinical trials

In most industry trials, the responsibilities of the sponsor as laid out in the Clinical Trials Directive (CTD)/Clinical Trials Regulation (CTR) will be carried out by the pharmaceutical company.[2] This will include ensuring that the clinical trial is carried out following the International Conference on Harmonisation of Technical Requirements for Registration of Pharmaceuticals for Human Use (ICH) Guideline for Good Clinical Practice (GCP).[3] Increasingly, companies are delegating some or all of the sponsor tasks to contract research organisations, although it is clear in the CTD/CTR that the ultimate responsibility for the quality and integrity of the data remains with the sponsor.

In addition, although many of the larger pharmaceutical companies may identify a potential product and take it through the complete product life cycle, it is now becoming increasingly common that several companies/ sponsors will be involved in the development of a paediatric medicine during its life cycle.

Industry supports paediatric clinical trials in various ways

The pharmaceutical industry does not act as a monolith. A number of scenarios are possible, depending on the nature of the molecule and the clinical environment. A company can:

- act as the sponsor, financing all paediatric trial work
- supply an investigational product, e.g. to an investigator-initiated trial
- collaborate with an advocacy group, e.g. Vertex and the Cystic Fibrosis Foundation
- collaborate with one or more other companies, e.g. ViiV Healthcare – a collaboration between Pfizer and GSK to develop HIV medicines.

More than one sponsor may be involved in development of a medicine

- A start-up or small biotechnology company may carry out the initial development of a compound which is then licensed by a larger company at the end of phase I.
- A large company may sell off an investigational compound to a small biotechnology company for development in an orphan indication, e.g. after previous clinical development for another indication.

Requirements on industry during trials

Industry is committed to collecting high quality data during clinical trials. This scientific commitment is supplemented by two other reasons. Firstly, each trial has to comply with GCP. Secondly, all the data that support an MAA will be scrutinised by regulators. A failure to meet either requirement can mean the failure of the drug development programme and waste of the investment in the programme. Accordingly, sponsors invest in maintaining the quality of the trial's conduct and the data collected by checking some or all data points against the patient's hospital records (source data verification).

Alternative ways to collect evidence on medicines for children

Registries

A registry differs from a clinical trial in that it selects patients either on a particular disease or condition or on exposure, e.g. to a medicinal product. This may be a more feasible way to collect the information/evidence required to support development of a paediatric medicine than a classical randomised controlled trial.

Use of registries may be helpful in the following:

- A situation where a child has a life-threatening or severely debilitating disorder, there is no available licensed treatment and/or the child is not eligible for a clinical trial; e.g. could be the case if the child has severe or rapidly progressive disease
- Collection of data after licensure of a medicinal product, e.g. in relation to a specific safety concern
- Looking at long-term safety, e.g. a medicinal product that has been used in premature neonates
- Collecting information on rare diseases when a medicinal product has been licensed on the basis of a relatively small trial or to comply with requirements of the Early Access to Medicines Scheme (EAMS), which was launched by the Medicines and Healthcare products Regulatory Agency in the UK

Compassionate use protocols

A compassionate use protocol is set up to provide an unlicensed or investigational product in cases of unmet medical need. There are similarities with registries, but a protocol will be set up giving, e.g., the dosage of a product to be used and some criteria that a child has to fulfil to be eligible. Situations in which a compassionate use protocol may be appropriate are:

- to treat a child with a life-threatening or severely debilitating disorder when there is no licensed treatment available
- to treat a very rare disease when there are not sufficient numbers of patients to carry out a clinical trial
- to provide a medicinal product to patients after clinical trials for registration have been completed but before the granting of a product licence.

Evidence collection after licensure

There are many reasons why it might be necessary to collect further evidence after licensure of a paediatric medicine, in addition to the usual pharmacovigilance requirements.

Further clinical trials and/or evidence collection may be required after licensure:

- to investigate a safety signal
- to fulfil any deferred requirements of a PIP
- to extend the indication to a different population/age group
- to apply for a new indication
- if a new formulation is being developed
- in the case of a new manufacturing process for a biologic.

How clinicians and pharmaceutical companies can work together

Clinicians (academics and others) can work with pharmaceutical companies on the shared goal of developing appropriate medicines for children by:

- obtaining and sharing information about unmet clinical needs and populations that would benefit from further research
- contributing to clinical trials efficiently through well established and experienced networks
- reporting suspected adverse events during development and once a medicine is on the market.

Working as a pharmaceutical physician is interesting and diverse, and can include involvement in the medical monitoring of clinical trials, drug safety, regulatory affairs and scientific advice.

Conclusions

New children's medicines developed by industry can be developed solely for children or for both adults and children. The pharmaceutical industry carries out clinical trials in children to obtain evidence on safety and efficacy both pre and post marketing and to assist with health technology assessments. Several sponsor companies may be involved in a product's life cycle. Alternative ways to collect evidence on medicines for children include registries and compassionate use protocols.

References

1 International Conference on Harmonisation of Technical Requirements for Registration of Pharmaceuticals for Human Use (ICH). E11: *Guideline on Clinical Investigation of Medicinal Products in the Paediatric Population*. 2000.
2 *European Union Directive 2001/20/ec of the European Parliament and of the Council of 4 April 2001 on the approximation of the laws, regulations and administrative provisions of the member states relating to the implementation of good clinical practice in the conduct of clinical trials on medicinal products for human use.* https://ec.europa.eu/health/sites/health/files/files/eudralex/vol-1/dir_2001_20/dir_2001_20_en.pdf
3 International Conference on Harmonisation of Technical Requirements for Registration of Pharmaceuticals for Human Use (ICH). *Guideline for Good Clinical Practice E6*. 1996.

Further recommended reading

Cystic Fibrosis Foundation. CF Foundation Venture Philanthropy Model. www.cff.org/About-Us/About-the-Cystic-Fibrosis-Foundation/CF-Foundation-Venture-Philanthropy-Model
European Commission. Guideline on the format and content of applications for agreement or modification of a paediatric investigation plan and requests for waivers or deferrals and concerning the operation of the compliance check and on criteria for assessing significant studies. 2014/C 338/01. ec.europa.eu/health/files/eudralex/vol-1/2014_c338_01/2014_c338_01_en.pdf
European Medicines Agency (EMA). www.ema.europa.eu/ema
Medicines and Healthcare products Regulatory Agency. www.gov.uk/government/organisations/medicines-and-healthcare-products-regulatory-agency
US Food and Drug Administration. www.fda.gov
ViiV Healthcare. www.viivhealthcare.com

23

Paediatric drug formulations

T Dennison, A Al-Khattawi, AR Mohammed and D Terry

Introduction

Over the past two decades there has been an effort to increase the number of prescription drugs designed specifically for use in the paediatric population, both in the EU and the USA. This chapter reviews the importance of developing age appropriate formulations of medicines for children and the difficulties faced.

The learning objectives of this chapter are:

➤ to understand why age appropriate formulations are important
➤ to recognise the practical and financial challenges in paediatric formulation development
➤ to be aware of relevant guidelines and legislative changes that aim to improve the development of medicines for children.

There are many reasons for the lack of medicines that are licensed for paediatric use, but primarily this arises from a significant knowledge gap. For example, there may be limited understanding concerning the acceptability of dosage forms and their size, volume of administration, and even taste. From a clinical perspective it is also important to define safe dosage levels of both the active drug and also all excipients included in a formulation, and how these safe dosages change with patient age. The lack of suitable licensed paediatric medicines means that unlicensed formulations are often used by healthcare professionals. Improving our understanding of the effect of medicines on children is therefore of vital importance. However, this is complicated by the requirement to protect the wellbeing of children in clinical trials and by fears over ethical issues and the potential to cause actual harm.[1,2]

Background

There are a number of reasons why paediatric formulations must differ from those for adults. Infants experience rapid growth and development with different rates of growth of organs and maturation of active transport systems, metabolic pathways and body systems. These differences mean that infants cannot be viewed as young adults, as response to medications will vary between paediatric subsets and between paediatric and adult populations. These may include differences in pharmacokinetics, pharmacodynamics and adverse effects to different formulations. Paediatric doses change throughout childhood, with doses usually calculated by body weight or surface area. As a result, paediatric formulations must be flexible enough and accurate enough to allow for this large dose range. A child's mental development will also determine its ability to tolerate different dosage forms, with many young children being unable to swallow conventional tablets or capsules. Indeed, the dosage must be in a form that can be accepted by a child or administered to that child by a caregiver.[3,4]

Oral formulations

Palatability of oral medication is crucial for paediatric compliance, since taste acceptance differs between adults and children, and children will be less willing to tolerate a medicament they find to have an unacceptable taste. The oral route is the most favoured for long term dosing, with liquid formulations being the most popular and prevalent in the market due to dose flexibility and difficulties in swallowing tablets and capsules. Taste-masking of oral formulations requires careful selection of excipients and can drive up costs, lead to long term instability, and may not even be completely achievable (especially for bitter drugs). Nonetheless some technologies exist to enable liquids to be flavoured according to the individual child's preferences at the point of dispensing, e.g. FLAVORx (see https://www.flavorx.com/about/). Although technologies such as encapsulation or complexation can be employed in taste masking, they can be difficult to achieve and costly.[5] Selection of a suitable vehicle, most often water, can also present significant formulation challenges. Limitations of dose and volume due to drug solubility are also common issues, as are chemical, physical and microbial stability, which must be controlled by the addition of antioxidants, buffers, suspending agents and preservatives. However, before prescribing a liquid for a child of 6 years of age or more, consider whether the patient can take a tablet at an appropriate dose, or another solid oral dosage form.

A range of solid oral dosage forms suitable for children are available. Multi-particulates such as, e.g., granules and pellets can be administered directly into the mouth or mixed with certain food or drink. These offer advantages like ease of swallowing, dose flexibility and the possibility of drug combination. However, the issue of incomplete ingestion, and therefore reduced dose, adds complications, as do packaging and stability issues.[3,6-8] Chewable tablets and gums have also been developed for paediatrics. They do not require water, offer stability and ease of transport, and are palatable. However, taste masking is difficult to achieve, especially when taste masking strategies in adults, such as the use of cyclodextrins, may not be acceptable for children. Oral wafers are also suitable dosage forms for children. These are small thin strips that adhere to the mucosa and dissolve, negating swallowing and avoiding the problem of spitting out. They benefit from containing small amounts of excipients, however have a limit for drug incorporation of around 50 mg and are also highly dependent on taste masking.

Excipients

It is not just the active pharmaceutical ingredient that is of concern in paediatric formulations. In order for a formulation to be successful, a wide range of functional excipients are included, the choice of which will be determined by the dosage form and delivery method. Despite the traditional view that excipients are inert, no substance is completely free from toxicity. As excipients (chapter 25) tend to make up a substantial portion of a formulation, care must be taken to select excipients that offer as little harm as possible to the patient. Guidelines concerning the use of excipients in paediatric formulations have been published both in the EU and USA and in the International Conference on Harmonisation Guidelines on Pharmaceutical Development.[9] These guidelines confirm that the selection of excipients for paediatric formulations should be done with special care and with consideration of different sensitivities between the different age groups. The inclusion of any excipient in a formulation should be justified by its function, and the excipient should be included at the lowest possible concentration for the desired effect. Ideally, excipients must be of high stability, purity and quality and adhere to Good Manufacturing Practice (GMP). (There are European, US and WHO versions of GMP.) The decision to use a specific excipient should also be underpinned by using as much information from toxicological data, scientific guidelines, food legislation and literature as possible. Information about the compatibility of excipients with the active ingredient, and with other excipients, should be considered. It is also agreed that any new excipient be examined in preclinical and clinical trials to ensure safety.

Relevant legislation

In 1994, the US Food and Drug Administration (FDA) introduced the Pediatric Labelling Rule, which was designed to encourage manufacturers to draw upon existing data to support modification of a drug's licence for paediatric use. (Note: in the USA, the drug 'label' refers to the product's data sheet, equivalent in the UK to the summary of product characteristics (SPC). The term 'off label' therefore indicates that the product is being used outside its licence. A common situation is to use a medicine licensed for adults (only) in children. This is an example of off-label use.) A few years later, the Food and Drug Administration Modernization Act (FDAMA) and the Pediatric Rule were both introduced. The Pediatric Rule was enforced to ensure that new drugs and biological products suitable for paediatrics have appropriate licensing (or labelling), by requiring manufacturers to submit mandatory safety and effectiveness information from suitable paediatric age groups.[10] The FDAMA was introduced to encourage drug studies in certain paediatric therapeutics. This was done by offering the incentive of an extra 6 months of patent exclusivity if the sponsor conducted the studies as stipulated in a written request from the FDA and in a timely manner. Importantly, this did not include generics.[11]

The Best Pharmaceuticals for Children Act (BPCA) (USA) in 2002 addressed this drawback and others, by extending the incentives programme for 5 years, allowing and encouraging off-patent (paediatric) drug studies and requiring public transparency of study results.[12,13]

Regulations for paediatric formulations in Europe are similar to those in the USA, although perhaps more streamlined. In 2007, the European Medicines Agency (EMA) introduced the Paediatric Regulation. The aims were to improve research into medicines for children, increase evidence concerning paediatric medication without delaying adult authorisation, avoid needless risk to children, and make authorised medications more accessible. This regulation requires manufacturers to submit a drug development plan, known as a paediatric investigation plan (PIP) in order for a drug to be considered for approval for use within the paediatric population. A PIP is analogous to a written request in the USA, although there are several differences. PIPs are required earlier in the drug regulatory process than in the USA – upon the availability of pharmacokinetic studies in adults. Manufacturers must provide a study description as well as formulation information, and focus on a range of paediatric population subsets from 0–17 years.

This earlier approach also requires consideration of details such as taste for oral formulations, different formulations for each age group, suitable delivery methods and the acceptability of excipients. In circumstances where children are not the intended target population for a drug, a waiver must be obtained from the EMA Paediatric Medicines Committee (PDCO) to forego a PIP. The Paediatric Regulation also differs from the US system in that both regulation and incentive are combined into a single piece of legislation. These incentives include a 6-month patent extension for new drugs upon PIP approval. There are also incentives to ensure older off-patent drugs are considered for paediatric use.

European manufacturers can also apply for a paediatric use marketing authorisation (PUMA). This incentivises the holder with 10 years of data protection (or 12 years of protection for orphan drugs). Another incentive is also provided by the EMA through free advice for development questions. Similar to the US system, the European system also comprises a committee of experts, similar to the FDA Pediatric Review Committee (PeRC), called the PDCO. The PDCO's remit is to assess PIP submissions. It also has the added authority to make binding decisions.[2,14]

Conclusions

Guidelines and legislation over the past two decades have thus far been successful in starting to narrow the paediatric knowledge gap. In particular, incentives have been a driving force for improving knowledge of the safety and efficacy of children's medicines, and this trend is set to continue. In order to improve effectiveness, however, more must be done to ensure that paediatric studies are made an integral part of a manufacturer's drug development plan, as with adults, instead of a separate consideration. There is now an increased awareness that excipients offer their own risk, and that responses in children will not necessarily mimic those of adults. It is encouraging that organisations are actively working to improve on this; the European Paediatric Formulation Initiative (EuPFI), for example, is developing an online Safety and Toxicity of Excipients for Paediatrics (STEP) database, seeking input from research and industry. The development of different dosage forms suitable for paediatrics is a major focus and will supply a new generation of safer, more flexible medicines that cause fewer problems with patient compliance. A range of different dosage forms is vital, since each drug has different characteristics and limitations which will dictate the formulation. Central to this is the development of novel solid dosage forms that offer advantages over traditional liquid dosage forms.

References

1   Food and Drug Administration. *Guidance for industry. E11 Clinical Investigation of Medicinal Products in the Pediatric Population.* 2000.
2   Drakulich A. *European Requirements for Pediatric Formulations.* 2009.
3   Nunn T, Williams J. Formulation of medicines for children. *Br J Clin Pharmacol* 2005; 59(6): 674–676.
4   Walsh J. Excipients for the formulation of medicines for children. *Eur Ind Pharm* 2012; 13: 14–16.
5   Cram A *et al.* Challenges of developing palatable oral paediatric formulations. *Int J Pharm* 2009; 365(1): 1–3.
6   Thomson SA *et al.* Minitablets: new modality to deliver medicines to preschool-aged children. *Pediatrics* 2009; 123(2): e235–e238.
7   AlHusban FA *et al.* Recent patents and trends in orally disintegrating tablets. *Recent Pat Drug Deliv Formul* 2010; 4(3): 178–197.
8   Stoltenberg I *et al.* Solid oral dosage forms for children – formulations, excipients and acceptance issues. *J Appl Ther Res* 2011; 7: 141–146.

9   International Conference on Harmonisation of Technical Requirements for Registration of Pharmaceuticals for Human Use (ICH). *ICH Harmonised Tripartite Guideline: Pharmaceutical Development Q8.* www.ich.org/products/guidelines/quality/quality-single/article/pharmaceutical-development.html

10   Zisowsky J *et al.* Drug development for pediatric populations: regulatory aspects. *Pharmaceutics* 2010; 2(4): 364–388.

11   Roberts R *et al.* Pediatric drug labeling: Improving the safety and efficacy of pediatric therapies. *JAMA* 2003; 290(7): 905–911.

12   Congress U. Pediatric Research Equity Act of 2003. *Public Law* 2003; 108(155): 117.

13   FDA. Draft Guidance. Pediatric Study Plans: Content of and Process for Submitting Initial Pediatric Study Plans and Amended Initial Pediatric Study Plans Guidance for Industry. 2016. Available at: https://www.fda.gov/downloads/drugs/guidancecomplianceregulatoryinformation/guidances/ucm360507.pdf [last accessed 2 March 2018].

14   Breitkreutz J. European perspectives on pediatric formulations. *Clin Ther* 2008; 30(11): 2146–2154.

24

Extemporaneous preparations of medicines for children

A Al-Khattawi, T Dennison, AR Mohammed and D Terry

Introduction

Adapting licensed medicines for use in children is widespread. This practice results from a lack of licensed medicines that are appropriate for children. Children's ability to take particular dosage forms (tablets, capsules, etc.) depends on their development and/or clinical condition. This variation is not accounted for during drug development for a number of reasons, including ethical, commercial and regulatory problems.[1] Constraints on resources may also mean that licensed medicines are not available. In 2010 the World Health Organization (WHO) drew attention to this issue and stated: 'Children should have access to authorized, ready-to-use, age-appropriate preparations of medicines.' According to the European Medicines Agency (EMA), 'The manipulation of adult medicinal products for paediatric use should be the last resort, but at the same time it is recognised as an unavoidable and necessary operation in many cases.'[2]

People who prescribe medicines for children need to be aware of the adaptations that will be needed to fulfil many of their prescriptions. A prescription that is often fulfilled using a licensed product for adults may result in an unlicensed product for a child. For example, a prescription of omeprazole 20 mg daily for an adult is likely to be dispensed using a licensed product. A similar prescription for a child may result in an unlicensed liquid. It is not the active ingredient that is licensed (in this case omeprazole), but rather the formulation. In this example, omeprazole capsules of 20 mg are licensed, but omeprazole liquid with 5 mg in 5 mL is unlicensed.

An awareness of adaptations to medicines is important, because the adaptation may have unexpected consequences on adherence and the efficacy and safety of the medicine. This chapter outlines the key issues so that prescribers can discuss the options with pharmacists.

The learning objectives of this chapter are:

> ➤ to recognise that medicines sometimes need to be modified or adapted for children
> ➤ to understand what is meant by compounding and extemporaneous preparation
> ➤ to know that such modifications may affect drug bioavailability, pharmacokinetics, stability and safety.

The scope of adaptations to medicines

While there is no consensus on the age at which children should be able to swallow tablets, it is generally accepted that below the age of 6 years young patients are likely to have difficulties in swallowing adult dosage forms (tablets, capsules, etc.). Modifying existing medication is often necessary to maximise the potential for use in children. In practice, this includes splitting or crushing tablets, sprinkling capsule contents over food or adding them to drinks, or giving by the oral route medicines designed (and licensed) to be injected. When these steps are done at the point of care, they are manipulations. When these steps are done in advance of care (e.g. in bulk), they are compounding procedures. If licensed medicines (those that carry a marketing authorisation from the regulator body) are manipulated or compounded in this way, they are used off label, with ethical, legal and clinical implications. Manipulated and compounded preparations may lack the safety profiles of the original (licensed) products, due to invalidated reformulation procedures performed outside the marketing authorisation framework. Efficacy may also be altered (e.g. because of altered bioavailability), but it may not be clear to what extent; see below. Manipulation is usually done at the bedside or in the home, while compounding is done in pharmacies or dedicated facilities. These procedures should be carried out consistently so that the prescriber and family can assess the effects of the medicine.

There are other risks associated with manipulation of dosage forms that may adversely impact on the safety of patients and their carers. Administration of medicines at home may require cutting or crushing of tablets or opening capsules. The lack of parent–carer expertise in the preparation of liquids from solid forms may introduce unacceptable risks, and this activity should be considered by prescribers and pharmacists when choosing the best therapeutic option, or families should be trained.

Unlicensed/off-label use and formulation options

Sometimes information about compounding or manipulation can be found in the summary of product characteristics (SPC). It may be preferable to source a licensed medicine from another country than to formulate an unlicensed preparation, e.g. importing chlorothiazide liquid, which is available in some countries, as opposed to local manufacture from the licensed tablets. However, significant difficulties arise when substituting products in this way, particularly when the product information (both for the healthcare professionals and the patient) is in a foreign language.

One form of compounding involves a process undertaken by an individual pharmacist who creates a medicine from an active drug substance and excipients or from an authorised dosage form and excipients. This is commonly known as extemporaneous compounding. One way to do this is to use suitable suspending agents, or standardised vehicles, that may help to improve uniformity and palatability. In UK practice, about 90% of extemporaneous preparations are made using relatively expensive diluents such as Ora-Plus or Ora-Sweet rather than simpler readily available excipients such as methyl cellulose. The use of multifunctional novel ingredients such as cyclodextrins in oral liquid preparations may be preferable, due to their superior taste masking and solubility enhancing properties (although note that cyclodextrins may also have safety issues such as renal toxicity in some animals). However, the high price of these ingredients limits their application in paediatric formulations, and there are safety concerns relating to the kidneys.[3]

In liquids prepared as adaptations of other dosage forms, the active ingredient may not be as uniformly distributed as in licensed medicines and quality control tests are unlikely to have been carried out to verify their homogeneity, stability and pharmacokinetic properties.

Other alternatives to liquid medicines include: oral-dispersible dosage forms, such as orally disintegrating tablets (ODTs); effervescent tablets; and thin films that disperse into a liquid when placed in the mouth. Some of these dosage forms may be prepared from commercially available ready-to-use powder blends. They offer better stability and dosing accuracy over liquids, and are promoted by the WHO for paediatric use.

In the UK, authorised manufacturers can prepare a variety of liquid formulations by special order. These products are often referred to as 'specials'. But these formulations may be expensive due to market demand and only rudimentary price control. It is not unusual for unlicensed liquid medicines to be 10–20 times more expensive than solid dosage forms (tablets and capsules).

Not all facilities will be compliant with national standards, e.g. Good Manufacturing Practice (GMP), and hence prescribers and pharmacists must accept greater responsibility for these (now) unlicensed products.

Issues and risks related to extemporaneous preparations

It is important that prescribers understand the risks associated with paediatric extemporaneous compounding. Potential hazards include dosing inaccuracy or errors, modified bioavailability and excipient toxicities.

Unknown bioavailability and pharmacokinetics

Unlike licensed medicines, extemporaneous preparations do not undergo clinical testing to verify their bioavailability. Product efficacy may be altered, and some preparations may not be clinically effective.[4]

In some cases, the safety of these medicines for children is compromised due to 'dose dumping', which may have clinical consequences. Dose dumping occurs when the bioavailability of a manipulated preparation is higher than that expected from the adult dosage form.

When preparing an extemporaneous liquid, the bioavailability cannot be predicted on a milligram-to-milligram basis and complicates dose estimates based on body surface area/weight of the child. This may be due to:

- *Different routes of administration:* e.g. intravenous injection of preparation administered as an oral liquid, which could have lesser absorption or undergo degradation in the gut. Alternatively, pregastric absorption may result in an abrupt increase in plasma concentration.
- *Different release profiles:* e.g. crushing/splitting of enteric-coated or sustained release matrix tablets may result in altered drug absorption profiles, which can lead to underdosing or overdosing respectively. Dispersion of omeprazole multi-unit pellet system (MUPS) tablets into a liquid prior to administration to children was found to result in the formation of 'poppy-seed' like particles in their stomach, due to degradation of the proton pump inhibitor in an acidic pH.[5]

Furthermore, splitting of tablets gives inconsistent dosing, even when commercial splitters are used, due to non-uniform distribution of the contents in tablet segments. One study revealed that less than 50% or more than 150% of the expected dose was administered after splitting tablets.[6]

Clinical pharmacological issues caused by inconsistent pharmacokinetics not only impact on the efficacy of medicines, but also increase the risk of toxicity.

Safety of extemporaneous preparations and excipient related toxicity

As described above, extemporaneous preparation is one of the highest risk activities in paediatric pharmacy practice and is often supported by poor quality evidence.[7,8] In addition, the subjective nature of extemporaneous preparation may result in medication errors. These may include incorrect (or even unfamiliar) strengths of the active drug or other ingredients and, more seriously, the use of toxic or sensitising excipients.[9] A mistake in an extemporaneous preparation of 'peppermint water' for colic in 1998 resulted in the death of a 4-day-old baby. The pharmacy used concentrated chloroform water (which requires dilution prior to use) instead of the intended double-strength chloroform water.[10]

Stability of extemporaneous preparations

Stability is a significant factor that determines the efficacy of extemporaneous liquid preparations.[11] Stability problems can be attributed to chemical, physical or microbiological causes, and are influenced by the physicochemical properties of the active ingredient, the type of excipients used and the storage conditions. The following factors need consideration when developing liquid preparations.

pH of the preparation

Stability of preparations depends on the pH of the medium and the dissociation constant of the active ingredient. Suitable buffering systems should be used to maintain the pH of the preparation. The addition of other excipients, such as suspending agents, preservatives and flavours, may alter the pH and in turn the stability profile. Careful assessment of the stability of the drug in the final formulation should be undertaken before dispensing. Extra care should be taken to manage the pH of formulations made from lyophilised injectables. Young infants have different gastric pH to older children and adults, and this should be taken into consideration when formulating medicines for this age group.

Solubility profile

Soluble drugs show better physical stability, as they have a lower tendency for sedimentation and caking; however, they are more susceptible to oxidation and chemical degradation.

Volume

In general, volumes of liquid medicines for young children should be small enough not to affect nutrition requirements. However, small volumes may introduce solubility issues, and so a balance must be struck between these competing needs.

Storage conditions

Extemporaneous preparations should be prepared and used freshly or within a predetermined shelf life. The expiry date is often determined empirically due to the lack of stability studies that determine its length. Some reports suggest that extemporaneously prepared medicines should not be stored for more than 2 weeks, although no published evidence currently supports that opinion. The longer an extemporaneous preparation is left on the shelf, the more it is prone to microbiological contamination. However, the use of preservatives should be avoided in children's formulations. When a preservative is used, the concentration should be the lowest feasible concentration according to the EMA.[12] Formulations that are prepared extemporaneously based on published data from literature may not result in an equivalent shelf life. This is due to inter-laboratory variability and the difficulty of reproducing studies carried out elsewhere under different conditions and using different suppliers of materials.

Compatibility of drug and ingredients

The active drug is a chemical molecule that may interact with other molecules if the conditions are suitable. Stability of the drug in food, drinks or milk (including breast milk) should ideally be evaluated to avoid administering ineffective or degraded medicine. Ideally these studies could be carried out in formulation laboratories, due to the availability of quality control facilities and *in vitro* tools for testing compatibility. Excipient interactions with the drug are also important, especially in liquid preparations. Tests should also consider how the drug will be administered to the patient. Children may not be able to swallow the drug with a large amount of water as may be assumed for an adult.

As highlighted by the EMA, it would be helpful to make available to pharmacists short term stability data and stability-indicating methods suitable for testing of extemporaneous preparations.[13]

Outlook

The development of licensed paediatric formulations is the best solution to avoid the disadvantages of extemporaneous preparations. Since 2007, pharmaceutical manufacturers in Europe have been able to apply for a paediatric investigation plan to introduce a new formulation for children. For certain medicines it is unlikely that there will be child appropriate licensed products, because the market is too limited. Therefore it continues to be necessary to prepare medicines extemporaneously in some cases. However, multiple stakeholders are involved in collaborative projects to produce more licensed products for children, and this is supported by research activities concerning paediatric formulation in the UK and across Europe.

Conclusions

Where clinically appropriate, use licensed medicines according to their licensed (labelled) indication and dosing recommendations. Discuss complex prescriptions with a pharmacist and/or specialist nurse, if available. As a first resource, the *British National Formulary for Children* (BNFC) provides information on unlicensed use of medicines and gives guidance on special orders and extemporaneous preparation.

References

1   Standing JF, Tuleu C. Paediatric formulations – getting to the heart of the problem. *Int J Pharm* 2005; 300(1–2): 56–66.

2 European Medicines Agency. *5-year Report to the European Commission: General Report on the Experience Acquired as a Result of the Application of the Paediatric Regulation.* 2012. EMA/428172/2012.

3 Shabir A, Mohamed AR. Exploring the use of cyclodextrins as carriers in paediatric formulations. *Br J Clin Pharm.* 2010; 2: 275–278.

4 Nahata MC, Allen LV, Jr. Extemporaneous drug formulations. *Clin Ther* 2008; 30(11): 2112–2119.

5 Tuleu C *et al.* 'Poppy seeds' in stomach aspirates: is oral omeprazole extemporaneous dispersion bioavailable? *Eur J Pediatr* 2008; 167(7): 823–825.

6 Cook TJ *et al.* Variability in tablet fragment weights when splitting unscored cyclobenzaprine 10 mg tablets. *J Am Pharm Assoc (2003)* 2004; 44(5): 583–586.

7 Pifferi G, Restani P. The safety of pharmaceutical excipients. *Farmaco* 2003; 58(8): 541–550.

8 Jackson M, Lowey A. *Handbook of Extemporaneous Preparation: A guide to pharmaceutical compounding.* London: Pharmaceutical Press, 2010.

9 Choonara I. WHO wants safer medicines for children. *Arch Dis Child* 2008; 93(6): 456–467.

10 Anon. Baby dies after peppermint water prescribed for colic. *Pharm J* 1998; 260: 768.

11 Brion F *et al.* Extemporaneous (magistral) preparation of oral medicines for children in European hospitals. *Acta Paediatr* 2003; 92(4): 486–490.

12 European Medicines Agency. Committee for Medicinal Products for Human Use (CHMP). *Reflection Paper on the Use of Methyl and Propylparaben as Excipients in Human Medicinal Products for Oral Use.* 2012. EMA/CHMP/SWP/272921/2012.

13 European Medicines Agency. Committee for Medicinal Products for Human Use (CHMP). *Reflection Paper: Formulations Of Choice For The Paediatric Population.* 2006. EMEA/CHMP/PEG/196810/2005.

Further recommended reading

Briggs H. Third baby in feed probe dies. 2014. www.bbc.co.uk/news/health-28113157

FDA. This Week in FDA History - Nov. 16, 1937. 2006. www.fda.gov/aboutfda/whatwedo/history/thisweek/ucm117880.htm

Lajoinie A *et al.* Solid oral forms availability in children – a cost-saving investigation. *Br J Clin Pharmacol* 2014; 78(5): 1080–1089.

MHRA. *MHRA/Department of Health Strategy on Medicines for Children.* London: MHRA, 2004.

Rocchi F *et al.* Prospective surveillance of extemporaneous dispensing of medicines for children. *Paediatr Perinat Drug Ther* 2001; 4(4): 152–155.

WHO Expert Committee on Specifications for Pharmaceutical Preparations. *WHO Technical Report Series No. 970,* 46th report. Geneva: WHO Press, 2012.

WHO. Working Document QAS/11.399/Rev. 1. *Provision by Health-care Professionals of Patient-Specific Preparations for Children that are not available as Authorized Products – Points to Consider.* Geneva: WHO Press, 2010.

25

Excipients in medicines for children

G Nellis, J Lass and I Lutsar

Introduction

Pharmaceutical products contain pharmacologically active ingredients and a range of other chemicals known as excipients. Excipients are used to improve the quality, stability, bioavailability and patient acceptability of medicines. They function as diluents, fillers, solvents, emulsifiers, binders, lubricants, glidants, sweeteners, preservatives and flavouring or colouring agents and make up, on average, about 90% of each product.[1] Therefore, administration of medicines entails an exposure to pharmaceutical excipients.

Under ideal conditions, excipients should bring little or no therapeutic value to the product and engender no pharmacological activity. However, not all excipients are inert substances; excipients have specific pharmacokinetic properties, as active ingredients do.

Paediatric medicines present particular complexity due to the diverse patient population, compliance challenges and safety considerations. When excipients are necessary, it is important to have a clear rationale for this so that drug development is expedited and clinicians know what they are working with, including any related risks.[2]

The learning objectives of this chapter are:

> to understand the role of excipients in paediatric medicines and their benefits
> to recognise the safety issues associated with excipients
> to be aware that polypharmacy increases excipient exposure.

Benefits of excipients

It is clear that the benefits of medicines would not be possible in the absence of excipients in many cases. Excipients: (1) aid processing of the system during manufacture; (2) protect, support or enhance stability, bioavailability or acceptability of a medicine to patients; (3) assist in product identification; and (4) enhance any other attribute of the overall safety and effectiveness of the drug delivery system during storage and use.

Children versus adults

Similar to the effect for active ingredients, biopharmaceutical differences between children and adults can affect administration, distribution, metabolism and elimination (ADME) of excipients. Pharmacokinetics and pharmacodynamics (PK/PD) in the paediatric population can also be affected by underlying medical conditions.[3]

Nowadays it is generally accepted that in paediatric pharmacology:

- Drugs should have acceptable palatability.
- Drugs should be easily swallowed (e.g. syrups and suspensions instead of solid forms).
- Drugs should be soluble in small volumes.
- Parenteral preparations should contain small dose volumes and be administered via small needles or cannulae.

All these are related to appropriate choices of excipients.

Excipients used for adults may behave differently in children, especially in the youngest groups, due to the physiologically immature functions of most organs, differences in body composition and activity of metabolising enzymes. The degree of immaturity may be aggravated due to prematurity or intrauterine growth retardation in neonates or any potential pathological condition affecting the child. Similar to active ingredient absorption, excipient absorption can be influenced by gastric pH variability and gastrointestinal transit time in childhood, with the greatest changes occurring during the neonatal period.[4] Further, children may not be able to metabolise or eliminate an ingredient in the same manner as adults, due to the altered PK/PD. Therefore, careful screening and selection of excipients is critical in the development of paediatric formulations, as certain excipients acceptable for adult medicines may not be appropriate for paediatric use.

The safety of excipients in children

Safety is one of the most important requirements of the pharmaceutical compound, including its excipients. Based on the safety profile, excipients can be classified as potentially safe (e.g. water, hydrochloric acid, starch) or potentially harmful or known to be harmful (Table 1), and as excipients with no safety data available (e.g. sodium carmellose) or with non-specific description (e.g. flavourings, colourants).[5]

Excipient	Reported adverse effects	
	Newborns (<28 days old)	Children >28 days old
Propylparaben	Hyperbilirubinaemia, hypersensitivity reactions, oestrogenic effects[10,11]	Allergic reactions, bronchospasm[10]
Polysorbate 80	E-Ferol syndrome – thrombocytopenia, renal dysfunction, hepatomegaly, cholestasis, ascites, hypotension, metabolic acidosis[11]	Hypersensitivity following topical and intramuscular use[11]
Propylene glycol	Skin irritation, central nervous system depression, cardiovascular, hepatic, respiratory adverse events, hyperosmolality; lactic acidosis[3,10,11]	Large volumes associated with adverse effects most commonly on the central nervous system[11]
Benzoates (benzyl alcohol, benzoic acid and sodium benzoate)	Hypersensitivity, kernicterus in benzoic acid and sodium benzoate; metabolic acidosis, seizures, gasping, fatal toxic syndrome in premature infants, kernicterus, intraventricular haemorrhage, death in benzyl alcohol[3,10,11]	Skin and eye irritation; benzyl alcohol may cause toxic and allergic reactions in children up to 3 years old[10]
Saccharin sodium	Urticaria, photosensitivity reactions	Generally regarded as safe; skin hypersensitivity[11]
Sorbitol	Diarrhoea, nutrient malabsorption	Mild laxative effect[10]
Ethanol	Lactic acidosis; hypoglycaemia; central nervous system effects[3,11]	Harmful for those with liver disease or epilepsy; skin irritation; may alter the effects of other medicines; hypoglycaemia; central nervous system effects[8,10]
Benzalkonium chloride	Ototoxic when applied to ear, skin irritation and hypersensitivity, eye irritation[3,10,11]	Skin and eye irritation, bronchospasm[10]

Table 1 Reported adverse effects of some commonly used excipients in neonates and older children

Children are routinely given medicines with no specific paediatric information because of the lack of clinical trials in this population. Much less attention has been devoted to the safety of excipients. While the need for excipients is indisputable, some of them are known to be toxic, and uncertainty about others, especially in specific age groups, exists.[2] Due to the differences in ADME, intake of a certain excipient in children may result in higher than intended circulating concentrations, which may cause adverse effects not seen in other age groups.[6]

Excipients have been associated with specific toxicity issues such as allergic reactions, intolerance, interference with absorption of the active ingredient and interactions with the active ingredient.[3] For example, ethanol is commonly used as a solvent and preservative in paediatric liquid formulations (e.g. some iron and furosemide formulations) and is frequently found in over-the-counter medicines.[7] Newborns, infants and children are not able to metabolise ethanol as efficiently as adults can, and are thus at higher risk of acute and chronic alcohol related toxicities.[8] Benzyl alcohol, used as a preservative in parenteral medicines, is metabolised to benzoic acid, which is conjugated to an excretable compound. Preterm neonates and children up to 3 years old are unable to conjugate benzoic acid efficiently due to an immature metabolic capability, and thus accumulation of benzyl alcohol may occur.[9]

There are elevated toxicological risks in children and particularly in neonates from various excipients (Table 1).

The use of sweeteners and flavouring agents is particularly important in paediatrics in order to improve palatability.[3] The use of carbohydrates with potential to raise plasma glucose, such as fructose, glucose or sucrose, should be limited or avoided in diabetic children. A number of allergic reactions have been associated with flavouring agents, the problem being the lack of data on exact composition of these complex mixtures.[12]

Selection of excipients

The selection and use of excipients in paediatric formulations should be justified. Consider the following factors:

- The functionality and safety/ toxicity profile across the proposed population
  - Efficiency of excipient
  - Metabolism and elimination pathways of the excipient
  - Toxicity in the specific age group
- Therapeutic indication and criticality of the condition to be treated
- Dosage regimen, i.e. exposure
  - Acceptable daily intake (acute toxicity)
  - The frequency of dosing
  - The duration of treatment (chronic toxicity)
  - Polypharmacotherapy (additive toxicity)
- Route of administration

Extent of exposure to excipients

It is generally accepted that oral medicine administration should be used when possible and appropriate in children. However, oral medicines often contain more excipients than parenteral formulations. Liquid preparations in particular are the most common source of excipients in children. Svirskis et al. identified 47 paediatric liquid medicines in New Zealand containing ethanol, with concentrations that ranged from 0.6% v/v to 76% v/v. The medicines were indicated for both acute and chronic use in patients of all ages, including preterm neonates.[7]

There are limited data available about the extent to which children are exposed to excipients. A few recent observational studies suggest that neonates are exposed to significant amounts of excipients, including potentially harmful amounts, with the doses occasionally exceeding internationally recommended limits of exposure.[5,13] Neonates in neonatal intensive care units may be exposed to over 20 different excipients per day during hospitalisation.[13] Lass et al. described the use of 123 different excipients in Estonian neonatal units, with 88% of neonates receiving at least one of the eight excipients known to be harmful to neonates.[5] Similar numbers were shown in a Brazilian neonatal unit: 86 different excipients with 87% of neonates exposed to harmful ones. Nellis et al. described the administration of potentially harmful excipients to 63% of neonates in a point prevalence study including 89 neonatal units from 21 European countries.[14] The exposure to excipients differed geographically, with some excipients administrated more frequently in one European region compared with others.

Polypharmacotherapy

Polypharmacy may lead to multiple sources of excipients; for some of them exposure will be additive. Cumulative exposure is one of several factors that determine whether a given excipient is likely to have toxic effects. Shchab et al. observed a wide range in the cumulative dose of benzyl alcohol and propylene glycol received by neonates, with potentially toxic doses registered during routine medication administration. However, acceptable daily and cumulative intake of excipients is not yet clearly defined for different paediatric age groups.

Avoiding toxic excipients

Excipients are necessary components of many formulations and thus cannot be totally avoided. If some excipients cause harm, or are likely to cause harm, it may be necessary to develop age specific formulations that avoid using them. Many excipients can be avoided with changes in manufacturing processes without altering the pharmaceutical quality of the medicine.[2] On the other hand, this has direct costs for reformulation and regulatory procedures, as well as opportunity costs; if existing medicines have to be reformulated, this may prevent other new medicines from being studied.

Substitution possibilities

Another way to reduce the exposure to unwanted excipients is to use medicines available on the market that do not contain harmful excipients. To facilitate this, alternative medicines with an identical active ingredient, route of administration and dosage form should be identified. For example, regional variations in neonatal administration of harmful excipients suggest it would be possible to reduce exposure to parabens, polysorbate 80, propylene glycol and saccharin sodium through product substitution.[14] Here, knowledge of at least the qualitative composition of any excipients included within a formulation is essential – quantitative data would save time and resources by aiding selection of only those products where replacement is really necessary.

Qualitative versus quantitative data

It is accepted that excipients may only show an effect above a certain 'dose'.[10] However, usually only qualitative data are presented in the summary of product characteristics (SmPC), and collecting information on the amount of excipients in drug formulations remains a challenge.

Adding quantitative information in the related section of the SmPCs may help health professionals to provide relevant advice. For example, Allegaert *et al.* showed that propylene glycol administration with median of 34 mg/kg/day (World Health Organization recommended limit for adults is 25 mg/kg/day) for a maximum of 48 h seems to be well tolerated in neonates and does not affect short term postnatal adaptations.[15] Thus having the quantitative data for excipients may spare time and resources, as many medicines with appropriate excipient concentrations can be safely used without any need for substitution or reformulation.

Conclusions

Pharmaceutical excipients are intended to improve the quality of medicines and patient acceptability. Although excipients should be pharmacologically inactive, they may indeed cause adverse effects. Children, including neonates, are exposed to excipients through many commonly used medicines.

Some excipients may not be safe for children. The different physiology and PK/PD of children compared with adults, as well as variations between different age groups, should be considered. Therefore, marketing authorisation applicants and holders should ensure that excipients are used appropriately; inclusion of excipients into the paediatric dosage forms should be appropriately justified, with minimisation of the number and quantity of excipients to be used. When excipients cannot be avoided, physicians, pharmacists and patients should be aware of their quantitative composition in the medicine and possible excipient related safety issues.

The gold manufacturing standard should be providing an age appropriate formulation ensuring that any excipients in the formulation do not pose unacceptable risks to the recipients of the medicine. Manufacturing 'one size fits all' formulations is suboptimal and is not an acceptable approach for the paediatric population.

References

1 Haywood A, Glass BD. Pharmaceutical excipients – where do we begin? *Aust Prescr* 2011; 34(4): 112–114.
2 Turner MA *et al*. Risk assessment of neonatal excipient exposure: lessons from food safety and other areas. *Adv Drug Deliv Rev* 2014; 73C: 89–101.
3 Fabiano V *et al*. Paediatric pharmacology: remember the excipients. *Pharmacol Res* 2011; 63(5): 362–365.
4 Batchelor HK *et al*. Paediatric oral biopharmaceutics: key considerations and current challenges. *Adv Drug Deliv Rev* 2014; 73: 102–126.
5 Lass J *et al*. Hospitalised neonates in Estonia commonly receive potentially harmful excipients. *BMC Pediatr* 2012; 12: 136.
6 De Cock RFW *et al*. Developmental pharmacokinetics of propylene glycol in preterm and term neonates. *Br J Clin Pharmacol* 2013; 75(1): 162–171.
7 Svirskis D *et al*. The use of ethanol in paediatric formulations in New Zealand. *Eur J Pediatr* 2013; 172(7): 919–926.
8 Zuccotti GV, Fabiano V. Safety issues with ethanol as an excipient in drugs intended for pediatric use. *Expert Opin Drug Saf* 2011; 10(4): 499–502.
9 LeBel M *et al*. Benzyl alcohol metabolism and elimination in neonates. *Dev Pharmacol Ther* 1988; 11(6): 347–356.
10 European Commission. Excipients in the label and package leaflet of medicinal products for human use. 2003; 3B(July). www.ema.europa.eu/docs/en_GB/document_library/Scientific_guideline/2009/09/WC500003412.pdf
11 Rowe CR *et al*. *Handbook of Pharmaceutical Excipients*. 7th edn. Pharmaceutical Press and American Pharmacists Association; 2012.
12 Walsh J *et al*. Playing hide and seek with poorly tasting pacdiatric medicines: do not forget the excipients. *Adv Drug Deliv Rev* 2014; 73: 14–33.
13 Whittaker A *et al*. Toxic additives in medication for preterm infants. *Arch Dis Child Fetal Neonatal Ed* 2009; 94(4): 236–240.
14 Nellis G *et al*. Potentially harmful excipients in neonatal medicines: a pan-European observational study. *Arch Dis Child* 2015; 100(7): 694–699.
15 Allegaert K *et al*. Prospective assessment of short-term propylene glycol tolerance in neonates. *Arch Dis Child* 2010; 95(12): 1054–1058.

Further recommended reading

Duro D *et al*. Association Between Infantile Colic and Carbohydrate Malabsorption From Fruit Juices in Infancy. *Pediatrics* 2002; 109(5): 797–805.
European Medicines Agency. *Guideline on Pharmaceutical Development of Medicines for Paediatric Use*, 2013. www.ema.europa.eu/docs/en_GB/document_library/Scientific_guideline/2013/07/WC500147002.pdf
European Medicines Agency. *Questions and Answers on Benzyl Alcohol in the Context of the Revision of the Guideline on 'Excipients in the label and package leaflet of medicinal products for human use' (CPMP/463/00)*, 2014. www.ema.europa.eu/docs/en_GB/document_library/Scientific_guideline/2014/02/WC500162032.pdf

European Medicines Agency. *Questions and Answers on Ethanol in the Context of the Revision of the Guideline on 'Excipients in the label and package leaflet of medicinal products for human use' (CPMP/463/00)*, Draft 2014. www.ema.europa.eu/docs/en_GB/document_library/Scientific_guideline/2014/02/WC500162033.pdf

Hiller JL *et al*. Benzyl alcohol toxicity: impact on mortality and intraventricular hemorrhage among very low birth weight infants. *Pediatrics* 1986; 77: 500–506.

Kaye JL. Review of paediatric gastrointestinal physiology data relevant to oral drug delivery. *Int J Clin Pharm* 2011; 33(1): 20–24.

Miszkiel K *et al*. The contribution of histamine release to bronchoconstriction provoked by inhaled benzalkonium chloride in asthma. *Br J Clin Pharmacol* 1988; 25(2): 157–163.

Pifferi G, Restani P. The safety of pharmaceutical excipients. *Farm* 2003; 58(8): 541–550.

Sam T *et al*. A benefit/risk approach towards selecting appropriate pharmaceutical dosage forms - An application for paediatric dosage form selection. *Int J Pharm* 2012; 435(2): 115–123.

Shehab N *et al*. Exposure to the pharmaceutical excipients benzyl alcohol and propylene glycol among critically ill neonates. *Pediatr Crit care Med* 2009; 10(2): 256–259.

Ursino MG *et al*. Excipients in medicinal products used in gastroenterology as a possible cause of side effects. *Regul Toxicol Pharmacol* 2011; 60(1): 93–105.

Warner A. Drug use in the neonate: interrelationships of pharmacokinetics, toxicity, and biochemical maturity. *Clin Chem* 1986; 32(5): 721–727.

26

The role of parents and children in paediatric medicines research

J Preston, C Prichard, H Bagley, S Stones and R Challinor

If you were a business developing a new soft drink, would you bring the product to market without consulting your target audience?

Should it be any different when developing and delivering neonatal and paediatric medicines studies and trials?

Introduction

It is commonplace for researchers to believe that by introducing patient and family involvement to their project, by which we mean research activities undertaken 'with' rather than 'to', 'about' or 'for' them, the timeline for research will extend rather than shorten, and the process of involvement will be time-consuming to coordinate.[1] This viewpoint has resulted in many trials and studies making a token gesture of inclusivity, e.g. patient representatives merely being invited to comment on a patient information leaflet. However, as a minimum, patient and family involvement can and should, like consumer involvement in generic market research, be invoked right at the very beginning at the prioritisation stage (identifying questions and outcomes) and ideally throughout the entire research process. Patient and family involvement is essential when investigating the likelihood of compliance and acceptability, e.g. when designing a sample collection method, hospital attendance regime or post-evaluation follow-up. The added insights from patients and their families prior to the project funding application may not only strengthen the application but can help to prevent unjustified investment in commencing a trial that might fail to recruit sufficient participants or might lose too many participants before each of the trial components has completed.

In this chapter, we would like to draw attention to the value of patient and family involvement to research design and delivery. The chapter will highlight how parents and young people within the UK's National Institute for Health Research (NIHR) Clinical Research Network (CRN) Children's theme have contributed to and impacted upon the design and delivery of research studies in children since it was established in 2005. To put this into context, the NIHR CRN: Children (originally known as the Medicines for Children Research Network, MCRN) provides researchers with the practical support they need to make paediatric studies happen in the National Health Service (NHS), so that more research takes place across the country and more participants can take part. The rationale of the network is that high quality research, growth and retention rates, and improved outcomes for children and young people depend on listening to the voices of families, carers, and children and young people themselves. This is done by listening to their experiences, priorities and perspectives. The network has been at the forefront of patient and public involvement (PPI) for some time, and has achieved this through the delivery of a PPI strategy.

The network involves parents and young people in a variety of ways. Primarily, this is via a national young person's advisory group set up in 2006, and via parent and patient representatives on the network's 14 clinical studies groups (CSGs), whose membership also includes active researchers (clinical and other professions), nurses, charity representatives and formulations experts. The remit of the CSGs is to help direct and develop the future research portfolio within each of the network's specialties.[2]

The learning objectives of this chapter are:

> to understand what patient and public involvement entails in paediatric research
> to recognise the benefits of PPI to patients, researchers and science
> to appreciate the importance of public engagement within clinical research activities.

Where does involvement happen and how does it benefit research?

Families and young people can become involved in research right from the early stages of study development through to the dissemination of study results. Within the NIHR CRN: Children, there are many examples of the different ways in which parents and young people have become involved in particular activities and the benefits of this involvement.[3,4] In the following section, we will highlight a series of questions to consider when designing research, followed by examples of how parents and young people have contributed to addressing each question.

Are you asking the right research question?

At the stage of identifying your research idea and study objectives, have you considered asking parents and young people with that particular condition whether your question is the right one to ask? One of the roles of parent and patient representatives on the CSGs is to contribute to priority setting, in partnership with researchers. All 14 CSGs have been working with the NIHR Evaluation, Trials and Studies Coordinating Centre (NETSCC) to identify research priorities to feed into the NETSCC funding programmes. Over 30 research questions, prioritised following consultation with the broader specialist clinical communities and parents, have been submitted to NETSCC, and more will be developed in this ongoing relationship with the funding body.

Additionally, some parent and patient members of CSGs have undertaken their own priority setting activities. For example, the parents and young person representative members of the Rheumatology CSG have been working over many years with fellow parent/patient representatives in proactively identifying patient-parent-driven research priorities and key concerns that feed into the research strategy of the CSG. An initial survey conducted by Douglas et al.[5] identified the top concerns of parents across the UK of children with rheumatological conditions. Building upon this activity, Douglas et al.'s current survey, identifying top concerns in children with rheumatological conditions, has been disseminated to children and young people aged 8 to 24 across the UK, through collaborative partnerships with charities and rheumatology centres across the country. This is an excellent example of how consumer-led research can be recognised as a quality contribution to current evidence and best practice. The survey has revealed key themes, which have been grouped and will soon be published in a PPI journal for wider dissemination. The themes identified will formulate research questions for future research in the paediatric rheumatology field.

Are you measuring the right outcomes?

Asking young people and parents about which outcomes are important to them will help to ensure your study is successful, as it will meet the needs of patients. An example of patient involvement in commenting on outcomes is a study that was looking at the development of a new formulation of metformin for the treatment of polycystic ovary syndrome (PCOS) in young people. METFIZZ was a project focusing on the development of a soluble, effervescent formulation of metformin for the treatment of PCOS in adolescent girls. METFIZZ received funding from the Seventh Framework Programme of the European Union and was coordinated by EffRx Pharmaceuticals SA, a speciality pharmaceutical company.

The METFIZZ patient and public involvement/engagement workstream team, led by the University of Liverpool/Alder Hey Children's NHS Foundation Trust, UK, approached young people to get their views on important outcomes to be used in this study. This was the first time young girls with this condition were asked their views of what it was like living with PCOS and how it impacted upon their lives. Importantly, they identified an additional outcome, that of pain, which had not originally been included in the trial. This outcome has since been included. A member of the PCOS Young Person's Group highlighted what this meant for her:

'*To be able to work alongside industry professionals and be taken seriously is really motivating. Having lived with this condition for several years, it is great to see that industry is open to involving young people in their research to develop a more patient friendly end product.*'

Another example that demonstrates the importance of patients and families in identifying outcome measures is a study that was looking at the quality of life of children and young people with increased tone (neuromuscular tone associated with cerebral palsy). The proposed randomised controlled trial was investigating oral medication for children with cerebral palsy. A group of affected young people and their parents discussed how they often differed in opinion to doctors when prioritising outcomes. For example, clinicians seemed to be more focused on primary clinical outcomes (e.g. the measure of tone); however, parents and carers were more concerned with 'secondary' outcomes relating to young people's experiences and quality of life (e.g. pain and participation). The study team reported that involving this group had improved the value of the research, because it identified and addressed the outcomes that mattered most to patients themselves, including factors that hadn't initially been considered important by the researchers.

Do your research tools and instruments make sense?

Gaining the views of patients and families about the appropriateness and effectiveness of research instruments and tools (such as patient information leaflets, consent and assent forms, questionnaires and interview schedules) is invaluable, as it enhances the acceptability of the study to the target group through improvements in design and child/family appropriate terminology. Young people and parents within the network have reviewed a significant number (approximately 200) of patient information leaflets for both publicly funded and industry funded studies. As a result, the young person's advisory group developed its own guidance for researchers on how to develop patient information for young people (www.hradecisiontools.org.uk/consent/examples.html). This guidance included advice on the content and format of patient information sheets, and the importance of gaining the views of patients and families when designing patient information sheets.

How participant friendly is your study?

Obtaining patient and family insights into the practical elements of a study, such as the amount and frequency of blood samples, and the length and frequency of hospital visits, will ensure a more participant friendly protocol, resulting in higher recruitment and retention to your study.

One particular example is when members of the young person's group were consulted as a means of informing a planned study to compare new and existing treatments for children who have low levels of vitamin D. The young people commented that if they were feeling well, they might forget to take the daily dose of the vitamin. They suggested ways that children could be reminded to take the medication if it was to be taken daily, such as via text reminders, sticker charts or rewards. The young people also raised that compliance with the two extra blood tests might be a challenge for some young people, but that this was not necessarily impossible to overcome. In particular, they said careful consideration should be made with regards to the timing and location of the blood tests to help ensure accessibility. The group suggested offering blood tests at home or at convenient locations such as walk-in surgeries instead. The study team reviewed its protocol to incorporate the views of young people, specifically regarding the collection of additional blood samples and the inclusion of age appropriate tools (e.g. sticker charts or text reminders) to aid medication compliance. Revised protocols also included costs to allow for home visits for blood sampling, to minimise the impact on participants, in response to comments made by the children, young people and their parents or carers.

In another study, young people were responsible for a major change in how a saliva sample would be collected from children, as highlighted by a study coordinator:

'*As a result of the young person's comments, we changed the information sheets accordingly; for example we changed the font size, reduced the writing and inserted more relevant pictures. We also made a few changes to the study procedures, for example how it made us reduce the number of saliva samples and have a look at other methods for collecting the samples. Partly because of the children's concerns, we changed the methodology to use a very small swab on a stick instead of chewing on cotton wool – children got on very well with these and they are about to be used at another site routinely for this procedure.*'

How best can you inform people about your research?

There are many ways to inform people about your research, but until fairly recently this was predominantly achieved via dedicated study websites, which in most cases where not very patient friendly or accessible. Patients, parents and carers are now frequently using social media platforms to network with other individuals living with their condition as well as to find out information about their condition, treatments and current research. Mobile applications developed for children and young people with long term conditions are also on the rise and will become a common tool to highlight research opportunities in the future.

How can you get people talking about research?

It is important that those working in health research create a dialogue with patients and the public to inform them of what research means and what it means to them, and to help researchers understand what research means to the public. There are many examples of how the NIHR CRN has achieved this in collaboration with patients and families. One particular initiative is called the Patient Research Ambassador Initiative (see www.nihr.ac.uk/patients-and-public/how-to-join-in/patient-research-ambassadors), and has been set up to ensure that people using local NHS care have the best opportunities and choices about taking part in research studies. Patient research ambassadors are patients, carers and lay people who promote health research from a patient point of view. Their roles vary from raising awareness of research via events and health awareness days to being an independent advisor and resource for patients thinking about taking part in research.

Another example is via the development of a website entitled GenerationR (R for Research; http://generationr.org.uk), whose target audience is predominantly young people and parents, with the purpose of improving understanding of the reasons for doing fair tests of treatments, what fair tests look like, and how everyone has some role to play in promoting better research for better healthcare. Members of the young person's group have been integral in developing this and have editorial responsibility for blogs and news stories.

How best can you disseminate your research findings?

All health researchers in the UK are encouraged to disseminate the findings of their research to participants who took part in the study. Previously, most research findings were reported in academic high impact journals, out of reach to the majority of patients and families who took part in the research. Researchers are now encouraged to produce summary information of the key findings of their research for patients. Young people and families can help with this process if researchers invite them to be involved in the analysis or interpretation of the findings, and they can also then help the research team to adapt study reports into child- and parent-friendly information.

Conclusions

To conclude, this chapter has highlighted some key questions to consider when you embark on a research study, and the importance and value of involving patients and families in this process. As consumers of publicly funded (e.g. government, funding councils, charity) and/or industry generated and sponsored medical research, parents, children and young people with experience of health conditions are already 'experts' on their most distressing symptoms, medicine side-effects, palatability issues, and any medical regimen incompatibility with normal daily life. By giving young people and their parents greater involvement in planning and executing trials, they are encouraged to contribute views on how the trial would be logistically most successful, and the 'buy in' explodes exponentially. When research excludes its consumers, it can fail to deliver meaningful outcomes. When it adopts patient and/or family involvement from its earliest inception, it can result in gold standard research that positively impacts every child that might need that medical intervention and whole communities involved in caring for the young people with that condition.

References

1 Coulter A. Participating in research. In: *Engaging Patients in Healthcare*. 2011: 138.
2 Lythgoe H *et al*. NIHR Clinical research networks: what they do and how they help paediatric research. *Arch Dis Child* 2017; 102: 755–759.
3 Preston J, van't Hoff W. GenerationR 2013 Meeting Report. National Institute for Health Research, 2013. http://generationr.org.uk/wp-content/uploads/2017/08/GenerationR-report2013.pdf
4 Eustace A, Wallace E. Evaluation of Consumer Involvement in the NIHR Clinical Research Network: Children 2013–2014. London: National Children's Bureau, 2014. http://generationr.org.uk/wp-content/uploads/2017/08/CRN-Children-CI-summary-evaluation-report.pdf
5 Douglas SL. A consumer perspective on embedding research in paediatric rheumatology. *Rheumatology* 2014; 53(11): 1915–1916.

27

The ethics of medicines research in children

A Altavilla and A Ceci

Introduction

Clinical research involving children is essential to increase understanding of childhood conditions and improve children's healthcare. The USA, the EU and Canada have all introduced initiatives and specific legal frameworks to stimulate the development of paediatric research. At the same time, the recognition of the vulnerability of children has led many countries to develop specific regulations/guidelines related to the ethical issues surrounding such research in order to ensure adequate protections of minors.

The learning objectives of this chapter are:

➤ to recognise the ethical challenges associated with paediatric medicines research
➤ to understand the importance of informed consent and the role of assent
➤ to learn the need for careful communication of the risks and benefits of study participation.

Inclusion criteria based on the principle of beneficence

According to the principle that the interests of science and society never prevail over the interests of individual research subjects, the 'scientific necessity' can be considered the first ethical pillar of paediatric research. This principle holds that children should not be enrolled in a clinical investigation unless necessary to achieve an important scientific and/or public health objective concerning the health and welfare of children.

A globally recognised corollary of this principle is that children should not be enrolled in studies that are duplicative (i.e. repeating previous research or based on an identical hypothesis) or unlikely to yield important knowledge applicable to children about the product or condition under investigation.

US Food and Drug Administration (FDA) regulations require that risks to subjects are minimised by eliminating unnecessary procedures and that the selection of subjects must be equitable. The EU Paediatric Regulation asks for developing medicinal products to meet the specific therapeutic needs of the paediatric population without subjecting children to unnecessary clinical or other trials.[1,2] To this aim, the information gained in any trial, whether positive or negative, should be made available both to researchers and the public.

The principle of equitable selection requires that subjects who are capable of informed consent (i.e. competent adults) should be enrolled prior to subjects who cannot consent (e.g. children), assuming there are no significant scientific reasons to enrol younger children in preference to older children and/or adults. Furthermore, it is broadly agreed that paediatric research should only be undertaken when the research serves the interests of minors, either by generating a direct benefit for the child concerned or by yielding benefit to the population of minors or the group of patients to which the minor belongs.

Differences in nomenclature exist between the US and EU regulations that require direct benefit. The 'direct benefit to the group' category allows studies to proceed in the EU that would be approved in the USA under the 'minor increase over minimal risk' category. Despite such differences, the US and EU approaches are in practice aligned, even if implementing associated regulations can be so challenging that experts need to debate their interpretation.

An appropriate – and favourable – balance of risk and potential benefit, as well as direct benefit, have a crucial position in the assessment of research protocols by ethics committees (ECs) or institutional review boards (IRBs).[3] The standard is used to weigh the acceptability of risks, based on the rationale that the greater the potential benefit involved, the lower the risk threshold should be. Major legal regulation requires that, basically, non-beneficial research does not exceed a stringent minimal risk and minimal burden threshold. While there is international consensus on the use of 'minimal risk' as a criterion of participation, its practical application lacks precision. A number of definitions of minimal risk exist. Minimal risk is defined in the Canadian guidelines (TCPS2) from an individual perspective as risks that are 'no greater than those encountered by participants in those aspects of their everyday life that relate to the research'.[3] Minimal risk has also been defined in guidelines from the Council for International Organizations of Medical Sciences (CIOMS) and World Health Organization (WHO) (2002) in a more objective manner as 'no more likely and not greater than the risk attached to routine medical or psychological examination of [the] persons'.[4] US research regulations define minimal risk in a way that combines these two perspectives (the daily life risks and the routine test standards), while the Additional Protocol on Biomedical Research (COE-2005) defines it on the basis of the concept of the 'very slight and temporary negative impact on the health' of the person concerned.

As a result of this ambiguity, different researchers and IRBs may interpret the concept differently. Some commentators regard the ambiguity (or flexibility) of minimal risk as a virtue of the concept. Others regard the ambiguity as a weakness, arguing that the lack of clarity concerning the interpretation of minimal risk can have an adverse impact on the consistency, fairness and integrity of human research. In addition, ethical norms do not mention whether the evaluation of risks and benefits should be conducted from a minor's perspective. Being inappropriate to extrapolate the adult experience to minors, researchers should think about how a child or adolescent may perceive the interventions and procedures proposed, in order to conduct an appropriate evaluation of the risks. Researchers should also think about the cumulative burden of research risks.

The determination of the levels of risk (including harms linked to the research intervention) and burdens (including those linked to the research participation itself) and the associated benefits are the basis for ethical approvability. As the assessment of the risk and the benefit may be based on probabilities and assumptions, respectively, this should also be balanced with the severity of the condition or diseases to be studied and the risk and benefit of alternative treatments. Clinical trials must also be designed to minimise pain, discomfort, fear and any other foreseeable risk in relation to the disease and developmental stage. The risk threshold and degree of distress must be specifically defined and constantly monitored.

The respect of autonomy in the informed consent procedures

Another ethical principle for consideration in paediatric research is the respect for persons, which includes respect for autonomous decision-making. It requires attention to the three main elements of informed consent: adequate information, voluntariness and capacity to understand the information.

Responsibility for consent to participation in research involving children (who cannot legally provide full consent themselves) is appointed to parents or guardians, who are assumed to choose according to the best interests of the child. Children, however, may develop the ability to fully consent during the course of a study or be able to consent to some aspects of the research. The (preferably) written authorisation of a competent adult (parent or legal guardian), acting as a surrogate decision maker, is required to enrol a minor in a clinical trial. The right of the responsible adults to refuse consent should be respected, once those adults have been informed that their consent may be revoked at any time without negative consequences to the minor concerned. Furthermore, depending on the type of research conducted, additional elements may need to be included in the information/consent form (e.g. in genetic research, it may be necessary to state the policy on the disclosure, to the participant and family, of results of genetic tests and their familial implications).

Children should also be involved in the decision to take part in research, as far as their developmental capacity permits. They should be provided with age-appropriate information regarding the trial, including the risks and the benefits, by an investigator or team member experienced in working with children. If a minor is deemed capable of forming an opinion, then their explicit wish or refusal to participate in research (whether expressed verbally or physically) should be respected.

Furthermore, ethical norms stress that consent is a continuing process that should be maintained throughout the course of research. This is especially true in longitudinal studies where changing circumstances or the need for additional information or samples necessitate additional contact with minors and/or their parents.

In order to respect children's developing autonomy and self-worth, international guidelines and some national legislation introduced the concept of assent, defined as a child's agreement to participate in research. It is recommended that assent be sought for participation in research at an age appropriate level and as suitable to the complexity of the project under consideration. If during a clinical trial the minor reaches the age of legal competence to give informed consent, as defined in the law of the state concerned, then that minor's express informed consent should be obtained before that subject can continue to participate in the clinical trial.

Many differences exist regarding the informed consent procedure.[4] Several EU member states specifically define age criteria or an age cutoff (e.g., at the time of writing, 12 years in Spain, 15–17 years in Denmark, 7–17 years in Estonia, and 12 years in The Netherlands) with regard to the decision-making capacities of minor research subjects.[5]

In the USA, it is the IRB that plays a crucial role to determine whether children provide assent, and to determine the form and value of their assent. In particular, the IRB decides when the assent of the participating children is not required for proceeding with the research (e.g. if the capability of some or all of the children is so limited that they cannot reasonably be consulted, or if the intervention or procedure involved in the research holds out a prospect of direct benefit important to the health or wellbeing of the children and is available only in the context of the research).

Confidentiality issues

Children participating in a trial are entitled to know any information collected on their health. Other personal information collected for a research project will need to be made accessible to them in conformity with national laws on the protection of individual data. Additionally, regarding the need to guarantee the confidentiality of personal data, it is established that where personal information on a child is collected, stored, accessed, used or disposed of, a researcher should ensure that the privacy, confidentiality and cultural sensitivities of the subject and the community are respected. The need to implement appropriate measures to protect information on the basis of the assessment of 'privacy risk' is also important, in accordance with modern information governance rules. Nevertheless, the analysis of existing guidelines/legal texts showed a considerable mixing of terminology and concepts applicable in the research area, which can lead to ambiguous interpretations and different understanding of conditions for processing paediatric personal data. Therefore, to avoid legal, ethical and technical problems, specific provisions for paediatric research need still to be implemented in data protection policy and regulations, in accordance with the fundamental rights of children.

Other specific ethical requirements

All international and EU ethical guidelines agree on the necessity to minimise the possibility of coercion or undue influence, particularly when children (and their families) are invited to take part in research studies. Some countries prohibit incentives in paediatric trials, either for the parents, legal representatives or the child. EU guidelines permit only parents'/legal representatives' compensation for their time and expenses. In the USA, the amount and schedule of all payments should be presented to the IRB at the time of initial review to assure that neither are coercive or present undue influence (21 CFR 50.20).[6] Canadian guidelines underline that 'incentives should not be so large or attractive as to encourage reckless disregard of risks'.[7]

With reference to the insurance that is required before starting clinical trials, the EU ethical recommendations (2017)[8] underline that insurance companies' contracts should not waive liabilities regarding long term effects, or limit the liability period, and ethics committees should pay careful attention to the insurance contract regarding this issue, in particular with respect to long term effects on development.

Finally, before research in children can start, the research protocol must be reviewed and endorsed by the competent authority and at least one ethics committee/IRB. To guarantee an adequate assessment of issues that are specifically related to the conduct of clinical research in minors, ethics committees require paediatric expertise – from within the ethics committee or by taking external advice – requested case by case, about the relevant paediatric clinical, ethical and psychological issues that pertain to each study.[8]

Conclusions

In conclusion, while some consensus has been reached on ethical standards of paediatric research, many differences still exist in regulations and guidelines. In particular, the new EU Regulation 536/2014, which came into force in 2016, confirms some existing ethical requirements (e.g. relating to inclusion criteria and the consent/assent procedure) but leaves many ambiguities on key aspects such as the risk–benefit assessment (e.g. the notion of minimal risk) left to an individual reporting member state chosen by the sponsor. Furthermore, the new regulation does not fully clarify important operational aspects concerning the role of ethics committees in the authorisation procedure that could impair the ethical review of trial protocols. To foster ethically sound paediatric research, it can be argued that further crucial clarifications are still needed, especially during the implementation process of the new regulation.

References

1   Regulation No 1901/2006 of the European Parliament and of the Council of 12 December 2006 on medicinal products for paediatric use and amending Regulation (EEC) No 1768/92, Directive 2001/20/EC, Directive 2001/83/EC and Regulation (EC) No 726/2004. Available at: https://ec.europa.eu/health//sites/health/files/files/eudralex/vol-1/reg_2006_1901/reg_2006_1901_en.pdf [last accessed 28 June 2018].
2   Regulation No 1902/2006 of the European Parliament and of the Council of 20 December 2006 amending Regulation 1901/2006 on medicinal products for paediatric use. Available at: https://ec.europa.eu/health//sites/health/files/files/eudralex/vol-1/reg_2006_1902/reg_2006_1902_en.pdf [last accessed 28 June 2018].
3   Government of Canada. TCPS 2 (2014)—the latest edition of Tri-Council Policy Statement: Ethical Conduct for Research Involving Humans.
4   Council for International Organizations of Medical Sciences (CIOMS) in collaboration with the World Health Organization (WHO). International Ethical Guidelines for Health-related Research Involving Humans. Available at: https://cioms.ch/wp-content/uploads/2017/01/WEB-CIOMS-EthicalGuidelines.pdf [last accessed 28 June 2018].
5   Council of Europe Treaty Series - No. 195. Additional Protocol to the Convention on Human Rights and Biomedicine, concerning Biomedical Research. Strasbourg, 25.I.2005. Available at: https://rm.coe.int/168008371a [last accessed 28 June 2018]. Available at: www.pre.ethics.gc.ca/pdf/eng/tcps2-2014/TCPS_2_FINAL_Web.pdf [last accessed 28 June 2018].
6   Department of Health and Human Services. Food and Drugs. Chapter 1: Food and Drug administration. PART 50. Protection of Human Subjects. Subpart B: Informed Consent of Human Subjects. Available at: https://www.accessdata.fda.gov/scripts/cdrh/cfdocs/cfcfr/CFRSearch.cfm?FR=50.20 [last accessed 28 June 2018].
7   Government of Canada. TCPS 2 (2014)—the latest edition of Tri-Council Policy Statement: Ethical Conduct for Research Involving Humans. Available at: www.pre.ethics.gc.ca/pdf/eng/tcps2-2014/TCPS_2_FINAL_Web.pdf [last accessed 28 June 2018].
8   European Commission. Ethical considerations for clinical trials on medicinal products conducted with minors. Recommendations of the expert group on clinical trials for the implementation of Regulation (EU) No 536/2014 on clinical trials on medicinal products for human use. Revision 1. 2017. Available at: https://ec.europa.eu/health/sites/health/files/files/eudralex/vol-10/2017_09_18_ethical_consid_ct_with_minors.pdf [last accessed 28 December 2018].

Further recommended reading

Gennet E, Altavilla A. Paediatric research under the new EU regulation on clinical trials: old issues new challenges. *Eur J Health Law* 2016; 23: 325–349.

Giannuzzi V *et al*. Clinical trial application in Europe: what will change with the new regulation? *Sci Eng Ethics* 2016; 22(2): 451–466.

Altavilla A. Paediatric clinical trials and Ethical standards for clinical trials. In Beran R, ed. *Handbook of Legal and Forensic Medicine*. Springer, 2013: 1117–1136.

Altavilla A *et al*. European survey on ethical and legal framework of clinical trials in paediatrics: results and perspective, *J Int Bioéthique* 2008; 19(3): 17–48.

Altavilla A *et al*. Impact of the new European paediatric regulatory framework on ethics committees: overview and perspectives. *Acta Paediatrica* 2012; 101(1): 27–32.

Lepola P *et al*. Informed consent for paediatric clinical trials in Europe. *Arch Dis Child* 2016; 0: 1–9.

28

Evidence-based prescribing

ES Starkey, S Conroy and HM Sammons

Introduction

An evidence-based approach to clinical practice can aid rational prescribing. There are, however, many challenges to evidence-based prescribing, including a lack of relevant clinical information and time for busy clinicians to identify, review and interpret the evidence, and translate this into clinical practice. In paediatrics, this is heightened by the fact that larger numbers of medications are used in an unlicensed (UL) or off-label (OL) manner, due to a paucity of drug trials in children.

The objectives of this chapter are:

➤ to highlight the incidence and nature of UL and OL drug use in children
➤ to understand the practical challenges faced in paediatrics because prescribing UL/OL drugs is unavoidable
➤ to describe key issues relating to evidence-based prescribing, including the role of paediatric formularies
➤ to become aware of the EU Paediatric Regulation.

What is OL or UL prescribing?

For a specific drug to be licensed, evidence to demonstrate safety, efficacy and quality must be presented by the drug company to the national licensing regulatory bodies (in the UK this is the Medicines and Healthcare products Regulatory Agency) or the European Medicines Agency. Following detailed scrutiny and approval of the information, the drug company is granted a marketing authorisation (formerly called a product licence; also known as a label in the USA). Information that will support prescribing is presented in a summary of medical product characteristics (SmPC). SmPCs are an essential guide to the optimal use of medicines (see eMC; www.medicines.org.uk/emc). This licensing system was introduced following a number of high profile historical cases where drugs caused significant toxicity. These included chloramphenicol causing grey baby syndrome and thalidomide producing

Table 1 OL medicines prescribed routinely in paediatrics		
Drug	**Prescription**	**Market authorisation**
Morphine sulfate	Intravenous bolus dose in a 10-year-old in severe pain	Not licensed for children under 12 years
Salbutamol	1 mg (10 puffs) via spacer for acute exacerbation of asthma in a 5-year-old	100–200 micrograms (1–2 puffs) for an exacerbation
Diclofenac	25 mg tablets for pain in an 8-year-old post tonsillectomy	Licensed only for juvenile idiopathic arthritis in children 1–9 years
Cyclizine	15 mg intravenously 8 hourly in a 5-year-old for postoperative nausea and vomiting	Injection not licensed for use in children

phocomelia in newborns. By definition, a UL drug is one where there is no marketing authorisation for a medicinal product in either adults or children, as the product has not been subjected to regulatory approval. An example is clonazepam suspension, which is usually prepared extemporaneously in a pharmacy department or by a pharmaceutical company under a special licence, as there is no commercially licensed form available.

OL prescribing describes using a drug outside the terms of its marketing authorisation. This may be in terms of:

● patient age
● therapeutic indication
● dosage
● route of administration
● contraindications.

Studies in the 1990s highlighted this problem by showing that 90% of babies on a neonatal unit and 36% of children on a general paediatric ward received UL or OL medication.[1,2] The most common reasons for OL use are doses outside licensed recommendations, use in a non-licensed indication, and use outside the licensed age range. In paediatrics, a large number of medications that are prescribed routinely are OL, as shown in Table 1.

Is using OL/UL drugs a problem?

Practicalities

Prescribing UL or OL in children can be problematic on a daily basis, due to the challenges of finding information and evidence on doses. This has improved with the use of national medicine databases, formularies and drug helplines.

Another challenge is the lack of age appropriate formulations. A large number of medications are only commercially available in preparations designed for adults, which may require significant manipulation to obtain a practical dose and an acceptable form, such as a liquid, for children. This is often carried out without knowing the physical and chemical properties of the drug, and so possibly altering its stability. This also leads to the drug being more difficult to source for families, with higher costs for health services. In addition, many such products have a short shelf life, making them inconvenient for families. Other options are to use different preparations, such as intravenous forms orally, and cutting or dissolving tablets to obtain fractions for the paediatric doses. Such manipulations may lead to inaccurate dosing and potentially to drug errors and adverse events.

Adverse drug reactions and medication errors

There is some debate as to whether OL and UL medications increase the risk of adverse drug reactions (ADRs). Various studies have been performed in different clinical areas (inpatients, intensive care units, outpatient settings) with conflicting results. Some have shown a higher relative risk of ADRs associated with UL/OL prescriptions, and a higher percentage of more severe reactions were found to be associated with these drugs. Other studies have not confirmed this increased risk but have highlighted that the children treated with UL/OL medicines are often also those receiving multiple medications, which is known to give an increased risk of ADRs.

One study has shown that the use of UL drugs increases the risk of medication errors in children. The risk appears particularly high in neonates and in those under 2 years, although it applied across all age groups. It appears to be particularly associated with dispensing errors, but was also prevalent in prescribing and administration errors. OL drug use does not appear to increase the risk of errors, although it was prominent in errors causing moderate harm.[3]

OL or UL use of a medicine does not always imply off-evidence use. Some medicines commonly used in children have been studied extensively without the data generated by those studies being incorporated into the SmPC. What is less commonly known is that the data to support a paediatric extension to a marketing authorisation have traditionally not been extensive. Some older SmPCs may provide incomplete information, so that evidence-based prescribing will require work to gather the information that is not included in the SmPC.

Paediatric regulation

Over the last decade, there has been a drive to provide safe and effective medication for children by improving the legislation around paediatric research and drug licensing requirements. In 2007, an EU regulation came into force making it mandatory for pharmaceutical companies to submit a paediatric investigation plan (PIP) (chapter 22) outlining how they will study their new drug in children. This is gradually starting to increase the number of paediatric trials, allowing more defined paediatric dosing regimens for new drugs.

Another aim of the regulation was to stimulate research into existing drugs used in an OL manner, by introducing a paediatric use marketing authorisation (PUMA). This provides incentives for drug companies to develop new paediatric indications or formulations appropriate for children. In the first 10 years of the regulation, there have been only three PUMAs granted, the first of these being buccal midazolam for seizures in 2011. The apparent lack of interest by drug companies in studying 'old' drugs is said to be due to the ethical, practical, cost and technical complexities of performing clinical trials in children. The European Commission funded 19 consortia to study 24 off-patent drugs, and the results of this programme are awaited.

Formularies and prescribing

There is provision within UK law for clinicians to prescribe, pharmacists to dispense, and nurses to administer UL or OL medicines. Prescribing a UL or OL drug may increase a prescriber's responsibility and potential liability. This means the prescriber needs to be able to justify and feel competent in using medicines in this way. Drug formularies, such as the *British National Formulary* (BNF) and *British National Formulary for Children* (BNFC), are invaluable sources of information and support for this. They inform the reader of a drug's licence status as well as providing advice on UL medicines and OL use. This advice considers the current treatment options available as well as weighing up current evidence on the UL or OL drug. When a drug is used outside its licence and is not in this formulary, patients and/or parents should be informed, with a discussion about the associated benefits and risks.

Rational prescribing

One of the main challenges of evidence-based medicine faced by paediatricians is the lack of data from rational drug development programmes. That is, prescribing should be supported by information gathered from a process that ideally starts from what is known about a drug in animals, adults or children with other conditions and fills information gaps. Commonly, a programme will start with evidence of a relevant effect (proof of concept), then select the optimal dose, then conduct trials of efficacy. While randomised controlled trials are said to be the gold standard of evidence, they are less likely to be informative if the dose has not been adequately defined before the RCT is done. This is compounded by the relative lack of RCTs in many conditions affecting children. Paucity of data leads to either the use of evidence from adult studies or the use of low quality paediatric evidence.

Use of adult evidence

Problems can arise when extrapolation occurs from adult studies. Empirical scaling from adults to children continues to be a main method for dose selection in children, with adjustment for body weight as the most commonly used approach. This, however, fails to consider the physiological and developmental differences that occur within the paediatric population, which can impact on the safety and efficacy of a drug. This can be illustrated with the historical example of chloramphenicol. Chloramphenicol was used to treat neonatal infections, using adult doses of 12.5–25 mg/kg four times a day. Large numbers of patients developed cardiovascular collapse and irregular respiration and died, features known as grey baby syndrome. Neonates have immature levels of the enzyme that converts chloramphenicol to the excreted water-soluble chloramphenicol glucuronide. This causes a build-up of chloramphenicol, resulting in grey baby syndrome. Consequently, dosing in neonates has been reduced to 12.5 mg/kg twice daily for those less than 1 month old.

Poor paediatric evidence

Intravenous salbutamol for use in severe asthma is an example where paediatric dosing used in practice is based on limited clinical evidence. Intravenous salbutamol is currently only licensed for adults and children 12 years and over. The dosing schedule in adults is founded on pharmacokinetic–pharmacodynamic (PK–PD) data from numerous studies and defined in the SmPC. The bolus dose recommended is 250 micrograms over 5–10 minutes and at an infusion rate of 3–20 micrograms/minute. In children, the British Thoracic Society (BTS) asthma guidance and the BNFC recommend an IV bolus dose of 15 micrograms/kg (to a maximum of 250 micrograms) over 5–10 minutes and a continuous infusion (CI) dose of 1–5 micrograms/kg/minute. These doses are based on small paediatric studies and case reports. Clearly, IV salbutamol doses for children are an order of magnitude higher than those recommended for adults when based on weight. This is inconsistent with the predicted similarity in their salbutamol PK–PD relationship. More importantly, higher doses could translate to an increased risk of toxic reactions, and inconsistencies in dosing regimens are liable to cause uncertainty and confusion among clinicians.

Evidence-based practice

Sometimes, ample studies show poor clinical evidence of a drug's safety and efficacy, and it is necessary to reconsider recommending further research. An example of this is the use of proton pump inhibitors (PPIs). An existing literature review showed a lack of evidence for many of the PPIs, e.g. omeprazole, for the treatment of gastroesophageal reflux disease in children.[4] PPIs are currently OL in infants under 1 year of age, yet continue to be prescribed readily by many clinicians in the management of reflux disease.

Despite the limited evidence to support prescribing in much of routine paediatric clinical practice, it can be helpful to follow a structured approach when faced with challenging prescriptions:

- Make use of national paediatric formularies (such as the BNFC) as well as local prescribing guidelines.
- Discuss drug, dosing or formulation queries with a paediatric clinical pharmacist or paediatric clinical pharmacologist.
- Liaise with the local medicines information service.

Conclusions

UL and OL drugs are used still commonly in neonatal and paediatric patients. The use of UL and OL treatments causes practical problems and may increase the risk of medication errors and adverse reactions. However, truly evidence-based prescribing in paediatrics can be challenging, due to the lack of robust paediatric studies. Identifying common UL/OL prescribing scenarios that are widespread in paediatric practice can help to identify research priorities for the future.

References

1 Conroy S *et al*. Unlicensed and off label drug use in neonates. *Arch Dis Child Fetal Neonatal Ed* 1999; 80: F142–F145.
2 Turner S *et al*. Unlicensed and off label drug use in paediatric wards: prospective study. *BMJ* 1998: 316: 343–345.
3 Conroy S. Association between license status and medication errors. *Arch Dis Child* 2011: 96: 305–306.
4 Tafuri G *et al*. Off-label use of medicines in children: can available evidence avoid useless paediatric trials? The case of proton pump inhibitors for the treatment of gastroesophageal reflux disease. *Eu J of Clin Pharm* 2009: 65: 209–216.

29

Improving training in prescribing

A Long

Introduction

This chapter aims to identify the need for improved training in prescribing for doctors, both within the undergraduate and postgraduate curriculum, while recognising that responsibility for safe prescribing is not solely an issue for doctors but for the whole multiprofessional team. There are examples of good practice, which have been referenced, and opportunities for quality improvement within this area of critical practice.

The learning objectives of this chapter are:

➤ to recognise the need for improved training in prescribing
➤ to identify, create and utilise learning opportunities
➤ to understand the purpose of current training initiatives
➤ to recognise the importance of assessing safe prescribing skills
➤ to be able to promote a safe prescribing environment.

While the chapter focuses mainly on training within the structure of undergraduate medical and postgraduate training in the UK, the principles will translate to similar training schemes in other countries that involve paediatric residency programmes.

Background

Medication errors are probably one of the most common types of medical error. They are estimated to result in harm to 1–2% of adult patients admitted to hospital in the UK and may occur in 10–15% of all childhood prescriptions, but the true incidence and harm to children is not known, as no mandatory reporting system is in place within the UK. The cost to the NHS of preventable medication errors is estimated to be in the region of £750 million per year. Studies of prescribing errors in children have largely been limited to the hospital setting; however, considering at least 18% of all GP consultations concern children less than 16 years of age, the potential for medication error is also considerable within the primary care setting.

The causes of medication errors are multifactorial and include simple dosing errors, dispensing and administration errors, which are compounded by the widespread use of unlicensed and off-label drugs as well as confusion over age related and weight related prescribing. Available formulations and compliance add further complexity in this age group. Further detailed information about medication errors is available in chapter 31.

A number of strategies have been established to reduce medication errors in children.[1] While the evidence base suggests that electronic prescribing reduces the risk of prescribing errors, the reality of paediatric specific systems – and their limited availability – makes this solution aspirational. The use of ward-based paediatric clinical pharmacists, pre-printed structured prescription order forms, 'protected' prescribing areas and clinical decision support systems all have their advocates; however, their use is sporadic and their incorporation into routine practice has been sparingly evaluated.

UK medical students' confidence in their own prescribing skills for all patients has been reported to be low, and it has been recognised that there is a need to improve undergraduate teaching in safe drug prescribing and administration.[2] There has also been a move to introduce a national prescribing safety assessment (PSA) examination aimed at ensuring prescribing competence in final-year medical students. At the time of writing, this has been introduced in all UK medical schools, five Irish medical schools and one in Malta (approximately 800 students); however, its use in terms of whether it was used formatively or summatively initially varied between medical schools. The PSA has also recently been piloted in some foundation schools across the UK.

This chapter will review some of the educational opportunities available to improve prescribing practice, some of which are specifically for children's prescribing, although recognising that the underlying principles need to be taught and evaluated before a purely paediatric approach is adopted.

Creating learning opportunities

Undergraduate

While recognising that undergraduate training in the UK is largely focused on adult medicine and surgical specialties, there is increasing recognition within the undergraduate curriculum that children are not just small adults. At the current time, the child health attachments in most UK medical schools are too short to teach safe paediatric prescribing; however, there have been some excellent examples of interprofessional teaching and shared learning workshops to teach knowledge, core competencies, communication and team working skills in paediatric prescribing. The recognition that this is an international problem for all medical students has led to a focus on improved teaching in safe prescribing for adults and children utilising a number of different learning methodologies.

A number of studies have been undertaken to review the effectiveness of different educational interventions aimed at changing prescribing practices. The majority of the studies were designed to cover teaching of general prescribing principles, demonstrating practical applications through the use of problem solving clinical scenarios. The World Health Organization (WHO) *Guide to Good Prescribing*[4] was the most frequently studied. Use of this guide, with a supported teacher guide, yielded the most positive results across a range of medical schools internationally studying students of different seniorities. The main criticisms were the limited range of clinical scenarios available to be used and the perceived lack of complexity; however, further work has suggested that augmentation with tutorials led by pharmacists has additional benefits in knowledge and skill retention.

The implementation of the PSA examination has resulted in the introduction of a range of interventions designed to increase the first time pass rate as well as offering remedial opportunities to those students who fail the assessment before they complete their medical school training. There has been a significant investment in e-learning at both a national and local level. The British Pharmacological Society has made a significant investment in Prescribe, an online resource for prescribers in training (Table 1). The intention is to support a curriculum-based approach with interactive learning sessions and an information resource, including the ability to develop a student formulary. It offers the opportunity to practise key skills using online simulators. E-Learning for Healthcare has also developed a Safe Prescribing resource in partnership with the Academy of Medical Royal Colleges, designed to support doctors from qualification throughout their foundation training to become expert prescribers.

While self-motivated learning has an important role in developing core knowledge, there is good evidence to support the role of group learning, especially with multiprofessional involvement in embedding skills. A range of interventions have been studied, including the use of simulation with tutorial support, the use of interprofessional workshops between medical and nursing or pharmacy students, and teaching programmes conducted by hospital pharmacists. All methodologies are dependent on high quality feedback and the opportunity to practise skills within a non-threatening environment. While these interventions did not result in significant differences in acquisition of skills or knowledge, there were significant attitudinal changes towards learning and working with other professionals.

	Name	E-learning	Teaching resources
Table 1 Examples of prescribing training resources			
Undergraduate	Prescribe	https://www.e-lfh.org.uk/programmes/clinical-pharmacology-and-prescribing/	
Foundation	e-Learning for Healthcare	www.e-lfh.org.uk/programmes/safe-prescribing	
	Script	www.safeprescriber.org	
	WHO *Guide to Good Prescribing*		http://apps.who.int/medicinedocs/en/d/Jwhozip23e
Postgraduate paediatrics	RCPCH Prescribing Tools	https://www.rcpch.ac.uk/training-examinations-professional-development/quality-training/paediatric-prescribing-tool/paediatr	www.rcpch.ac.uk/training-examinations-professional-development/examinations/assessment-tools/safe-prescribing-tool/p
	Hands-on Guide to Practical Paediatrics	www.wileyhandsonguides.com/paediatrics/scenarios.asp	
General practice	Prescribing in General Practice	http://elearning.rcgp.org.uk/course/info.php?id=136&popup=0	

Postgraduate

While it is recognised that undergraduate teaching has a critical role in developing knowledge and skills required to practise safe prescribing, the behaviours developed do not have an impact until there is a need to develop independent prescribing after qualification. Much as the PSA may demonstrate achievement of a certain level of competence, the risks associated with prescribing errors will not materialise until an individual is required to write prescriptions without close supervision. Since most paediatric attachments take place relatively early within undergraduate clinical training, the drivers to develop safe paediatric prescribing skills that are assessed close to the end of training are limited.

Most of the educational interventions associated with safe prescribing for children have been aimed at students entering paediatric training. However, it is recognised that many foundation posts for junior doctors in both medical and surgical specialties include a responsibility for prescribing for children or young adults. Doctors then entering general practice training in the UK may not necessarily undertake a paediatric training post despite the fact that approximately 25% of their workload may involve seeing children and young people. A number of interventions have therefore been focused on doctors during their foundation training years (the first 2 years after graduating from university).

There has also been a sustained drive within many foundation programmes to ensure that doctors required to prescribe for children have specific training. The interventions used vary between lectures, workshops and a period of 'shadowing' before taking on the full responsibilities of prescribing. There are varying degrees of success, depending on the importance that is attached by foundation programme directors and supervising consultants. The best interventions seem to involve practical workshops delivered by paediatric pharmacists; however, some success has been attributed to courses that are designed and delivered by other junior doctors, notably other paediatric trainees.

The main thrust of educational interventions for those entering paediatric training has been focused on the selection processes and induction of trainees into their working environments. It is widely asserted that assessment drives learning and that the introduction of a safe prescribing 'station' into the national recruitment process into paediatric training does ensure that those entering have a defined level of competence requiring a minimal knowledge and skill level on assessment.

Current training initiatives

The majority of educational interventions are still focused around the process of induction. Given the variety of experiences of doctors prior to entering paediatric training, it is generally considered unsafe to assume a specific level of knowledge or skill. Clinical governance dictates that the responsibility for individual performance rests with the employer, and therefore both an understanding of the skill level as well as a safe prescribing environment is essential for good paediatric practice. While some schools of paediatrics undertake regional induction programmes for all ST1s entering paediatric training (ST1 is the first year of the UK paediatric specialty training programme), all NHS trusts and departments also have their own induction programmes.

In order to facilitate standardised minimal levels of induction training in safe paediatric prescribing for all UK paediatric trainees, the Royal College of Paediatrics and Child Health (RCPCH) has made freely available an electronic presentation (developed in the London School of Paediatrics and Child Health) intended for use in induction (Table 1). This has been evaluated in practice and has been found to improve understanding in the principles and practice of safe prescribing in paediatrics. This has been further supported at a national level by a suite of e-learning modules on safe prescribing developed by the RCPCH.

Different organisations have taken a variety of approaches to ensure the safety of prescribing within their own paediatric units. Many larger trusts have introduced a mandatory assessment of paediatric prescribing skills before allowing doctors to prescribe unsupervised. The Joint RCPCH and NPPG (Neonatal and Paediatric Pharmacists Group) Medicines Committee has developed an assessment paediatric prescribing tool (PPT), which is available to all trusts that do not have a separate assessment tool in place. However, the responsibility still rests with the trust to ensure that trainees who fail to meet an acceptable level of safe prescribing skills are either offered remedial training or are closely supervised until they show that they can prescribe safely.

Assessing effectiveness of training

While the responsibility for patient safety rests with the employing organisation, the RCPCH has a responsibility to ensure that trainees are meeting minimum standards of competence. This responsibility has largely been devolved to schools of paediatrics, which are required to undertake annual reviews of trainee competence. The standards for training are defined within the training curriculum, and the requirement for safe prescribing skills is set within that context. While basic prescribing skills are assessed at entry to paediatric training (both at ST1 and ST4), these assessments are not designed to be pass/fail but rather to verify previous training and provide reassurance that the trainee has the necessary arithmetical skills as well as demonstrating an understanding of the complexity of prescribing in children.

All paediatric trainees are required to pass the membership examination of the RCPCH (the MRCPCH) during their first 3 years of training. The RCPCH has introduced safe prescribing questions within the three written parts of the examination. While this largely tests knowledge rather than prescribing skills, the applied knowledge paper does test clinical reasoning and provides context around issues of safe prescribing. In addition, there are several clinical scenarios within the communication section of the clinical examination that test application of prescribing skills; examiners are also encouraged to question aspects of safe prescribing within the other stations (clinical, history and management).

Since trainees are unable to progress to level 2 training (previously known as the registrar grade) without passing MRCPCH, there has been a natural assumption that trainees at this grade (ST4+) are safe prescribers. However, a number of serious incidents, reported at a national level, have shown this assumption to be flawed. All trainees are required to undertake an external formalised assessment towards the end of training (Structured Assessment of Readiness for Tenure – START) before becoming a consultant. It was decided that a prescribing station should form part of this final assessment. Experience to date, since the assessment has been implemented, has revealed a number of serious concerns raised about trainee performance in prescribing. This has led to individual trainees being required to have remedial training and be reassessed in their prescribing skills.

As a result, the RCPCH has considered introducing regular formative assessment in prescribing skills throughout training. Workplace-based assessments (structured learning events) seem to be well placed to identify prescribing weaknesses, offering the opportunity for further remedial work to be undertaken during training. The RCPCH is reviewing the potential value of using either case-based discussion (CbD) or mini clinical examination (mini-CEX) assessments to demonstrate safe prescribing skills, which might involve paediatric pharmacists evaluating trainees' performance. However, it was also recognised that formative development might be equally well achieved through encouraging reflection on prescribing errors and adverse drug reactions (ADRs), which should be documented in trainees' e-portfolios and might be discussed at the annual review of trainee competence.

Developing a safe prescribing environment

Research has suggested that, while education has an important role to play in preventing serious prescribing errors in children, the most effective means of preventing error is through local systems.[4] E-prescribing (see chapter 30) can reduce prescribing and dispensing errors, but there has been little investment in child specific systems; the current systems have largely been designed for prescribing for adults, with modifications made for paediatric practice which are often suboptimal.

Many organisations have developed other systems to ensure safe prescribing for children. While pharmacy mentoring, which has the capacity to offer formative feedback to trainees, is well established, some departments have produced 'pocket guides' for prescribing, introduced limited list prescribing, or have developed their own e-learning programmes. The use of simulation methodology in paediatric prescribing is also becoming more formally established. Some organisations have introduced a protected prescribing area for prescriptions to be completed in, where doctors are not to be disturbed.

Many organisations have active quality-improvement systems: they have invested in systems to review 'near misses' in prescribing or dispensing errors within a non-punitive incident monitoring system. This has resulted in other systematic changes, which include double checking for potentially harmful drugs, modifying medication charts, and employing ward-based pharmacists to undertake regular drug chart inspections.

Decision support tools that provide prompts to help prescribers avoid errors when writing prescriptions have been shown to be beneficial either as part of e-prescribing systems or as standalone systems. The increase in smartphone applications demonstrates a growing demand among trainees for this type of support, but these applications have not been evaluated scientifically.

Conclusions

Prescribing errors are, unfortunately, common in the routine care of children both within and beyond the hospital setting. Although education alone is not the whole solution, it is clear that training in safe prescribing is an important component of good paediatric practice. Teaching of the principles of safe prescribing should start within medical school and should include paediatric content as well as generic principles. Continuing training should include some self-directed learning, either through e-learning or alternative resources, preferably then augmented with practical workshops and multiprofessional learning. Assessment of prescribing skills is an essential component of patient safety, and close supervision should be encouraged where skills are in doubt. Reflection on prescribing errors is a powerful tool in preventing further mistakes; however, systems should still be designed to minimise the risk to patients (see Box 1).

Box 1 A prescription to improve prescribing

- Education, to be taken as often as possible (a repeat prescription – learning should be lifelong)
- Special study modules for graduates and undergraduates, to be taken as required
- Proper assessment in the final undergraduate examination, to be taken once or twice, and in postgraduate appraisal, to be taken occasionally; this could be linked to a licence to prescribe
- A national prescription form for hospitals, to be applied uniformly and used as a training tool
- Guidelines and computerised prescribing systems, to be taken if indicated (their roles and proper implementation are currently unclear)
- A national prescribing council to integrate these activities

Adapted from: Aronson[5]

References

1 Conroy S *et al*. Educational interventions to reduce prescribing errors. *Arch Dis Child* 2008; 93: 313–315.
2 Maxwell S, Walley T. Teaching safe and effective prescribing in UK medicalsSchools: a core curriculum for tomorrow's doctors. *Br J Clin Pharmacol* 2003; 55(6): 496–503.
3 World Health Organization (WHO). *Guide to Good Prescribing. A practice manual*. 1994. Available at: http://apps.who.int/medicinedocs/pdf/whozip23e/whozip23e.pdf [last accessed 2 March 2018].
4 Evidence Scan: *Reducing Prescribing Errors*. London: The Health Foundation, 2012. www.health.org.uk/sites/health/files/ReducingPrescribingErrors.pdf
5 Aronson JK. A prescription for better prescribing. *Br J Clin Pharmacol* 2006; 61: 478–491.

30

Electronic prescribing

NA Caldwell and OJ Rackham

Introduction

By the time our current neonatal patients become adults, paper prescription charts will probably have become historical artefacts. Electronic prescribing for children and neonates will happen, and debates about the pros and cons of electronic prescribing will be redundant.[1] Consequently, in the future, all medication orders will be legible. However, other challenges remain, and to overcome these will present a significant test.

Electronic prescribing impacts on the entire medicines-use process and the multidisciplinary team. It is not just about ordering medicines or exclusively of relevance to prescribers. For example, nurses administer medicines, pharmacists and technicians review orders and manage medicine supply, and children, parents and carers give and receive medicines. Although no longer in existence, *Connecting for Health* prepared useful resources outlining challenges and lessons learned from electronic prescribing in hospitals.[2] This chapter will outline some key considerations during development and maintenance of electronic prescribing and medicines administration systems for children. We will outline some of the major challenges now and in the future.

The learning objectives of this chapter are to:

➢ appreciate the advantages and disadvantages of electronic prescribing
➢ be aware of the role of clinical decision support
➢ recognise the challenges of electronic prescribing in a mixed healthcare setting with both adults and children; system design is often not specific to the needs of children
➢ understand the importance of dose rounding in electronic prescribing.

Does e-prescribing eliminate medication errors?

Medication errors within e-prescribing systems differ from those observed with paper prescribing processes, and there is considerable variation between different systems.

Obvious benefits of electronic prescribing include:

- All prescriptions are legible, signed, date and time stamped.
- Prescriptions can be accessed at a distance.
- Prescriptions when viewed are up to date and complete.

There are also drawbacks:

- Screen size and text layout may not suit all users.
- Prescriptions may be truncated to allow more information to be displayed in one view.
- Currently, many prescribers are more familiar with and therefore quicker at handwriting clinical entries than typing them.

Further differences will be explored through this chapter.

Two main groups of errors, comprising 22 types of medication error risks, have been reported with electronic prescribing:[3]

- Information errors due to data fragmentation and integration failures – examples include prescribers completely relying on the system to guide dosing, failure to chart or delayed charting of stat orders, gaps in antibiotic therapy due to failure to renew treatment, and incorrect diluents for parenteral therapies
- Human–machine interface flaws – examples include errors with selecting the correct patient, loss of data, and time when the system was non-functional

Great attention must be paid to the very serious consequences of wrong patient selection when prescribing. Children are often treated simultaneously with their siblings. Neonatal intensive care units may have multiple siblings without forenames. Systems must have near perfect identity management.

Experience at Wirral suggests that clinicians may over-rely on technology and assume that if the computer gives the option, or allows order creation, it must be correct. Sometimes gram (g) and milligram (mg) are not so obviously wrong when viewed electronically.

Selection error, from drop down lists, where electronic data are poorly constructed is another risk. Clinicians may inadvertently prescribe the wrong drugs by selecting a medicine directly above or below the intended medicine in the alphabetical catalogue. 'Tall man' lettering may be a useful preventative measure for selection error, e.g. to distinguish DOPamine from DOBUTamine. Systems should be designed to make the right choice the easiest one to make. Prescription information must always be clear, consistent and without truncation.

Consideration of the consequences of predefined stop dates, particularly of antibiotics, is essential. A review date, or no defined course length with daily senior review, may be appropriate in an intensive care setting. In emergency department settings, defined course lengths may be more appropriate. Care must be taken when introducing prompts, to ensure they are not overly intrusive while ensuring that they are always read. If the system is able to automatically cease a medication prescription when reaching the stop date, care must be taken during the design process to ensure that it remains clearly visible to the clinical team.

Combined electronic prescribing and medicines administration systems can reduce risk. If well designed, they can incorporate detailed administration instructions to support nurses and carers to correctly administer medicines and minimise missed doses.

Clinical decision support

Clinical decision support (CDS) ranges in complexity from the use of a single drug dictionary right through to checking the suitability of drug doses and combinations based on a thorough review of existing comorbidities and allergies. Decision support can also be applied on a continuum and work in the background to support prescribers to change drugs or alter dosing schedules if clinical parameters such as renal function, weight or diagnosis change.

An advanced dosing model that interacts with existing e-prescribing systems has been proposed.[4] This model takes account of the following factors and uses dose rounding functionality to prescribe practical doses:

- **Indication:** A condition that makes a particular medication dose advisable
- **Care area:** Physical location of patient within institution, which is used to infer intensity
- **Chronological age:** Age of patient in years, months and days since date of birth
- **Post-conceptual age:** Age of patient in years, months and days since clinician estimated date of conception
- **Dosing weight:** A user-defined weight that will be used to dose medications; this may not reflect the patient's current weight
- **Renal impairment:** Qualitative assessment of renal impairment by the ordering provider, i.e. 'impaired' or 'not impaired'

A danger with CDS, if alerts are perceived to have low specificity, is that they may simply be overridden. When an alert is repeatedly triggered, clinicians are more likely to 'click through' the alert.[5] Repeated alerts may result in high override rates ('alert fatigue'). However, override rates may not fully reflect the clinician's response to the information contained in an alert. Instead, clinicians may have noted the information when they first viewed it, and thus the subsequent presentation may be considered irrelevant.

Care must also be taken, when designing systems, to decide whether these messages are alerts that must just be acknowledged or actual 'stops' that do not allow an action.

Many electronic prescribing systems are developed with 'order sentences' containing suggestions for dose, route and frequency based on locally developed rules. Prescribers then either accept or change these suggestions. Alerts may be developed that must be acknowledged and the order either:

- changed
- cancelled or
- prescribed as is with no change.

A challenge with CDS is the relevance of the underpinning evidence to the patient cohort. For example, rifampicin induces metabolism of fluconazole by enhancing cytochrome p450 enzymes. These enzymes are not fully developed in preterm neonates. Therefore the clinical relevance of a CDS alert highlighting a potential drug interaction must be considered in context. This may not be appreciated by a trainee clinician, who may erroneously follow the 'computer's' advice. The challenge is therefore to ensure that CDS alerts are carefully tailored to the correct patient cohort. Prescribers must also recognise that the computer is not always right.

A personal view of the authors is that CDS should be developed to guide the clinician to select an appropriate medicine, dose, route and frequency seamlessly and invisibly. It is much better to offer limited and appropriate choices rather than ask, 'Are you sure you want to do this?' As an example, if a patient is allergic to penicillin, why allow selection of a penicillin and then ask the prescriber, in view of the documented allergies, 'Do you want to continue?' Surely a safer option would be to filter access to penicillin-containing preparations so they do not appear? One must also consider the accuracy of an allergy status and consequence of withholding effective treatment based on an erroneously documented allergy. The electronic allergy status is always there, unlike a paper prescription chart which is completed on each new episode of care. In addition, one must consider grey areas where there needs to be a clinical evaluation of the potential consequences of overriding an allergy alert, e.g. prescribing a cephalosporin in a child with penicillin anaphylaxis.

Limiting the prescriber's options must be balanced with the need for the flexibility for an experienced prescriber to prescribe against the CDS advice.

Challenges of e-prescribing in a mixed setting

Prescribing for children often takes place in mixed settings, with adults, children and neonates within a single healthcare facility. This introduces design challenges in determining the best way to present order sentences.

Great care must be taken to ensure that options are suitable for paediatric specialists and trainees as well as those in other specialties who also care (and prescribe) for children (e.g. general surgeons). Prescriptions generated by non-paediatric specialists may require careful review to ensure patient safety.

The American Academy of Pediatrics has defined key electronic health record functional areas of electronic prescribing systems for children:[6]

- **Immunisation management:** Ability to record immunisation data and link to immunisation information systems and decision support.
- **Growth tracking:** Allow access to results graphically and calculate percentile value against defined distribution. This should feed into decision support functions.
- **Medication dosing:** To include dosing by body weight with dose range checking. Dose rounding to safe and convenient doses to express dose in volume of medicine to be administered rather than just mass of drug. Include age-based dosing decision support and dosing for the school day.
- **Patient identification:** Newborn identification, and link prenatal data to postnatal record. Accommodate name change and ambiguous sex.
- **Norms for paediatric data:** Include both numeric and non-numeric data and complex normative relationships and gestational age.
- **Privacy:** Adolescent privacy, children in foster or custodial care, consent by proxy, adoption, guardianship and emergency treatment.

Prescribing for neonates has aspects of both high and low risk. It is low risk because of the small number of medicines used compared with adult general medicine; prescribing guidance and default doses can therefore be readily constructed. It is simultaneously high risk because of the use of multiple continuous infusions, often starting, stopping and restarting over short time periods, and the potential for dose calculation errors (e.g. mistakenly using a weight in grams instead of kilograms).

Dose rounding

Medication errors in children are recognised internationally as a significant problem. None of the commercially available electronic prescribing dose rounding solutions are specifically designed to meet the needs of children. Most do not take account of available medicinal products and do not round doses to ones that can be easily and safely administered. Ideally, liquid medicines should be measurable within a single syringe. Syringes have different graduations and enable doses of:

- less than 1 mL to be measured to the nearest 0.01 mL
- 1–2.5 mL to be measured to the nearest 0.1 mL
- 2.5–5 mL to be measured to the nearest 0.2 mL
- 5–20 mL to be measured to the nearest 0.5 mL.

Clinicians tend to round doses intuitively to the nearest 5 or 10 mg. Liquid medicines are available in various concentrations, and commonly prescribed doses of medicine are not physically measurable. For example, co-amoxiclav injection is reconstituted as 60 mg/mL. A dose of 20 mg is 0.3333 mL, which cannot be measured and must be approximated. A dose of 21 mg, which initially appears over-precise, is actually a better dose, equal to 0.35 mL, because it can be measured accurately. Development of an electronic dose rounding and volume rounding calculator would realise an innovative solution to a common problem. If this were incorporated into all electronic prescribing systems, it would improve safety and reduce risk from medication use in children and neonates.

Commonly asked questions with rounding are: 'Do you round up or down?' and 'By how much?' Recommended rounding tolerances have been defined for commonly prescribed medicines for children.[7] Medicines can be split into four main groups:

- Medicines where rounding is used judiciously to retain intended effect
- Medicines where rounding takes particular account of potential unintended effect
- Medicines that are rarely rounded because of the potential for toxicity and
- Medicines where there is insufficient data to provide rounding recommendations

Using a Delphi process to achieve consensus, dose rounding tolerances that consider avoiding unintentional adverse effects, controlling intended effects and avoiding toxicity have been defined for 102 medicines.[7]

An added complexity to dose rounding for children is the fact that recommended doses are often disease specific. Doses may be calculated on weight or body surface area, or both, depending on the clinical indication. Therefore it is not simply a matter of defining the dose of each medicine. Order sentences must be flexibly presented to enable diagnostic specific prescribing. If too many options for dose are presented, then prescribers may choose the wrong one. This creates a significant challenge for electronic data display.

Conclusions

Electronic prescribing for children and neonates will be implemented in many clinical environments. Its successful development will reduce many risks. Medication orders will in future be clear, legible and accessible at multiple sites and will show the most up-to-date entry. A major challenge will be to ensure that medication orders have appropriate CDS to help prescription and administration of appropriate dose and volume of drugs.

Great care must be taken with deployment of CDS to ensure it is age appropriate and guides staff to the safest practice without undue obstacles.

References

1 Caldwell NA, Power B. The pros and cons of electronic prescribing for children. *Arch Dis of Child* 2012; 97: 124–128.
2 NHS Connecting for Health. Electronic prescribing in hospitals – challenges and lessons learned. 2009. www.connectingforhealth.nhs.uk/systemsandservices/eprescribing/ challenges/Final_report.pdf
3 Koppel R *et al*. Role of computerized physician order entry systems in facilitating medication errors. *JAMA* 2005; 293: 1197–1203.
4 Ferranti JM *et al*. Using a computerized provider order entry system to meet the unique prescribing needs of children: description of an advanced dosing model. *BMC Med Inform Decis Mak* 2011; 11: 14.
5 Sheehan B *et al*. Cognitive analysis of decision support for antibiotic prescribing at the point of ordering in a neonatal intensive care unit. *AMIA Annu Symp Proc* 2009; 2009: 584–588.
6 Spooner SA. Council on Clinical Information Technology, American Academy of Pediatrics. Special requirements of electronic health record systems in pediatrics. *Pediatrics* 2007; 119(3): 631–637.
7 Johnson KB *et al*. Automated dose rounding recommendations for pediatric medications. *Pediatrics* 2011; 128: e422–e428.

31

Avoiding medication errors

A Fox

Introduction

The use of medication to treat disease, alleviate symptoms and prevent illness is the most common intervention utilised in healthcare. The vast majority of medication does not cause harm. However, all medicines carry some level of risk, and medication errors are a significant cause for concern. The true extent of medication errors in the National Health Service (NHS) is not known. Estimates for medication error rates in both adults and children are difficult to compare, due to the wide range of definition and data collection techniques used.[1]

In the UK, medication error has been defined by the National Patient Safety Agency (which is now within NHS England) as:

'A medication error is any preventable event that may cause or lead to inappropriate medication use or patient harm while the medication is in the control of the health care professional, patient, or consumer. Such events may be related to professional practice, health care products, procedures, and systems, including prescribing; order communication; product labelling, packaging, and nomenclature; compounding; dispensing; distribution; administration; education; monitoring; and use.'

Medication errors, therefore, are preventable, and most do not cause harm, e.g. a dispensing label describing the formulation as tablets rather than capsules. Some medication errors can cause an adverse drug reaction; e.g., if the wrong dose of a drug is prescribed and administered, there is an increased likelihood of a toxic effect if the dose is too high. These reactions, caused by a medication error, are preventable and are included within the definition above. However, a proportion of adverse drug reactions are idiosyncratic and therefore neither predictable nor preventable.

Medication errors are probably more common in children than in adults. The process of prescribing, dispensing and administering medicines to children has the added complexities of dose calculation, adult formulations and a greater use of unlicensed and off-label medicines.

This chapter will outline the causes of medication errors, focusing primarily on prescribing, and identify strategies for individuals to adopt in order to help avoid medication errors. Some organisational changes that can improve medication safety are also described; however, electronic prescribing and education are covered in other chapters.

The learning objectives of this chapter are:

➢ to understand the different types of medication error
➢ to recognise the core principles of good prescribing and their role in avoiding errors from the perspective of individual prescribers
➢ to identify important features that are specific to paediatric prescribing, such as dose rounding and complex calculations, which can be error prone
➢ to be aware that organisational changes can also improve medication safety.

Types of medication errors

To help understand how medication errors occur, it is important to have an understanding of their classification, which can be contextual, modal or psychological. Contextual classification relates to the time at which an error occurred and place where it occurred. Categories such as prescribing, dispensing and administration errors are commonly used to describe this. Modal classification describes the way in which an error occurs, e.g. by omission or substitution. The following psychological classification helps to explain events rather than being a pure description and is based on work by James Reason.[2] Some examples have been included along with simple strategies for prevention.

Knowledge-based error

A knowledge-based error is an error caused by lack of knowledge of the patient or drug (or both). Examples include prescribing gentamicin without taking into account the patient's reduced renal function, or prescribing a penicillin-containing antibiotic without knowing the patient's allergy status. These types of errors ought to be avoidable with adequate knowledge and access to reliable up-to-date information. Interception of such errors can occur by using computerised decision support and with cross-checking by pharmacists and nurses. Clearly, education and training have a major role to play in helping to avoid knowledge-based errors (see chapter 29).

Rule-based error

A rule-based error is the use of an inappropriate/bad rule or applying a rule in the wrong way. An example could be prescribing a solid formulation for a patient with a nasogastric tube when there is a suitable liquid alternative.

Action-based error

Action-based errors are often labelled as slips. The intended action is correct, but a slip in attention results in an error, e.g.: having the intention to prescribe cefotaxime but selecting cefuroxime on the electronic system drop-down menu; writing clonazepam instead of the intended clobazam; or picking up a bottle of sodium chloride oral solution instead of sodium bicarbonate. One way of helping to prevent these errors is to create conditions in which they are unlikely. In the example above, having different packaging and labelling for the two similar preparations, or stocking only the most commonly used preparation may help. Technical errors such as adding the wrong diluent to an injection or writing illegibly are also classed as action-based errors. They may be reduced by the use of checklists and reminders.

Memory-based errors

Often regarded as lapses, an example of a memory-based error might be forgetting to specify a maximum frequency for a prescription for paracetamol, or knowing a patient is allergic to penicillin but forgetting. These types of errors are hard to avoid and prevent, although some electronic prescribing systems have the functionality to reduce these types of errors.

Causes of medication errors in children

The most commonly reported medication error in children is wrong dose.[3] This is to be expected when the vast majority of doses need to be individualised using the patient's age, weight or in some instances body surface area. This increases the opportunity for error. In particular, the need to calculate a dose heightens the risk of mathematical errors and errors with decimal points, trailing zeros and various units of measure.

Added to this is the lack of appropriate commercially available formulations that enable children's doses to be easily administered. A lack of knowledge of these formulations and concentrations can also lead to significant dosing errors.

The lack of appropriate formulation can necessitate the use of an unlicensed medicine, or 'special'. These formulations may be used by a specific hospital, for example, and may not be readily available in the community. This can increase the risk of missed doses when the preparation is unavailable.

Unfamiliarity with the paediatric population has also been cited as contributing to medication errors in children.

Avoiding medication errors

This section details ways in which medication errors can be avoided both from an individual and organisational perspective.

Individual perspective

General principles of good prescribing

The following ten principles of good prescribing are included in a paper by Aronson.[4] They follow the natural process of prescribing and take into account the patient, the drug and the prescriber. They are completely generalisable to all prescribing.

1 **Indication:** Be clear about the reasons for prescribing, the risks and the benefits.
2 **History:** Take into account the patient's medication history (including over-the-counter medicines, alternative therapies (e.g. herbal remedies) and allergies).
3 **Diseases:** Take into account other factors/comorbidities that might alter the benefits and harms of treatment (renal function, etc.).
4 **Patient:** Take into account the patient's/carer's expectations and concerns.
5 **Effectiveness:** Select effective, safe and cost-effective medicine. Consider benefit versus harm, best formulation, dose regimen, individualisation, etc.
6 **Information:** Utilise national and local guidelines.
7 **Order:** Write clearly with an awareness of common mistakes that lead to error.
8 **Monitor:** Monitor the treatment.
9 **Communicate:** Ensure your prescribing decisions are clearly documented; take particular care in relation to healthcare interfaces.
10 **Knowledge:** Prescribe within the limitations of your knowledge.

Prescribing for children: additional measures

Bearing in mind the general principles above and the causes of medication errors in children, there are some specific points that must be considered when prescribing for children.

- **Age and weight:** Check that you have accurate and up-to-date information.
- **Dose rounding:** Round doses to an amount that can be easily administered yet is still suitable for the individual patient. Good knowledge of the available formulations is essential.
- **Units:** Prescribe using unambiguous units (e.g. micrograms not mcg). Avoid stating doses in volumes, since more than one concentration of a syrup/suspension may exist, increasing the chance of a dosing error.
- **Calculations:** Get complex calculations double-checked by someone else, and for critical or high risk medicines also document your calculations.

Administration

Nursing staff should utilise the six rights of medicine administration, ensuring the right:

- patient
- drug
- route
- dose
- frequency
- documentation.

In addition, responding to any patient queries in relation to the administration is paramount. Patients' concerns should be listened to and checks made with the prescriber.

Organisational perspective

Organisations can help to reduce the risk of medication errors by:

- Ensuring safe working environments (e.g. 'Do not disturb' signs during drug administration rounds)
- Having a paediatric clinical pharmacy service
- Providing access to regular training
- Using standardised equipment such as smart pumps
- Having a comprehensive medication error reporting system to allow recognition of local trends and learning
- Creating a safe culture in which questioning and checking are regarded as normal and in the patient's best interest
- Making available up-to-date prescribing information and resources

Conclusions

This chapter has defined medication errors and provided some background as to why they occur both generally and specifically in children. It has provided advice for individuals to help avoid prescribing errors and has outlined some organisational measures that can help to improve medication safety. In your own practice, it is recommended that you develop a habit of always following the principles of safe prescribing and encourage questioning and checking of your own and others' prescribing. It is also worth taking time to review your own prescribing and learn from errors, and ultimately take a role in leading organisational changes designed to improve medication safety.

References

1   Ghaleb MA *et al*. Systematic review of medication errors in pediatric patients. *Ann Pharmacother* 2006; 40(10): 1766–1776.
2   Reason J. Human error: models and management. *BMJ* 2000; 320(7237): 768–770.
3   National Patient Safety Agency. *Safety in Doses – Improving the use of medicines in the NHS*. London: National Patient Safety Agency, 2009.
4   Aronson JK. Medication errors: what they are, how they happen, and how to avoid them. *QJM* 2009; 102(8): 513–521.

Further recommended reading

Wong IC *et al*. Minimising medication errors in children. *Arch Dis Child* 2009; 94(2): 161–164.
Wong ICK *et al*. Incidence and nature of dosing errors in paediatric medications: A systematic review. *Drug Saf* 2004; 27(9): 661–670.

32

Intravenous medicines administration

J Haylor and N Christiansen

Introduction

Intravenous (IV) medicines are widely used in hospitalised children and increasingly common in ambulatory paediatric care as well. Knowledge about the safe and effective administration of IV medicines is therefore important for all those involved in paediatric healthcare, particularly doctors, nurses and pharmacists.

The learning objectives of this chapter are:

➢ to understand when IV drug administration is necessary in children
➢ to know the key factors that underpin the safety and efficacy of IV medications, including drug reconstitution, dilution, compatibility and stability, as well as rate and duration of administration
➢ to recognise the potential for serious drug errors when preparing or administering IV medications and the role of a centralised intravenous additive (CIVA) service in helping to prevent these.

Background

Preparations for IV administration are pyrogen free and contain the active drug as well as excipients to enable optimal manufacture and use. They may be in a form ready for administration, but often come as a concentrate or powder requiring reconstitution and dilution.

The decision to administer a drug intravenously is made if the enteral route is not available, if a rapid onset of action is required, or if a drug is not adequately absorbed or is destroyed when given enterally. In contrast to other routes, the IV route provides 100% bioavailability. Hence IV doses may be lower compared with those for other routes, particularly for drugs with high first-pass metabolism or low absorption. Absorption is immediate, leading to quicker onset of action and higher peak concentrations. For drugs with a short half-life or very narrow therapeutic index, a continuous infusion may be required. In general, IV access is more difficult in children compared with adults due to the smaller vessel size, and central lines rather than peripheral cannulas are used more commonly. Compared with other routes, parenteral administration is relatively costly as well as complex, and therefore should be limited to situations when other routes are not suitable. Especially in children, IV administration may also create pain and anxiety, and needle phobia is not uncommon. Distraction techniques, anaesthetic creams or cold sprays are therefore routinely used to minimise pain and discomfort during IV cannulation.

If IV administration is not possible, other parenteral routes of administration may be used to treat children. These include:

Subcutaneous (SC): The pain on administration is lower compared with IV access, but an access device such as an indwelling subcutaneous catheter may be used to reduce pain if repeat injections are required. For children, the appropriate size needle or pen tip must be used in order to ensure the drug is injected into the correct site.

Intramuscular (IM): The IM route can also be used if IV access is not possible, e.g. to deliver some systemic antibiotics such as ceftriaxone or when using adrenaline in an emergency. However, the muscle is less well perfused, resulting in slower absorption, particularly in neonates and infants, and due to the lower muscle mass IM administration can be particularly painful; therefore this route is mostly avoided.

Practicalities of administration

In order to deliver a medication intravenously, various factors need to be considered.

Access devices

Peripheral administration – This requires a device such as a cannula. Small amounts of fluid can be administered through this device, but if multiple injections or high flow rates are required, a more robust device is needed. The risk of harm on extravasation should be considered for each drug (see extravasation section later in this chapter).

Central administration – This requires a central venous access device such as a peripherally inserted central catheter (PICC), a tunnelled device (Hickman line) or a portacath. Central access should be used if there is a risk of harm on extravasation, if long term treatment is required or if multiple drugs are given concomitantly.

Duration of administration

Short bolus injections (3–5 minutes) for IV administration are preferable, as no infusion device is required. However, bolus administration is not possible if the drug has a very short half-life; the risk of adverse effects is increased with rapid administration or if constant drug levels need to be maintained.

Intermittent IV infusions are used when an injection would be likely to cause harm due to the high flow rate associated with a bolus, but where a constant drug blood level is not required. The duration of an infusion depends on the drug, but may range from 20 minutes to 8 hours and may be age dependent.

Continuous IV infusions are used for drugs with very short half-lives and where a constant level of drug is required to achieve the desired effect.

Rate of administration

The rate may be expressed in terms of dose over time (e.g. mg/min) or volume over time (e.g. mL/min).

Dose over time – This will be specified in dosage resources.

Volume over time – The patency of the venous access device and the accuracy of the infusion device should be taken into account here. The rate of drug administration is usually governed by local policies. For example, on a general paediatric ward, the local standard may be that a minimum volume rate of 10 mL/hour is required to maintain patency of the IV line. A standard volumetric pump may only be reliable down to 5 mL/hour. However, in paediatric or neonatal intensive care settings, the standard may be 1 mL/hour or 0.1 mL/hour respectively.

Reconstitution

Reconstitution is the addition of a solvent to a powder to form a solution. Instructions are provided by the manufacturer but differ among brands of the same drug, so it is important that the correct information is used.

On reconstitution, some powders will create a solution that has a greater volume than the volume of solvent added. The difference between the final volume of the solution and the volume of the solvent is called the displacement value. The relevance of the displacement value in clinical practice is dependent on the dose of the drug and what effect the displacement value may have on that dose.

Example (see Table 1) – a brand of vancomycin has a displacement value of 1.5 mL for a 500 mg vial and requires 10 mL solvent to be added to the powder during reconstitution. A dose of 180 mg is required.

Where the displacement value is used in practice, a 1.4% overdose is given due to rounding to measurable doses at each manipulation stage. Where the displacement value is not used, a 13% underdose is given to the patient.

Table 1 Example of reconstitution of vancomycin		
	Using the displacement value	Not using the displacement value
Volume of solution calculated	11.5 mL (correct)	10 mL (incorrect)
Concentration of solution calculated	43.5 mg/mL (correct)	50 mg/mL (incorrect)
Volume for 180 mg drawn up by IV giver	4.2 mL	3.6 mL
Actual dose given to the patient	182.5 mg	156.6 mg

There is some debate among paediatric hospitals about whether displacement values should be used or not. The answer lies in the clinical consequence of underdosing the patient unknowingly.

Dilution

Once reconstituted, the drug may need to be further diluted with an appropriate diluent before use. This may increase stability, reduce the risk of harm on extravasation, reduce side-effects or create a practical volume.

If appropriate, the manufacturer will specify a concentration range. In paediatrics, there are difficulties when the drug is not licensed for use in children, so the information provided by the manufacturer may not be sufficient. In these cases, the practitioner should seek advice from the local pharmacy department or other resources in order to obtain a concentration range.

Usually, sodium chloride 0.9% is used as a diluent, but other diluents may be specified by the manufacturer. Water for injections is unlikely to be used in practice as it can cause haemolysis and hyperkalaemia. Glucose may be preferred as a diluent where calorie input is clinically significant. Sodium chloride 0.18% with glucose 4% should not be used as a diluent in children, following a National Patient Safety Agency (NPSA) alert on hyponatraemia.[1]

If a very small dose requires a significant dilution, it may be necessary to carry this out in multiple stages. This is usually called a double dilution.

The IV access device should be flushed using a compatible flushing solution (usually the same as the diluent) pre and post administration, unless significant harm to the patient would be caused if the amount of drug left in the line post administration were flushed through too quickly.

Flushing solutions must be prescribed. Medication errors have included flushing high strength heparin instead of low strength heparin, and high strength potassium chloride instead of sodium chloride. Strategies are now in place to avoid these errors.[2]

Compatibility

Ideally, when giving multiple IV infusions at the same time, each infusion should be run through a separate lumen of the IV access device. If two different infusions are given through the same lumen, they mix, potentially resulting in loss of potency, toxicity or precipitation.

In paediatric practice, a child may require multiple infusions but have very limited IV access. Here concomitant infusion through the same lumen is often the only practical solution.

Manufacturers may provide some data on compatibility; however, this is often limited. Other resources on compatibilities are available (see references). Yet, data are often still scarce. In the absence of any evidence, an individual decision based on the best interests of the patient has to be taken. Some basic rules are that drugs should not normally be added to blood products, mannitol, sodium bicarbonate or parenteral nutrition.[3] Drugs that have opposing pHs should never be mixed, as it is likely a salt would be formed.

Stability

The stability of an IV drug is dependent on:

- temperature
- pH
- exposure to light
- concentration.

The manufacturer will specify how long a solution will be stable for once reconstituted or diluted. If a drug is prepared or stored differently to the manufacturer's instructions, advice should be sought from the manufacturer or local pharmacy department. If in doubt, the product should be discarded.

Infusion device

Available infusion devices include burette sets, infusion pumps and syringe drivers. Use will vary depending on local contracts and preferences.

In paediatric practice, in order to facilitate administration, the drug often needs to be further diluted or manipulated in some way to produce a solution in a syringe or bag that can be given via an infusion device. The accuracy of the infusion device should always be taken into account when deciding the rate and volume of the infusion. Further information on infusion devices is available at https://www.gov.uk/government/uploads/system/uploads/attachment_data/file/403420/Infusion_systems.pdf.

Adverse effects

Adverse effects associated with the administration of an IV drug that would not be associated with oral administration are usually rate dependent.

Rate dependent reactions include red man syndrome (vancomycin) or convulsions (very high dose penicillins). Premedications may be given, and the reduction in infusion rate will avoid the chance of a reaction.

Extravasation refers to the leakage of a vesicant drug out of the IV access device or vein and into the surrounding tissue. This causes harm (blisters, severe tissue damage or necrosis) if the drug has:

- high/low pH (below 5 or above 9)
- high osmolality (above 600 mOsmol/L)
- vasoconstrictive action (inotropes)
- cytotoxicity (some drugs can bind the DNA in the surrounding tissue, causing further harm).

The safest way to avoid harm on extravasation is to deliver the drug via a central venous access device. If this is not practical, some strategies can be used to reduce the risk of harm:

- **pH** – Excipients such as sodium bicarbonate or buffers can be added to increase the pH of the drug. However, the effect on the stability of the drug itself should be taken into account, as adding bicarbonate to an acidic drug could also create a salt and render the injection useless.
- **Osmolality** – Diluting the drug will reduce the osmolality; however, stability information on the concentration needs to be considered.

Excipients in IV preparations

As well as the active drug, IV preparations also contain excipients, e.g. solvents, preservatives and stabilisers (see chapter 25). These excipients are supposedly inert, and their use is regulated. The guidelines issued by the Committee for Medicinal Products for Human Use[4] state that the excipients to be used in formulations for the paediatric population should be carefully selected, taking into account different age groups. However, as many preparations used are not necessarily licensed in paediatrics or were licensed prior to the new EU Paediatric Regulation, IV preparations prescribed in the paediatric setting may contain excipients known to be harmful (such as benzyl alcohol, polyoxyl castor oil and propylene glycol). Additionally, available safety data are often based on adult data, and information relating to the suitability and safety of excipients in the paediatric population is often missing.[5] For example, the use of benzoic acid, sodium benzoate and benzyl alcohol as preservatives in IV preparations must be avoided in low birth weight infants, as it can result in severe metabolic acidosis and neurological deterioration and may be fatal.

IV drug errors

In most cases, preparation of IV medication takes place immediately prior to administration and involves a number of steps, including dissolving, dilution and transfer to other containers. Particularly in paediatrics, calculations based on the individual patient's weight and dose add further to the complexities, leading to the frequent use of part vials and serial dilutions. A UK study in paediatric inpatients has shown that 13.2% of all prescriptions written contain an error, and in 19.1% an administration error is made, with incorrect IV administration rates being the second most common error.[6] Additionally, incidents in the prescribing, preparation and administration of IV medication have been shown to be higher than for other routes.[7,8]

One way to minimise preparation errors is through the provision of a centralised intravenous additive (CIVA) service, delivering ready to use injections or infusions. Many pharmacy departments provide this, but often only for a limited number of drugs. (Medication errors are discussed in chapter 31.)

In recognition of the risks relating to injectable medicines, the NPSA issued an alert in 2007, providing guidance on how to minimise harm from IV medication.[9] Strategies to reduce harm from medication incidents related to IV drugs should be created and implemented at all levels. National strategies such as the 'never events' programme used within the National Health Service (NHS) ensure that local NHS trusts have protocols in place to avoid certain errors at all times.[10]

In the UK, the Neonatal and Paediatric Pharmacist Group has teamed up with Medusa, an injectable medicines guide, to develop and provide access to a resource of IV administration monographs for paediatrics, which is available online.[11] There are also books available with additional details on injectable medications, which can provide valuable supplementary information.[12]

Conclusions

Ensuring IV medicines are administered in a safe and effective way is essential in paediatric healthcare and requires that knowledge and skills are kept up to date through clinical practice. The advent of new technology, including so-called 'smart' infusion pumps, means continuing professional development and training is increasingly important. Standardised paediatric drug administration guidelines and monographs increase the safety of these procedures. It is recommended that healthcare professionals always seek senior supervision if asked to prepare or administer IV drugs that they are not familiar with.

References

1   National Patient Safety Agency. Reducing the risk of hyponatraemia when administering intravenous infusions to children, patient safety alert NPSA/2007/22. NPSA, 2007.
2   National Patient Safety Agency. Intravenous heparin flush solutions, Rapid Response Report NPSA/2008/RRR002. NPSA, 2008.
3   Paediatric Formulary Committee. *BNF for Children*. London: BMJ Group, the Royal Pharmaceutical Society of Great Britain and RCPCH Publications Ltd, 2017.
4   European Medicines Agency. Committee for Medicinal Products for Human Use (CHMP): Reflection paper: formulations of choice for the paediatric population, EMEA/CHMP/PEG/194810/2005. London: European Medicines Agency, 2006.
5   Strickley RG *et al*. Pediatric drugs – a review of commercially available oral formulations. *J Pharm Sci* 2008; 97(5): 1731–1774.
6   Ghaleb MA *et al*. The incidence and nature of prescribing and medication administration errors in paediatric patients. *Arch Dis Chil* 2010; 95: 113–118.
7   Taxis K, Barber N. Ethnographic study of incidence and severity of intravenous medicine errors. *Br Med J* 2003; 326: 684–687
8   Cousins DH *et al*. Medication errors in intravenous medicine preparation and administration: a multicentre audit in the UK, Germany and France. *Qual Saf Health Care* 2005; 14: 190–195.
9   National Patient Safety Agency. Promoting safer use of injectable medicines, patient safety alert NPSA/2007/20. NPSA, 2007.
10 NHS Improvement. Never Events policy and framework: Revised January 2018. Available at: https://improvement.nhs.uk/documents/2265/Revised_Never_Events_policy_and_framework_FINAL.pdf [last accessed 2 March 2018].
11 Medusa. *Injectable Medicines Guide*. Available at: http://medusa.wales.nhs.uk/HomeAbout.asp [last accessed 2 March 2018].
12 Trissel, LA, ed. *Handbook on Injectable Drugs*, 17th edn. American Society of Health-System Pharmacists. 2012.

Further recommended reading

Medicines and Healthcare products Regulatory Agency. Infusion systems. December 2013. Available at: https://www.gov.uk/government/uploads/system/uploads/attachment_data/file/403420/Infusion_systems.pdf [last accessed 2 March 2018].
NHS Improvement. Never Events list 2018. Available at: https://improvement.nhs.uk/uploads/documents/Never_Events_list_2018_FINAL_v2.pdf [last accessed 2 March 2018].

33

Team working in medicines administration

E Bolton and S Conroy

Introduction

Team working is essential to optimise paediatric medicines management and healthcare. It enables the skills and expertise of different healthcare professionals and family members to be combined and utilised to improve patient outcomes and provide seamless care.[1,2] For effective team working a clear understanding of the work of fellow healthcare professionals and how they contribute to medicines management is needed, thereby enabling a more holistic approach to patient care.

The learning objectives of this chapter are:

> to understand the distinct roles of each healthcare professional in improving medicines management for children
> to recognise the importance of all key individuals in the delivery of paediatric medicines management.

Team working

By working as a team, doctors, pharmacists, nurses, dieticians and other healthcare professionals can provide seamless patient care. The knowledge of each professional must be recognised as a key component of the whole healthcare package.

There are various factors that support team working, including:[1,2]

- keeping the patients at the centre of all healthcare delivery and involving them in the decision-making process
- having a common goal: provision of safe and effective drug therapy
- team members having a personal commitment to achieving the goal
- clear roles and responsibilities of individual team members
- all involved focusing on outcomes that are important to the patient
- recognising and valuing the roles of others.

Some barriers also exist that can reduce effective team working:

- Presence of hierarchical boundaries, where certain members consider their roles to be superior or inferior to those of others
- Poor communication and information sharing within the team

However, it is important to always remember the numerous benefits of team working:

- Accessibility to the expertise and contributions of different healthcare professionals, which should improve the patient experience and outcome
- The opportunity for co-working on medicines management improvement projects and clinical audits
- Sharing ideas and learning from each other
- Establishing trust and strengthening working relationships
- Seeing and tackling problems from different perspectives
- Working more effectively and efficiently with one another
- Breaking down organisational barriers and improving communication

Roles and responsibilities of team members

Pharmacists

The paediatric pharmacist's knowledge of pharmacokinetics, pharmacodynamics, dosing and toxicity of drugs in children is essential to being a key player in the paediatric multidisciplinary team. The pharmacist is equipped to lead on many aspects of medicines management.

Interventions by paediatric clinical pharmacists have been shown to reduce medication errors.[3,4] Such interventions may be made by a ward-based pharmacist either screening drug charts or reviewing computerised physician order entries remotely.

Ward-based pharmacists can influence clinical decisions at the point of prescribing during medical ward rounds,[5] and they can also be available to provide general medicines information or formulation and administration advice during nurse administration rounds.

Pharmacists working with doctors and nurses can develop paediatric drug formularies and guidelines to provide information on drug doses, administration and formulations available, based on the best current evidence, as discussed elsewhere in this book (chapter 28 and chapter 34).

The increased presence of clinical pharmacists on the wards provides direct access to other healthcare professionals, principally doctors and nurses, and the opportunity to provide proactive advice and training in real time rather than retrospectively.

Working together with clinical staff, parents and children, pharmacists can ensure that medicines supplied to their patients are in formulations suitable for administration and acceptable to the patients, with minimum impact on children's education and lifestyle. This is particularly important for children with chronic conditions.

Medicines prescribed for children are not always licensed for use in this population or often not available as suitable licensed formulations.[6,7] Licensed medications may also be prescribed off label, i.e. used for an indication outside the terms of the licence. Formulations of such drugs may not be always be suitable for administration in children, especially neonates; e.g. intravenous (IV) drugs intended for adult administration may contain excipients not suitable for neonates, e.g. benzyl alcohol (see chapter 23).[8]

Likewise, unlicensed or off-label oral medication may also contain unsuitable excipients or have a high sugar or ethanol content. Phenobarbital liquid BP contains 38% w/v alcohol, is very bitter and not appropriate for use in neonates or older children. In practice, solid dose formulations are crushed and dispersed in water for administration, or alcohol-free extemporaneous preparations may be compounded by a pharmacist or special manufacturing units. Medication with high sugar content can promote tooth decay, particularly in children with chronic conditions or where drugs have to be administered at night.[9,10] Where possible, sugar free formulations should be provided.

It is sometimes necessary to administer doses as fractions of solid dose medication such as capsules or tablets where a liquid preparation is not available. The pharmacist is key to providing advice on how to manipulate and administer such formulations, which may need to be crushed or divided, and also on the stability of resulting products. In addition, the resulting preparations are not always acceptable to the patient, and it may be necessary to mix them with suitable fruit juice, puree or a small amount of soft food, while retaining pharmacological activity. Pharmacists working together with medical and nursing staff play an important role in facilitating adherence in order to avoid treatment failure.

The preparation of IV infusions in children and neonates often requires complex calculations and the dilution of preparations designed for adults. Tenfold errors have occurred following wrong calculations or misplacement of decimal points during preparation of such infusions.[11] Pharmacists working with medical and nursing staff can provide practical information and simplified guidelines with standardised dilutions in order to minimise the calculations needed. Alternatively, or in addition, where there are manufacturing facilities available a centralised additive service can prepare IV doses in a controlled and clean environment.[11]

Discharge planning should also involve the whole team, including pharmacists, at an early stage to ensure that information on administration as well as supply of complex medication is provided. The pharmacist can counsel parents on drug administration and coordinate plans for further supply of medication for patients with chronic conditions.

Patients prescribed unlicensed medication may have difficulty in procuring supplies of the medication in the community after discharge. The pharmacist also has an important role to play to ensure continuing supply of medication and should ensure that this is discussed during discharge planning.[12] Information for the GP and community pharmacist regarding monitoring of therapy and information on how to procure medication should be communicated in a timely fashion in writing and also verbally if possible/appropriate. It is also important to counsel parents regarding drugs that are not easily obtainable and the importance of ensuring that new supplies are ordered in a timely manner.

Doctors

Doctors have clear responsibilities in ensuring safe and effective use of medicines in children. When selecting a drug, consideration must be given to possible effects on growth and cognitive development as well as other potential adverse effects. These possible risks must be weighed against the benefits of therapy.

The use of off-label and unlicensed medication must be based on current best clinical practice, the evidence base for which may be lacking (see chapter 28). In such cases, the pharmacist working with the prescriber should evaluate the drug based on current best practice or any anecdotal evidence to decide the safest and most effective dose.

Adverse drug reactions (ADRs) (chapter 10) can differ in children compared with adults. All healthcare professionals have a responsibility to report ADRs; in the UK this is done through the Medicines and Healthcare products Regulatory Agency (MHRA; www.gov.uk/government/organisations/medicines-and-healthcare-products-regulatory-agency). In the UK, parents can also submit reports. Spontaneous reporting of ADRs is an important source of information regarding safety of drugs in children, especially about unlicensed and off-label medications.

Nurses

Nurses maintain the most amount of contact time with the children and their parents. It is important to involve the family actively in the patient's care and endeavour to dispel any anxieties that parents may have about the treatment of their child.

The nurse also has a role in ensuring that parents understand what medication their child is having and the reason for prescribing the drug. A better understanding of the importance of the medication in treating chronic conditions can improve adherence.

During their hospital stay, the parents of the patient should be educated in the administration of the drugs to the child and observed when they do so. Where possible, children should be empowered to take responsibility for their own medication as well.[10] Working with the pharmacist, nurses should provide written information for patients, particularly regarding complex regimens.

Nurses can develop strategies to teach young children and even adolescents how to swallow tablets, where suitable palatable liquid preparations are not available. The nursing team can involve the play specialist for patients with needle phobias or patients struggling with complex medicine regimens.

Doctors, nurses and pharmacists work together to identify any patients who are having problems with their prescribed medicines and to work out means of overcoming such challenges. This sometimes requires dose adjustments or the choice of alternative drugs, formulations, brands or concentrations.

Discharge plans should include a review of the medications required at discharge, methods of administration and any compliance aids or measuring devices required for administration of medication. Advice and action plans on what to do in the event of a missed dose or if the patient vomits a critical drug, e.g. an anticonvulsant, should also be provided.

Nurses can discuss with the pharmacist if there are any issues around palatability, so as to source alternatives if available, and ensure timings of any drug administration do not interfere with the normal activities of daily living. Where a patient is to be discharged on a parenteral medication, e.g. an antibiotic, the nurse will provide training and ensure that parents are competent in administration before discharge.

Nurses should be trained on the importance of pharmacovigilance, as they are in a position to see ADRs when they occur.

Nurses must check prescriptions when administering medication, to ensure doses are correct and also that the appropriate drug has been prescribed and supplied – i.e. that the basic principles of drug administration are adhered to, the six 'rights': right patient, right drug, right dose, right route, right time and right documentation.

Nurses play a key role in identification and avoidance of errors made by other professionals, as they are often the final barrier in preventing a medication error reaching a patient.

Double-checking processes are often used in drug administration to children to reduce the risk of errors occurring; however, there is insufficient evidence to support or oppose this. It is vital that the roles and responsibilities of both checkers are clearly defined in order for this to improve safety.

Example scenarios

Below we illustrate some of the pertinent points using two scenarios.

Case presentation 1

A 12-year-old boy diagnosed with cystic fibrosis as an infant is admitted to the paediatric ward with a 2 day history of respiratory symptoms of increasing difficulty in breathing and pyrexia. On admission, he is started empirically on IV antibiotics according to the local policy agreed between microbiology, paediatricians and pharmacists.

On the second day of admission, he is reviewed by the medical team and a care plan is made which includes the duration of his antibiotic therapy. The pharmacist includes a plan for monitoring plasma drug levels, with advice for the levels needed and recommendations for dose adjustment if necessary. IV drugs are provided by the pharmacy's centralised IV additive service in a form that is ready to administer, in order to reduce the manipulations and calculations needed at ward level.

By day three, the boy has responded to treatment and has been apyrexial for 24 hours but needs to complete a 2 week course of antibiotics. His parents would like to complete this course at home rather than the boy stay in hospital. They have been trained to administer IV antibiotics by nursing staff and have done this in the past. The pharmacist will liaise with the nursing staff to ensure that the parents are still competent in administration.

The pharmacist is contacted to organise the supply of IV antibiotics and also other discharge medication required. The pharmacist organises for the medication to be supplied and delivered to the family by a homecare company as ready prepared doses in ambulatory infuser devices. These devices are non-electric, pump free and also needle free, allowing the safe administration of IV medication in the home environment. Pharmaceutical waste accrued during the course of IV antibiotics is disposed of by the homecare company.

Before discharge, arrangements are made by the specialist nurse team in liaison with the ward nursing and medical staff for the community team to visit the patient at home to take blood samples to monitor drug levels.

Case presentation 2

A 9-year-old boy with refractory epilepsy is admitted with increased seizure frequency and a 2 day history of respiratory symptoms with increased work of breathing. He is diagnosed with a lower respiratory tract infection and started on IV antibiotics. The medical team also requests plasma assays of one of his drugs – phenytoin – due to the increased seizure frequency.

A drug history taken by the pharmacist confirms that the patient is on several drugs for managing his seizure disorder and has been recently commenced on a ketogenic diet to manage his increasingly refractory disorder. Referral to a drug history taken during a previous admission indicates that the patient has inadvertently been provided with the lower strength of phenytoin formulation in the community. The patient normally has an unlicensed preparation of a higher strength of phenytoin. The results of the blood test show subtherapeutic levels of his medication. The medication is prescribed at the correct dose and the patient's mother is counselled on the importance of maintaining the same brand for all of her son's antiepileptic drugs.

The patient shows significant improvement after 2 days, and the medical team decides to switch his course of IV antibiotics to oral to complete a 7 day course and plans to discharge him. The pharmacist is contacted by the medical team to recommend the most appropriate oral formulation for administration, due to the patient's dietary requirements.

The ketogenic diet is a low carbohydrate, high fat and moderate protein diet that promotes ketosis. Oral antibiotic suspensions may contain large amounts of sugars, which may affect ketosis if taken regularly for a period of time. The pharmacist can provide information on antibiotics with low dosing frequency, i.e. twice daily instead of four times daily, and provide a sugar free formulation containing a non-nutritive sweetener if possible; where this cannot be done, the pharmacist working with the dietician will determine whether the carbohydrate content is significant enough to affect ketosis. Adjustments may be required to the diet while the patient is on oral antibiotics, with increased monitoring of ketosis. The alternatives may be to provide solid dose formulations if the patient is competent in swallowing tablets or capsules, as these have a lower carbohydrate content than liquid preparations. An oral formulation requiring once-daily administration is recommended by the pharmacist.

Conclusions

The cases above highlight the specialist and mutually beneficial roles that the different members of the multidisciplinary team play in the care of hospitalised children. The common goal of improved patient outcomes should drive positive team work in the healthcare setting, to optimise the safe and effective use of medicines in children. The key to effective team working is that all members understand their roles and also recognise and respect the roles of others.

References

1   Carson C *et al*. Medicines optimisation: the safe and effective use of medicines to enable the best possible outcomes. NICE Medicines and Prescribing Centre. 2015. Available at: https://www.nice.org.uk/guidance/ng5 [last accessed 2 March 2018].
2   Borrill C *et al*. *Team Working and Effectiveness in Health Care. Findings from the Health Care Team Effectiveness Project*.

3   Cullingham KJ. Analysis of clinical interventions and the impact of pediatric pharmacists on medication error prevention in a teaching hospital. *J Pediatr Pharmacol Ther* 2012; 17(4): 365–373.

4   Fernandez-Llamazare CM *et al*. Impact of clinical pharmacists interventions in reducing paediatric prescribing errors. *Arch Dis Child* 2012; 97(6): 564–568.

5   Miller G *et al*. Including pharmacists on consultant-led ward rounds: a prospective non-randomised controlled trial. *Clin Med* 2011; 11(4): 312–316.

6   Conroy S *et al*. Survey of unlicensed and off label drug use in paediatric wards in European countries. *BMJ* 2000; 320: 79–81.

7   Turner S *et al*. Unlicensed and off label drug use in paediatric wards: prospective study. *BMJ* 1998; 316(7128): 343–345.

8   American Academy of Pediatrics Committee on Fetus and Newborn, and Committee on Drugs. Benzyl alcohol: toxic agent in neonatal units. *Paediatrics* 1983; 72: 356.

9   Bigeard L. The role of medication and sugars in pediatric dental patients. *Dent Clin North Am* 2000; 44: 443–456.

10 Department of Health. *National Service Framework for Children, Young People and Maternity Services. Medicines for Children and Young People*. London: Department of Health, 2004.

11 Conroy S *et al*. Medication errors in a children's hospital. *Paediatr Perinat Drug Ther* 2007; 8(1): 18–25.

12 Barry M, Semple D. Impact of hospital pharmacists on the paediatric discharge process. *Arch Dis Child* 2014; 99: 1136.

Further recommended reading

Alsulami Z *et al*. Double checking the administration of medicines: what is the evidence? A systematic review. *Arc Dis Child* 2012; 97: 833–837.

Choonara I, Rieder MJ. Drug toxicity and adverse drug reactions in children – a brief historical review. *Paediatr Perinat Drug Ther* 2001; 5(1): 12–18.

Choonara I. Direct reporting of suspected adverse drug reactions by patients. *J R Soc Med* 2004; 97(7): 316–317.

Medicines and Healthcare products Regulatory Agency (MHRA) Commission on Human Medicines. Antiepileptic drugs: new advice on switching between different manufacturers' products for a particular drug. MHRA, November 2013.

Conroy S *et al*. Use of checking systems in medicines administration with children and young people. *Nurs Child Young People* 2012; 24(3): 20–24.

Department of Health. Building a safer NHS for patients – Improving medication safety. London: Department of Health, 2004.

Picton C, Wright H. *Medicines Optimisation: Helping patients to make the most of their medication. Good practise guidance for healthcare professionals*. London: Royal Pharmaceutical Society, May 2013.

Priyadharsini R *et al*. A study of adverse drug reactions in paediatrics. *J Pharmacol Pharmacother* 2011; 2(4): 277–280.

Walson PD *et al*. Principles of drug prescribing in infants and children. A practical guide. *Drugs* 1993; 46(2): 281–288.

34

Evidence-based formularies

A Gwee and N Cranswick

Introduction

Evidence-based formularies provide a one-stop, up-to-date resource for prescribers and are essential for achieving safe, effective prescribing. They allow comparison of efficacy and side-effects of medications, and provide treatment alternatives, typically including a minimum of two drugs in each class.[1] Currently, off-label prescriptions in children are common practice, and paediatric specific dosing and safety data are often lacking.[2] Some dosing recommendations provide information extrapolated from adult data, with the potential for errors.

The existing evidence to guide paediatric prescribing is limited, and dedicated research into drug pharmacokinetics, pharmacodynamics and safety of medications specifically in children is required. This concept underpins the 'better medicines for children' resolution passed by the World Health Assembly in 2007.

The objectives of this chapter are:

➢ to understand the principles of development of evidence-based formularies
➢ to understand the role of evidence-based formularies
➢ to know the key evidence-based formularies available for children.

Principles of development

What is a formulary?

Formularies are handbooks that contain up-to-date clinically relevant drug references. Included medications are usually tailored to country specific or institution specific disease prevalence and the availability and affordability of medications.[3] Formularies should include information on indications for treatment, dosing, adverse effects and potential drug interactions of medications, with alphabetised drug monographs.

Principles for evidence-based formularies

The development of drug formularies requires critical appraisal of the available evidence, specifically relating to efficacy, cost-effectiveness and quality of evidence:[1]

- **Efficacy:** Preference is given to drugs that confer a survival benefit or reduce morbidity. Drug efficacy must be consistent, accounting for intra-individual and inter-individual variability.
- **Cost-effectiveness:** Pharmacoeconomic models are used to determine cost-effectiveness of drugs. The lowest-cost medication is often recommended as first line therapy, with a higher-cost alternative provided for failure of first line therapy. Consideration must also be given to long versus short term indications for medications.
- **Quality of evidence:** Comparative studies and, specifically, those comparing the drug with a placebo or with the current standard therapy are preferred.

Processes for addition of new drugs to formularies

In many hospitals, drug and therapeutic committees oversee the development of hospital-based formularies and approve the addition of new drugs.[4]

Both nationally and internationally, these processes are not standardised, and studies have shown that the process is often hindered by inadequate documentation and limited evaluation of evidence, specifically pertaining to evaluation of bias and safety.[5,6,7]

If a medication has dosing information in an evidence-based formulary, most physicians can safely assume that the use of the medicine is evidence based, even if the recommendation is off label. Not all formularies clearly indicate which drugs are off label, and this is also country specific – i.e. labels vary between countries, depending on the national drug regulation.

A formulary leveraged improved prescribing tool (FLIP tool) has been developed to evaluate formulary drug applications.[8] This tool highlights six considerations when evaluating a new drug application:

1 **Evidence of need:** burden of disease and efficacy of existing therapies
2 **Efficacy:** comparative efficacy of the new drug compared with existing therapies as well as level of evidence
3 **Safety:** available safety data, monitoring and precautions required for use
4 **Misuse impact potential:** potential for widespread off-label usage
5 **Cost:** comparative cost of drug, including costs for drug monitoring
6 **Decision-making information, calculations, timing and process:** review by other formulary committees, awareness of committee bias, use restrictions required

This tool shifts the onus for providing efficacy and safety data onto the person applying for modification of the existing drug formulary, thus avoiding the addition of expensive drugs for which risk and benefit are as yet undetermined.

Role of evidence-based formularies

Drug formularies have a role in the following:[3]

Drug information/education resources

Formularies provide objective, accurate and up-to-date evidence. A formulary is developed by a panel of clinicians with expertise in drugs and therapeutics. For medications where data are lacking, guidance on the safe use of medications is provided. As prescribing is standardised through a rigorous process and an expert body of opinion, individual clinicians are protected from litigation.[9] Access to an impartial drug resource is also important, as the influence of physician interactions with the pharmaceutical industry on requesting addition of drugs to hospital formularies has been demonstrated in a number of studies.[10]

Safer prescribing

Emphasis on judicious prescribing is central to evidence-based formularies. Drug formularies have been shown to influence prescribing practice and, specifically, to limit the number of different drug prescriptions.[11] In many instances, there is more than one treatment option for common conditions. Therefore, choice of medication relates to the clinician's knowledge of the comparative effectiveness of drugs. This information is considered in drug formulary recommendations and, therefore, formularies regulate drug prescriptions. Furthermore, use of drug formularies and drug utilisation databases is vital in assessing post-marketing comparative effectiveness of drugs.

Up to 90% of prescriptions for children are off label.[2] As data for off-label prescriptions may be extrapolated from adults, the use of these medications carries the risk of exposing a child to adverse effects and potentially ineffective treatment. A US study reported that 73% of off-label prescriptions by office-based physicians were evidence based.[12] It is important to differentiate between off-label prescriptions with high quality evidence versus exceptional use of a drug for a serious underlying condition. Off-label prescriptions for exceptional use raise ethical issues and require approval by a drug and therapeutics committee. It is advised that in these cases, written informed consent from the patient and/or family is obtained.[2]

Cost-effective drug utilisation

Selection of drugs for inclusion in formularies takes into account availability and accessibility of drugs. Therefore, formularies restrict the use of expensive drugs for which safety and efficacy data are limited, to allow for access to essential evidence-based medicines.[1]

Careful implementation of drug formularies is required, as they have been criticised for increasing clinicians' workloads, inhibiting autonomy and placing too much importance on drug costs.[8] These are potential barriers to physician use. Acceptance of such a resource must be given by drug and therapeutic committees with paediatric expertise.

Key evidence-based formularies available for children

There are a number dedicated paediatric evidence-based formularies currently available, including:

- *WHO Model Formulary for Children 2010*, which was first developed in 2002. A paediatric specific formulary was developed in 2010. The model formulary includes information on dosing for medications listed on the World Health Organization Essential Medicines List 2009 and is used in children up to 12 years of age. This is available online at www.who.int/selection_medicines/list/WMFc_2010.pdf.
- *British National Formulary for Children* (BNFC), which was developed in 2005 and is updated every 4 months.[13] This evolved from the *British National Formulary* (BNF) *Medicines for Children*, which was the first evidence-based national formulary for the UK.
- *Pediatric and Neonatal Dosage Handbook* (American Pharmacists Association), which is primarily used in North America.
- *AMH Children's Dosing Companion* is the first Australian national formulary for children. (The AMH is the *Australian Medicines Handbook*.) It currently has a limited number of medications lists and is aimed at primary care physicians.

Conclusions

Evidence-based paediatric formularies are essential for safe, effective, and economic prescribing in children. The frequency of off-label prescriptions in paediatric practice can be addressed through the use of formularies, which highlight the areas in which further research is needed in children.

References

1 Simon GE *et al*. Principles for evidence-based drug formulary policy. *J Gen Intern Med* 2005; 20(10): 964–968.
2 Gazarian M *et al*. Off-label use of medicines: consensus recommendations for evaluating appropriateness. *Med J Aust* 2006; 185(10): 544–548.
3 Organization WH. *How to Develop a National Formulary Based on the WHO Model Formulary – A Practical Guide*. http://apps.who.int/medicinedocs/en/d/Js6171e/2.2.html.
4 Organization WH. *Drugs and Therapeutics Committees – A Practical Guide*. http://apps.who.int/medicinedocs/pdf/s4882e/s4882e.pdf.
5 Sinha YK *et al*. A national study of the processes and outcomes of paediatric formulary applications in Australia. *Medical J Aust* 2014; 200(9): 541–545.
6 Plet HT *et al*. Drug and therapeutics committees in Danish hospitals: a survey of organization, activities and drug selection procedures. *Basic Clin Pharmacol Toxicol* 2013; 112(4): 264–269.
7 Mittmann N, Knowles S. A survey of pharmacy and therapeutic committees across Canada: scope and responsibilities. *Can J Clin Pharmacol* 2009; 16(1): e171–177.
8 Schiff GD *et al*. A prescription for improving drug formulary decision making. *PLoS Med* 2012; 9(5): 1–7.
9 Stephenson T. The medicines for children agenda in the UK. *Br J Clin Pharmacol* 2006; 61(6): 716–719.
10 Chren MM, Landefeld CS. Physicians' behavior and their interactions with drug companies. A controlled study of physicians who requested additions to a hospital drug formulary. *JAMA* 1994; 271(9): 684–689.
11 Avery AJ *et al*. Do prescribing formularies help GPs prescribe from a narrower range of drugs? A controlled trial of the introduction of prescribing formularies for NSAIDs. *Br J Gen Pract* 1997; 47(425): 810–814.
12 Radley DC *et al*. Off-label prescribing among office-based physicians. *Arch Intern Med* 2006; 166(9): 1021–1026.
13 Lenney W. The development of a national children's formulary. *Br J Clin Pharmacol* 2013; 79(3): 441–445.

Further recommended reading

Glassman PA *et al*. Physician perceptions of a national formulary. *Am J Manag Care* 2001; 7(3): 241–251.
Lexchin J. Interactions between physicians and the pharmaceutical industry: what does the literature say? *CMAJ* 1993; 149(10): 1401–1047.
Rosenau PV *et al*. U.S. pharmacy policy: a public health perspective on safety and cost. *Soc Work Public Health* 2009; 24(6): 543–567.
Schiff GD *et al*. Principles of conservative prescribing. *Arch Intern Med* 2011; 171(16): 1433–1440.
Schneeweiss S. Developments in post-marketing comparative effectiveness research. *Clin Pharmacol Ther* 2007; 82(2): 143–156.

35

Therapeutic drug monitoring

NA Caldwell and OA Cuevas

Introduction

'*Treat the patient, not the level.*' Therapeutic drug monitoring (TDM) involves measuring drug concentrations, usually in plasma, serum or blood. The results are then utilised to adjust the patient's dosage regimen so that drug concentrations can be maintained within a target range.[1] The target therapeutic range gives an indication of a drug concentration that is more likely, but not guaranteed, to produce the desired pharmacological effect while minimising adverse effects.

'*Drugs don't have doses, patients do.*' The primary focus of dose individualisation must be on clinical effect, informed where appropriate by a serum drug concentration. While TDM increases the likelihood of selecting the correct dose of medicine for a child, you should only measure drug concentrations if it will influence how you treat a child; do not measure just because you can.

This chapter aims to provide background information on what to consider when reviewing serum drug concentrations in children and, by doing so, increase the chance of achieving the desired clinical effect.[2]

The learning objectives of this chapter are:

➤ to appreciate the necessity of an accurate dosing history when interpreting serum drug concentrations
➤ to be able to describe which drugs require serum concentration monitoring, and why, when, how and where to measure serum concentrations
➤ to recognise why predicted and measured drug concentrations often differ.

Why do you need an accurate history when interpreting serum drug concentrations?

'*All serum drug concentrations are historical and do not necessarily predict the future.*' If it were possible to accurately predict drug concentrations, it would not be necessary to measure them. Always take care to gather a comprehensive and complete picture of what preceded the reported serum drug concentration. High concentrations do not always require dose reduction, and low concentrations do not always require a dose increase.

All drug concentrations are sampled after administration of a dose or doses of a medicine. Each measurement is the sum of the doses of medicine given within the last 5 half-lives. Half-life describes the time required for the serum concentrations to fall by 50%. This influences the time for both drug clearance and accumulation.

Consider a drug with a half-life of 8 hours:

- A dose 8 hours ago will contribute 50% to a measured concentration.
- A dose 16 hours ago will contribute 25%.
- A dose 24 hours ago will contribute 12.5%.
- A dose 32 hours ago will contribute 6.3%.
- A dose 40 hours ago will contribute 3.1%.
- A dose 48 hours ago will contribute 1.6%.

Doses given more than 5 half-lives previously will contribute little to measured concentrations.

Note also that for this same drug it will reach steady state over the following time course:

- After 8 hours it will reach 50% of steady state.
- After 16 hours it will reach 75%.
- After 24 hours it will reach 87.5%.
- After 32 hours it will reach 93.8%.

Never make assumptions about dosing history and sample times. When interpreting concentrations, always check and consider:

- **Dose and formulation given**. All doses of medicine given within the previous 5 half-lives will contribute to the measured drug concentration.
- **Relevant clinical history,** which will influence absorption, clearance and distribution – such as diarrhoea, vomiting, dehydration, oedema, volume expansion, transfusion, double volume exchange transfusion, diuretics, shunts or drains.
- **Time doses given.** The best source of information is the parent/carer/child who, if forewarned of the importance of this information, will often give a detailed history. Medicine administration records (e.g. drug charts) often give detail of when doses should be given. Signed records do not always signify that a dose was actually given at the prescribed time.
- **Route and method of administration**. With neonates, it is important to consider the drug administration process. To illustrate the importance of flushing appropriately, consider a 0.67 kg neonate prescribed 15 mg/kg of vancomycin:
  - A 10 mg dose of vancomycin is given using a 5 mg/mL solution.
  - It is infused over 60 minutes into a giving set with a 1.5 mL (7.5 mg) residual volume.

- Only 2.5 mg of vancomycin reaches the neonate.
- An equal volume of sodium chloride must be infused at the same rate to flush drug in.
- Blood for peak concentrations should be sampled 2 hours after the flush is complete.
- All the 'facts' must be clearly documented.
- **Sample time**. The time the blood sample is obtained, both in relation to the last dose and, specifically, at what time, is critical. This detail is often difficult to obtain after the event. Laboratories will report results in the patient record system and assume the time of sampling is the same as the time the request was generated on the computer. Clinical staff may, however, generate requests some time before or after the sample is actually taken; this may lead to misinterpretation of reported concentrations. Again a useful source of information may be the parent/carer/child, who should ideally be forewarned and invited to participate in the TDM process.
- **Sample site**. Was there any contamination or haemodilution? The decision on how to flush a line is difficult and depends on rate, pressure and volume of flush. Basic physics suggests the central core of a line may be flushed but the periphery is not. Sampling from administration lines is therefore problematic. Capillary sampling may overcome such issues, but care must be taken to avoid 'hand/glove contamination'. When a pre-dose trough concentration is required, staff may prepare the sample tube while preparing the next injection. A droplet on a glove or hand may contaminate the sample tube. Children receiving nebulised tobramycin may have 'toxic' serum tobramycin concentrations if their skin is not properly cleansed before capillary blood sampling.
- **Line locks** may lead to haemodilution of samples and falsely low concentrations if locked with sodium chloride. Line locks may also cause high results if measuring antibiotic concentrations.

For which drugs and why, when, how and where should you measure and interpret serum concentrations?

Before considering whether to measure a drug concentration, ask:

- Is the patient already responding appropriately? Would you measure a theophylline concentration where a child receiving intravenous aminophylline was clinically improving and required fewer nebulisers?
- Does the patient show any signs of toxicity?
- Is efficacy better predicted by evaluating clinical response or measuring drug concentrations?
- Will a drug concentration change clinical management?

- Can the regimen be altered to minimise cost? Could the vancomycin dosing be changed from 20 mg every 6 hours to a continuous infusion to reduce waste from using and wasting four 500 mg vials each day?
- Is adherence erratic?

When clinical effect is readily measured, such as by measuring blood pressure or pain, the dose of a drug should be adjusted according to response. If a clinically important event happens rarely, such as a seizure, or is life-threatening, or if the beneficial effect of drug treatment is delayed, measuring drug concentrations may be appropriate.

Why?

An important question to ask before considering measuring serum drug concentrations is 'Why?' If it is for interest, because it can be measured, and is not going to change how the child is managed, do not do it. Valid reasons for measuring concentrations include the following:

- An immediate effect is needed
- Lack of clinical effect despite seemingly appropriate dosing
- Erratic or questionable compliance
- Possible toxic side-effect
- Narrow therapeutic index drugs where, due to patient idiosyncrasy, it is easy to cause toxicity at 'normal' doses

When?

With regard to 'When?' consider what the sampling aims to prove. Concentrations may be sampled as follows:

- Peak concentration sampled after a dose, allowing time for drug absorption and distribution into the tissues
- Pre-dose trough concentration sampled immediately before a dose is given
- Two timed samples following a single dose, which can allow calculation of individualised pharmacokinetic parameters such as elimination rate constant, half-life and volume of distribution
- At steady state, namely the time when drug into the body equals drug out, which occurs following repeated dosing (after approximately 4 to 5 half-lives)

Sampling blood after a loading dose will guide interpretation of the adequacy of that dose. Always consider clinical response simultaneously. Measuring concentrations at steady state, at least 5 half-lives after a dose change, when 97% of the final concentration will be achieved, will guide interpretation of the appropriateness of the maintenance dose.

It is not always necessary to wait for steady state to make an assessment of the adequacy of the maintenance dose. For example:

1 A 7-day-old baby receives a 20 mg/kg loading dose of phenytoin.
2 The 8 hour post-dose concentration is 15 mg/L.
3 A maintenance dose of 2.5 mg/kg twice daily is commenced.
4 After three further doses, the pre-dose concentration is 3.6 mg/L.

Drug concentrations must always be interpreted in the context of each individual patient, without rigid adherence to a hypothetical target range.

- If seizures continue, a further loading dose may be considered, perhaps of 15 mg/kg to create a concentration rise of 11 mg/L.
- The maintenance dose would also need to be increased, as with repeated dosing the concentration has fallen.
- However, if there have been no further seizures, a loading dose is not necessary and the maintenance dose may be increased.

Timing of sample collection is also critically important, because drug concentration changes throughout the dosing interval. The least variable point between dosing is just before the next dose is due. For many drugs, such as anticonvulsants, a pre-dose trough concentration is measured. Concentrations may be measured at different times, often informed by the time course of absorption. Digoxin concentrations do not need to be measured 6 hours post dose. The recommendation is to measure at least 6 hours post dose to allow absorption and distribution and an assessment of clinical effect. Sampling pre-dose is therefore entirely appropriate.

How?

Laboratories sometimes advise that blood sample bottles must be filled to the line, often 4 mL, to measure drug concentrations. This volume may be inappropriate for small babies and some children. Measurement of drug concentrations can sometimes be done from small capillary blood samples following discussion with the laboratory. This will be influenced by the method of analysis and whether the sample needs special preparation beforehand.

Where?

Pharmacokinetic review is ideally performed during the clinical consultation, either at the bedside or during clinic review. Individualised pharmacokinetic review within the pharmacy or at a computer, away from the patient, may not take account of the full clinical effect of drug treatment and the history. Patients and parents/carers should ideally be participants in the TDM process and can often provide insightful detail to explain why concentrations are not as predicted or expected.

Why do predicted and measured drug concentrations differ?

Dosing regimens may be based on population derived pharmacokinetic parameters of distribution volume, clearance and elimination half-life. These figures will probably not reflect the pharmacokinetic handling of the baby or child being reviewed. It is possible to define individualised pharmacokinetic parameters, but this often involves measurement of sequential blood concentrations.

When reviewing drug concentrations, always consider **whether** the value makes sense. Possible explanations for differences are shown in Table 1.

Table 1 Possible scenarios when reviewing drug concentrations		
Scenario	Problem	Solution
Peak concentration too high	Incorrect dose given.	Take measures so that correct dose is given next time and resample when/if appropriate.
	Sample drawn from administration line with contamination.	Request capillary sample.
	Sample drawn during distribution phase.	Request another level if still clinically appropriate. Document time of sample.
	Distribution volume smaller than predicted.	Bear in mind for future dose adjustments. Note if the change in distribution volume is due to a particular clinical issue (shunt blocking or unblocking) then, if that issue changes, this will alter the influence it may have on future concentrations.
	Clearance smaller than predicted.	[1] Bear in mind for future dose adjustments. Note if the change in clearance is due to a particular clinical detail (e.g. reduced renal perfusion due to hypotension and inotropic support) the influence this may have on future concentrations.
Peak concentration too low	Dose administered incomplete or less than prescribed or omitted completely.	[2] Take measures so that the correct dose is given next time. Ensure appropriate flushing method followed and resample when/if appropriate.
	Sample dilute: did the sample contain saline flush?	[3] Make sure staff discard appropriate volume of blood before filling sample bottle.

Table 1 (*Continued*)

Scenario	Problem	Solution
	Sample time incorrect, with sample drawn too late.	Unless a second level can be drawn before the next dose is due, you will not be able to use regression to calculate an earlier plasma concentration. Suggest resample.
	Distribution volume bigger than predicted.	Bear in mind for future dose adjustments. Note if the change in distribution volume is due to a particular clinical factor (e.g. hypoalbuminaemia with oedema) then alterations in this factor may also affect future concentrations.
	Clearance greater than predicted.	[4] Bear in mind for future dose adjustments. Note if the change in clearance is due to a particular clinical detail (e.g. profound diuresis) the influence this may have on future concentrations.
Trough concentration too high	Dose given previously too high.	Adjust to appropriate dose and resample.
	Sample drawn from administration line.	Ask for capillary sample.
	Dose given before the trough sample was drawn.	Resample.
	Previous dose given late.	Estimate what the concentration would have been using population kinetics (but acknowledge risks and limitation of using population data above) or resample.
	Clearance smaller than predicted.	See [1] above.
Trough concentration too low	Dose administered incomplete or less than prescribed or omitted completely.	See [2] above.
	Sample dilute: did the sample contain saline flush?	See [3] above.
	Sample time incorrect.	Resample.
	Last dose given earlier than predicted.	Estimate what concentration would have been using population kinetics (but see risks and limitation of using population data above) or resample.
	Clearance greater than predicted.	See [4] above.

Conclusions

TDM requires a critical evaluation of clinical effect. Drug dosing should be based on clinical effect whenever possible and informed by reported serum drug concentrations where appropriate, not the other way around. Treat the patient, not the 'level'. TDM helps neonates and children get better safely when delivered by expert practitioners who understand limitations, assumptions, uncertainties, ambiguities and consequences. Without an accurate history of what happened and when, the ability to get the dose right is limited. Predicted and measured drug concentrations may differ because of differences in both pharmacokinetic parameters and the administration process.

References

1 Birkett DJ. Therapeutic drug monitoring. *Aust Prescr* 1997; 20: 9–11.
2 Pai VB, Nahata MC. Drug dosing in pediatric patients. In: Murphy JE, ed. *Clinical Pharmacokinetics*, 5th edn. Bethesda, MD: American Society of Health-System Pharmacists; 2012: 29–44.

36

Medicines for children in low to middle income countries

A Ojoo

Introduction

Children in sub-Saharan Africa are over 14 times more likely to die before the age of 5 than children in developed countries.[1] Despite significant reduction in under 5 mortality, by 58% since 1990 (from 12.6 million in 1990 to 5.4 million in 2017),[1] there remains unacceptable disparity in where and when these children die. More than half of child deaths are still caused by diseases that are preventable or otherwise treatable using proven, cost-effective interventions. In 2015, 3.6 million children died from infectious diseases. Of these deaths, 99% occurred in low and middle income countries.[2]

The positive progress made during the Millennium Development Goals (MDG) era demonstrates that the knowledge of what needs to be done exists. How can we distribute these benefits to reach all?

Goal 3 of the 2030 Agenda for Sustainable Development states, 'Ensure healthy lives and promote well-being for all at all ages' and constitutes a major shift of focus from child survival to child thriving. While greater emphasis must continue on preventative services such as immunisation and provision of clean drinking water, sanitation and hygiene facilities, prompt treatment of infections remains crucial. No one should die for lack of life-saving medicines.

The learning objectives of this chapter are:

➢ to provide a background on essential medicines for children
➢ to outline challenges in meeting their pharmaceutical needs
➢ to reflect on opportunities to address these needs
➢ to offer proposals to address the related challenges.

This chapter assumes that the oral route of administration is most common for medicines for children.

Background

Essential medicines are those that meet the priority healthcare needs of the majority of the population. The concept of essential medicines was launched in 1977 and became one of the pillars of the Primary Health Care Alma Ata declaration of 1978.[3] Declaration II states, 'The existing gross inequality in the health status of people, particularly between developed and developing countries as well as within countries is politically, socially and economically unacceptable.' Declaration VII, item 3, states that primary healthcare includes at least (among others) 'provision of essential drugs'.

In 2007, the World Health Organization (WHO) passed World Health Assembly resolution WHA60.20, 'Better Medicines for Children', which outlined several strategies to improve access to essential medicines of adequate quality for children.[4] In 2007, the WHO and UNICEF launched the 'Make medicines child size' campaign to create awareness and advance action to address the need for child specific medications, and published the first WHO Model Essential Medicines List for Children. The first WHO Model Formulary for Children was published in 2010.[4] World Health Assembly resolution WHA69.20, 'Promoting Innovation and Access to Quality, Safe, Efficacious and Affordable Medicines for Children', was passed in 2016.

At the macro level, a multiplicity of factors unique to children, such as heterogeneity of developmental stages (variation in body size, composition and anatomy, maturity of body organs), limited safety and efficacy studies, and practical challenges such as palatability contribute to the complex nature of using medicines to treat children. Recognising that significant expertise for drug development resides with industry, legislation has been enacted and implemented in Europe[5] and the USA[6] with incentives for the pharmaceutical industry to develop medicines for children.

Despite recent global efforts to increase access to much-needed medicines for children, a significant number of medicines for diseases that predominantly affect children in resource limited settings are still missing. Some medicines for managing diseases that are predominantly in developing countries are not produced and, when available, are too expensive.

The campaign for access to essential medicines inadvertently reframed many pharmaceutical product issues as being about cost, yet the main challenge for medicines for children is their inherent complexity. Manipulating adult medicines for children may provide upstream cost savings, but most likely transfers the cost of healthcare from pharmaceuticals to other health budget lines such as hospitalisation for treatment failure, adverse events or medication errors.

Challenges

In 2001, I (the author) coined the phrase 'children are dying while on treatment' to focus attention on the fact that health professionals, caregivers

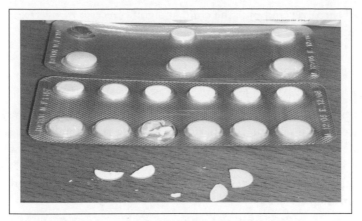

Figure 1 Split or crushed adult solid oral dosage. Source: *Picture courtesy of Atieno Ojoo*

and patients in developing countries were burdened with the responsibility of manipulating any adult dosage forms for use by children. The common practice of splitting or crushing adult solid oral dosage forms (see Figure 1) does not guarantee accurate dosing for children, since the active substance is often not uniformly distributed; neither is there due consideration for bioavailability. Manipulation that is not industry verified increases the risk of medication errors and treatment failure.

Other challenges are outlined below.

Knowledge and skill of healthcare workers and caregivers

Developing countries still have an imbalance in the delivery of health services where demand for healthcare professionals far outstrips supply. There are a wide spectrum of healthcare workers with varied levels of skills, literacy and numeracy. Caregivers for sick children range from elderly grandparents with vision impairment and dexterity limitations to children themselves as caregivers. Often, the one who brings the child to the healthcare facility is not necessarily the one who will administer the medication; education and information provided at the time of prescribing and dispensing may be conveyed inaccurately to the next caregiver.

Inadequate prescribing and dispensing information at the point of care

Increasing access to stable internet access and telephony has brought significant progress in access to health knowledge and information, but information asymmetry around medicines remains. While information asymmetry in healthcare is global, its effect is more pronounced in low resource settings; it is not uncommon for prescribers in busy healthcare settings to provide limited information to patients or caregivers. The dispenser may have limited training on the medicines, beyond simply interpreting the written prescriber instructions. A poorly informed healthcare provider leads to a poorly informed caregiver and puts the child at significant risk of overtreatment or undertreatment and medication errors.

Limited availability

Intellectual property

Medicines are a commodity of trade and public good at the same time. Pharmaceutical intellectual property plays a key role. Intellectual property rights are intended to incentivise inventions that benefit a majority of the population. However, the complex system to navigate the patents landscape and related flexibilities often leads to limited availability and prohibitive costs of medicines.

Regulatory and commercial barriers

Often, manufacturers of a suitable paediatric dosage form do not register it in developing countries, citing a limited, fragmented and highly regulated market.

Manufacturers are typically located far away from the beneficiaries, increasing the time to and cost of access.

Cost

On a dose by dose basis, the cost of children's medicines is often higher than that of adults' medicines; most of the cost of goods relates to underlying fixed costs such as more complex manufacturing processes and more packaging per unit dose as well as the cost of transport and storage. To optimise resources, medicines are procured in bulk containers. As an example, oral liquid medicines are often supplied in bulk containers and patients asked to bring their own bottles for repackaging. The cleanliness of the bottles cannot be guaranteed, and often there may be no labels to write instructions for use.

Many governments deprioritise procurement of medicines for children, due to their relatively higher costs, opting to manipulate adult medicines for use by children.

Dose measurement and administration devices

Oral medicines that are procured in bulk do not come with dosing devices to facilitate proper dispensing and administration by the patient or caregiver. Where dosage delivery devices are available, they may not be consistent with the dosing of the medicine. As an example, doses less than 1 mL cannot be accurately delivered with dosing devices with only 0.5 mL graduations. Often caregivers are instructed to use ungraduated household spoons. What is a teaspoonful?

Limited access to energy services and potable water

Limited access to energy services undermines access to medicines that require refrigeration. Over 1.3 billion people, or 18% of the global population, are without access to electricity. More than 95% are in sub-Saharan Africa or developing Asia, and 84% are in rural areas.[7]

Where electricity is available, electricity costs are prohibitive. The average citizen cannot afford a refrigerator.

This is a quote from a pharmacist:

'... *in a study (clinical trial) ... involving children and adolescents, one of the subjects, a 5-year-old boy, had to commute daily accompanied by either of his parents to the hospital to take the drug, which was a (oral) suspension that needed to be stored in a refrigerator. The family did not have a refrigerator and did not have an electricity connection either, so we could not even donate a refrigerator.*'

Limited access to potable water undermines access to oral medicines that require reconstitution before use. Among the global population, 783 million people, or 11%, remain without access to an improved source of drinking water, more than 40% being in sub-Saharan Africa. The quality and reliability of water supplies from boreholes, dug wells, open water pans, rivers, springs and rain water collection cannot be guaranteed.[8]

Poor healthcare and supply infrastructure

Products with less than 24 months' remaining shelf life are challenging to handle in the typical supply chain in a developing country.

Opportunities

Medicines for children can be practical and usable, without compromising on safety and efficacy. The challenges above offer an opportunity to capture the context of the user environment during drug development and as part of target product profiles. This is not a case of user preference, but user need.

The assessment of the quality of a finished pharmaceutical product (FPP) should include its usability in the target user environment. Minimising the requirement for cold storage and measurement of doses is a great step in simplifying use, reducing costs and optimising supply logistics.

Stability in tropical climates

For stability testing of pharmaceutical products, four different climatic zones are defined as follows: zone I, temperate; zone II, subtropical, with possible high humidity; zone III, hot/dry; zone IV, hot/humid. Developing countries, particularly in sub-Saharan Africa and Asia, would benefit from medicines formulated for and subjected to zone IV stability studies unless the active moiety is pharmaceutically unstable.[9] The incremental costs of performing zone IV stability studies instead of zone II or III only are minimal.

The products should be labelled with actual storage conditions. Label claims can be improved to be more specific; e.g. change from 'Keep in a cool, dry place' or 'This medicinal product does not require special storage conditions' to 'Do not store above 25°C or 30°C'.

Heat-stable products that do not require cold chain or end user refrigeration are ideal.

Cost considerations

Cost should not be a prime driver when making clinical decisions, but opportunities exist at the policy level for selecting paediatric dosage forms that optimise the overall acquisition, logistics and user related costs without compromising on safety, efficacy and quality.

Dosage forms that use simpler manufacturing technology generate time and cost efficiencies for the manufacturer, thereby eliminating a significant proportion of costs.

Minimising the need for accurate dose measurement

Dosing for medicines for children is often based on body weight and body surface area. Prescribing guidelines should provide for surrogates for weight that are easier to use, such as age. From a public health perspective, it may be necessary to accept some variability from the ideal dose.

In developed countries, the range of oral medicines for children is wide, the majority being liquids.

For developing countries, priority should be given to dosage forms that require the least accuracy in measurement and/or manipulation.

Flexible solid oral dosage forms for children

Flexible solid oral dosage forms (FSODs) offer a broader spectrum of options, often in one dosage form; they can be swallowed whole, chewed, placed on the tongue, sprinkled onto food or transformed from solid to liquid on a dose-by-dose basis at the time of use. The latter end of the spectrum brings the added benefit of easing supply logistics and represents crucial advances in reinvigorating the campaign to meet the pharmaceutical needs of children in developing countries.

FSODs embrace all age groups, accounting for the majority of socio-cultural settings and prescriber preferences for liquid oral dosage forms for younger children.

Other advantages of FSODs include:

- Onset of action similar to that for oral liquids
- Can be dosed across weight bands
- Require minimal manipulation that the end user can safely do
- Do not require accurate dose measuring devices

- Solid-state physical and chemical stability allows for longer shelf lives over higher temperatures
- No cold storage; only the required dose is reconstituted and consumed immediately
- Optimal for the supply chain because of reduced weight and volume of the FPP

FSODs have been instrumental in recent remarkable success in increasing access to treatment of HIV in children. Concerted efforts towards providing fixed dose combination dispersible tablets of antiretroviral medicines (ARVs) that are less costly and easier to transport than the previously available oral liquids have simplified paediatric ARV treatment by not requiring accurate dose measurement of several liquids, thereby ensuring complete dosing and improving adherence and overall quality of care. This success has prompted a similar campaign for FSODs of antibiotics for pneumonia, and should be replicated in other disease areas that contribute to the major causes of mortality in children.

Proposals for improvement

Research and development

1 Continue research that verifies safety, efficacy and dosing specific for children.
2 Conduct drug discovery, research and development that seeks stable active substances and cost-effective, age appropriate drug delivery mechanisms and contextualises the user environment very early in the process. Develop robust paediatric target candidate profiles and target product profiles.
3 Scientific journals and drug regulatory authorities should require clinical trials to be explicit about the formulations of medicines given to participants.
4 Develop collaborative dynamic knowledge clusters to carry out research to better understand the correlation between medicine formulations and child health outcomes.

Policy level

5 Offer public development support for essential medicines for children for diseases that disproportionately affect resource limited settings, with specific emphasis on age appropriate formulations. Public–private collaborations should be encouraged.
6 Ensure age appropriate dosage forms are specified and prioritised during drug registration and in treatment guidelines, essential medicines lists, procurement lists and drug budget lines.

7 Facilitate regulatory pathways that enable quick access to medicines for children.
8 Enable exchange of knowledge, evidence, standards and expertise, including guidance on regulatory matters.
9 Promote transfer of technology and knowhow to support manufacturers in developing countries to explore higher levels of technological innovation in the pharmaceutical industry.

Pharmaceutical industry

10 Prioritise platform technologies that support the physicochemical properties of an active pharmaceutical ingredient (API), typically API + excipient to give a base form (enabling formulations). This allows a secondary process to be applied to produce a final dosage form near to the point of use. The distinction between the platform technologies is less important as long as the formulation is uncomplicated, functional and cost-effective in resource limited settings.
11 Support industry verified formulations to allow manipulation of other dosage forms for use in children when this is the only option. For example, a manufacturer of valaciclovir has provided guidance on how to manipulate the adult formulation for use in children.
12 Develop other promising FSODs such as mini tablets or granules that can be sprinkled onto food, administered directly onto the tongue or swallowed with water.
13 Where liquids for dilution or powders for reconstitution are technically the most viable option, minimise the skill requirements by ensuring that:
   a bottles have a reconstitution mark in addition to the volume of liquid to be added
   b they are in patient pack sizes, with adequate labelling and information to eliminate the labour-intensive, often unhygienic repackaging from bulk
   c they are accompanied by suitable dose measuring and administration devices such as graduated medicine spoons and oral syringes
   d they are heat stable, even after reconstitution
   e they have sufficient shelf life, ideally for zone IV stability.

Health professionals

14 Prioritise the prescribing and dispensing of FSODs.
15 Before manipulating other dosage forms, such as adult tablets, consider another medicine with a suitable paediatric formulation (therapeutic/pharmaceutical interchange) or a different route of administration, e.g. from oral to rectal.
16 Follow extemporaneous preparation guidelines when manipulating other formulations.

Conclusions

For parents and caregivers, it is stressful enough that their child is sick. Make their lives easier by providing medicines suitable for them to use and with information they can understand.

Future drug discovery, research and development must plan for age appropriate drug delivery mechanisms that contextualise the user environment as early as possible in the process.

Research opportunities exist to look into robust active substances and drug delivery mechanisms that can withstand all climates yet remain affordable across all populations globally. Scientific possibilities are welcome but must be balanced with cost-effectiveness and dosage forms that a child can take and the caregiver can administer. The premise is simple yet compelling: user-centred design that addresses public health needs. Arguably, such innovations have the potential added benefit of contributing to saving the environment.

References

1   United Nations Inter-agency Group for Child Mortality Estimation. United Nations Children's Fund, World Health Organization, The World Bank, UN. *Levels and Trends in Child Mortality*. UNICEF: 2018. https://childmortality.org/wp-content/uploads/2018/12/UN-IGME-Child-Mortality-Report-2018.pdf

2   UNICEF's Strategy for Health (2016–2030). *UNICEF Programme Division*: 2015. www.unicef.org/health/files/UNICEF_Health_Strategy_Final.pdf

3   Declaration of Alma Ata. International Conference on Primary Health Care, Alma-Ata, USSR, 6–12 September 1978. www.who.int/publications/almaata_declaration_en.pdf

4   Zucker H, Rago L. Access to essential medicines for children: World Health Organization's global response. *Clin Pharmacol Ther* 2007; 82: 503–503.

5   European Commission. Regulation (EC) No 1901/2006 of the European Parliament and of the council on medicinal products for paediatric use and amending regulation (EEC) No. 1768/92, Directive 2001/20/EC, Directive 2001/83/EC and Regulation (EC) No. 726/2004.

6   Cohen IG. Therapeutic orphans, pediatric victims? The best pharmaceuticals for Children Act and existing pediatric human subject protection. *Food Drug Law J* 2003; 58: 661–710.

7   World Health Organization and United Nations Development Programme. The Energy Access Situation in Developing Countries. www.undp.org/content/dam/undp/library/Environment%20and%20Energy/Sustainable%20Energy/energy-access-situation-in-developing-countries.pdf

8   Strickley RG *et al*. Pediatric drugs – a review of commercially available oral formulations. *J Pharm Sci* 2008; 97(5): 1731–1774.

9   World Health Organization. Stability testing of active pharmaceutical ingredients and finished pharmaceutical products, Annex 2 to WHO Technical Report Series No. 953. 2009: 1–6.

37

Optimal prescribing in the resource-poor setting

A Gray and P Jeena

Introduction

Optimal prescribing is a challenge in all settings and for all patients. The problem is amplified in relation to paediatric and neonatal patients, where there are insufficient data to guide best practice. Making a diagnosis in a child who does not volunteer symptoms is difficult enough, but paediatricians also have to deal with a lack of evidence to support the use of many medicines, combined with an incomplete understanding of pharmacokinetics and drug–drug interactions in children. As a result, paediatricians are often forced to extrapolate from adult data and to use medicines in an off-label manner.[1] These challenges are further compounded in resource-poor settings.

The learning objectives of this chapter are:

> to understand that prescribing for children in resource-poor settings is influenced by many factors, including poor health infrastructure, lack of access to essential medicines, inadequate healthcare financing, and a high burden of disease

> to recognise that prescribers in these settings also need to consider the socioeconomic circumstances of their patients, including issues such as poor access to transportation, lack of funds to purchase healthcare, and lack of facilities to store medicines.

Access to medicines and prescribing information

Although efforts in developed country settings (largely in the USA and some European countries) have resulted in increased numbers of medicines being registered for paediatric age groups, with appropriate labelling and the development of age appropriate dosage forms, there is still a backlog.[2] All too often, paediatric registration implies an increase in the price of these medicines. As a result, such medicines may not be available in resource-poor settings, and off-label use of medicines in children will be the only option. Access to essential medicines and prescribing information may be difficult in resource-poor settings, due to the lack of human and financial resources.

Standard treatment guidelines

In many parts of the world, standard treatment guidelines are not available. It is important that, where possible, prescribers consult the standard treatment guidelines that are developed within their health system, as medicines availability may be based on such guidelines. Such guidelines should, however, be appropriately evidence based and be developed by multidisciplinary teams including personnel with the necessary paediatric clinical expertise. Ideally, local standard treatment guidelines will inform the essential medicines list that is followed in that health system, and will guide procurement and availability. Local guidelines need to be sensitive to local conditions. For example, in settings where venous access in neonates and children is challenging, alternative routes of administration might be considered. In particular, local guidelines need to take account of the available human resources for health. Care may depend on nurses and medical officers rather than trained specialists. Where no locally developed standard treatment guidelines are available, World Health Organization (WHO) guidance can be used as the starting point. An example is the WHO's *Pocket Book of Hospital Care for Children*.[3]

Recommendations

1 Start with a locally developed and appropriate standard treatment guideline, if available.
2 If a local resource is not available, consider whether another source (WHO or other) is applicable in your settings, and use the guidance with care and clinical judgement.

Medicines formularies

Choosing the right dosing regimen for a child or neonate requires access to good quality medicines information. In developed countries, there are a range of up-to-date resources that can be consulted, including online decision support software available in health facilities. Such resources are unlikely to be available in resource-poor settings. Where resources exist, access to even paper-based resources may be limited. Although many prescribers rely on resources such as the *British National Formulary for Children* (BNFC), the health authorities in such settings are encouraged to develop their own documents, drawing on the WHO Model Formulary for Children.[4] This model formulary was based on the 2nd WHO Model List of Essential Medicines for Children (2009). The most up-to-date version of the Model List of Essential Medicines for Children should be used (see www.who.int/selection_medicines/list/en).

Medicines information covers far more than dosing advice, and an up-to-date and locally relevant resource is needed on adverse effects and contraindications. Prescribers in resource-constrained settings may not always have access to the diagnostic technologies required to safely manage pharmacotherapy in children with hepatic and renal disease, for instance, let alone clinical pharmacokinetic services. Careful consideration of the available data on compatibility of injectable medicines and infusion fluids is needed, and in these cases, standard texts can be consulted. Many rely on Trissel's *Handbook on Injectable Drugs.*[5] Alternatives are available, but may not be as authoritative or reliable. These compatibility data may not always be reflected in local labelling (package inserts or summaries of product characteristics). Medicines information also needs to be appropriately packaged for the cadres of health workers that are available in resource-poor settings.

Recommendations

1 Paediatricians, medical officers, nurses and paediatric pharmacists need access to high quality information to guide safe medicines use, but this information must be simple, locally relevant and applicable.

2 Locally developed standard treatment guidelines can guide not only practice, but also rational procurement of medicines that meet the needs of children.

3 Treatment guidelines should be specific to the levels of care provided and the various categories of health professionals who will prescribe and dispense medicines for children.

4 Care needs to be exercised when using dosage guides (especially dose recommendations by age bands), which may not necessarily be based on locally applicable weight and height for age data.

5 Locally developed and printed formularies must be available in all healthcare facilities. While electronic versions are useful, unreliable electricity supply and poor internet connectivity need to be taken into account.

Selection and availability of medicines

The challenges that all prescribers face in relation to appropriate dosage forms for paediatric and neonatal patients are intensified in resource-poor settings.

While oral liquid dosage forms are needed for some age groups, and are also most appropriate for dosing via nasogastric or other feeding tubes, they are associated with serious disadvantages. The stability of many medicines is reduced when in aqueous solutions, and this may either shorten the shelf life or require that the medicine is stored under controlled temperature conditions (such as under refrigeration). Caregivers may lack access to such storage facilities. Oral liquid dosage forms are also considerably more expensive than the equivalent oral solid dosage forms. Large volumes and packaging in glass also present challenges for transport and storage. For these reasons, some health systems in resource-poor settings are reluctant to procure oral liquid dosage forms. Carers may also experience difficulties affording such medicines when out-of-pocket purchases are required.

While there is increasing development of divisible, dispersible oral solid dosage forms designed for paediatric age groups, these new products may not be available or accessible. Whenever medicines selection decisions are taken, there should be careful consideration of whether an oral solid dosage form will meet the needs of as many children as possible, and preference given to the selection and procurement of appropriate divisible, dispersible oral solid dosage forms. Care should be exercised when selecting oral solid dosage forms that will have to be divided, as dose accuracy and consistency may not always be guaranteed.

Manipulation and compounding of medicines for children

When an age appropriate oral liquid dosage form is not available, prescribers need to consult with the available pharmaceutical personnel and make a careful decision about manipulating or compounding a liquid form from available solid dosage forms or from active pharmaceutical ingredients (where these can be purchased). The decision to make an oral solution or suspension is never a simple one and requires access to quality information about the methods to be employed, the solvent or suspending agent/vehicle to the used, and the stability of the resultant product. It may be necessary to advise carers to prepare single doses for administration, including the administration of a fraction (aliquot) of a solution or suspension made from an oral solid dosage form. This has proved to be a practical approach in some settings. In general, sustained release and enteric-coated tablets cannot be divided or crushed. Where tablets are to be split, the use of commercial tablet splitters is advised. Withdrawing the contents of liquid filled capsules is not advisable. Splitting suppositories is also problematic, as the dose is seldom evenly distributed in such dosage forms. Care is also needed when administering injectable solutions by the oral route, as they may contain undesirable excipients, such as propylene glycol or ethanol, or have a pH that is unacceptable.

Making bulk quantities of oral liquids in a hospital or other pharmacy should only be done when the necessary quality standards can be met.[6]

Particular care is needed when manipulation of sterile products is contemplated, as the necessary laminar air flow or isolator facilities may not be available. Failure to ensure the sterility of such products has been associated with significant nosocomial sepsis events.

The International Pharmaceutical Federation and WHO have developed technical guidelines on extemporaneous preparation of age appropriate preparations when authorised products are not available.[7] Accessing the necessary information to guide safe practice is not always easy. Many formulae that have appeared in peer reviewed literature depend on the use of commercial suspending bases that may not be easily available. However, there are resources that can be of assistance.[8] A resource that is particularly useful in resource-poor settings is the eMixt database (www.pharminfotech.co.nz).

Recommendations

6 Paediatricians and paediatric pharmacists need to advocate for the selection and procurement of a full range of age appropriate dosage forms, avoiding the manipulation of adult dosage forms in pharmacies or by carers.

7 Preference should be given to the provision of divisible, dispersible oral solid dosage forms as far as possible.

8 Bulk compounding of oral liquid dosage forms should be avoided.

9 Extreme care should be exercised whenever medicines for children are prepared from oral solid dosage forms or active pharmaceutical ingredients, and every effort made to access information on the methods to be used and the stability of the resultant product. Particular care is needed with sterile products such as injectable medicines.

10 It must be noted that formulations for compounded medicines based on active pharmaceutical ingredients and crushed tablets are not interchangeable.

11 Compounded liquid formulations are susceptible to microbial growth, and therefore require the addition of a suitable preservative unless they are to be used within a short period (of a maximum of 3 days) and can be stored under refrigeration.

12 The same care should also be exercised when prescribing a medicine that will need to be manipulated at ward level in a hospital, as this is an important source of medication errors.

Clarity of prescribing and instructions

- Every prescription needs to be precise and allow for the provision of clear instructions to the patient and caregivers (whether in hospital or in ambulatory settings). This need is amplified in the case of paediatric and neonatal patients, in every setting.

- Prescribers in resource-poor settings need to be aware of the risk of medication errors that are associated with the use of abbreviations (including Latin and unapproved abbreviations for medicine names), poorly written dosing units and trailing zeroes.
- Prescribers should be precise about specifying doses and strengths, and avoid using fractions of tablets or spoons. They should also be specific about dosing intervals.
- The *British National Formulary for Children* (BNFC) provides a useful list of potential pitfalls in paediatric prescribing.
- In resource-poor settings, particular care should be exercised when safe administration will depend on the use of undertrained health personnel, as well as low-literacy carers.

Conclusions

Prescribing in a resource-poor setting is hampered by lack of access to appropriate medicines information and a restricted range of medicines. Careful use of locally relevant standard treatment guidelines, combined with clinical judgement, is required. Consideration needs to be given to the available dosage forms and whether they are suitable for the particular paediatric or neonatal patient. Manipulation of available dosage forms or the compounding of age appropriate products from available authorised medicines must only be done, with extreme caution, after accessing the necessary information and in consultation with available pharmaceutical personnel.

Paediatricians and paediatric pharmacists have an important advocacy role in such settings, and can contribute to rational medicines selection and procurement and the development of locally relevant guidance, as well as to safe and effective care of the individual patient. They can also contribute to continuing professional development programmes for medical officers, nurses and pharmacy support personnel who provide care for children and neonates in such settings. Calculation challenges for medical, pharmacy and nursing staff should be considered, in order to evaluate competence in prescribing, dispensing and administration.

References

1   Mason J *et al*. Off-label and unlicensed medicine use and adverse drug reactions in children: a narrative review of the literature. *Eur J Clin Pharmacol* 2012; 68: 21–28.
2   Hoppu K *et al*. The status of paediatric medicines initiatives around the world – what has happened and what has not? *Eur J Clin Pharmacol* 2012; 68: 1–10.

3 World Health Organization. *Pocket Book of Hospital Care for Children. Guidelines for the management of Common Childhood Illnesses*, 2nd edn. World Health Organization, Geneva, 2013. www.who.int/maternal_child_adolescent/documents/child_hospital_care/en/

4 World Health Organization. Model Formulary for Children. World Health Organization, Geneva, 2010. http://apps.who.int/medicinedocs/en/m/abstract/Js17151e/

5 Trissel LA. *Handbook on Injectable Drugs*, 17th edn. Bethesda, USA: American Society of Health-system Pharmacists, 2012.

6 Pharmaceutical Inspection Co-Operation Scheme. *PIC/S Guide to Good Practices for the Preparation of Medicinal Products in Healthcare Establishments*, PE 010-4. 2014. www.picscheme.org/publication.php?id=8

7 International Pharmaceutical Federation and World Health Organization. FIP–WHO Technical Guidelines: Points to Consider in the Provision by Health-care Professionals of Children-specific Preparations that are not Available as Authorized Products. WHO Technical Report Series, No. 996, 2016, Annex 2. Available at: http://apps.who.int/medicinedocs/documents/s22399en/s22399en.pdf [last accessed 5 February 2019].

8 Jackson M, Lowey A. *Handbook of Extemporaneous Preparation: A Guide to Pharmaceutical Compounding*. London: Pharmaceutical Press, 2010.

PART II

38

Gastrointestinal system

E Gaynor and L Howarth

Introduction

Gastrointestinal disorders are a common cause of paediatric presentations to primary and secondary care. There are a wide range of presenting symptoms and multiple treatment options for most conditions. It is important that mechanisms of actions and side-effects of medications are considered when making management plans for these children.

The learning objectives of this chapter are:

➢ to know the key therapeutic options available for common gastrointestinal conditions
➢ to develop awareness of common or important drug side-effects and complications
➢ to understand the role of stepwise management of constipation in children.

Dyspepsia and gastro-oesophageal reflux disease

- Gastro-oesophageal reflux disease (GORD) occurs when gastric contents regurgitate up the oesophagus, causing troublesome symptoms such as vomiting, dyspepsia, irritability, weight loss, cough and wheezing. Around 50% of children under 3 months of age regurgitate some of their gastric contents; most cases spontaneously resolve by 12–14 months of age.
- The diagnosis of GORD and associated dyspepsia is clinical (see joint NSPGHAN/ESPGHAN guidelines for diagnostic criteria[1]). The management options for gastro-oesophageal reflux (GOR) and dyspepsia are lifestyle changes, pharmacological therapy and surgery.
- Medications suppress acid secretions, buffer gastric contents or reduce regurgitation through thickening of gastric contents.

Antacids: (i) H2 receptor antagonists (H2RAs)

Ranitidine

- *Preparations:* liquid (75 mg/5 mL); tablets 150 mg, 300 mg
- *Pharmacokinetics:* rapid absorption with peak concentrations 2–3 hours after ingestion. Reduces acid production by H2 receptor blockade of gastric parietal cells. A single dose is found to increase gastric pH for 9–10 hours in infants. It also has an antisecretory effect. H2RAs are used to reduce the degradation of pancreatic enzyme replacement when used in the treatment of cystic fibrosis.
- *Side-effects: uncommon:* abdominal pain, diarrhoea, constipation, nausea
- *Advice:* excellent first line management of dyspepsia or irritability in children thought to be secondary to GORD – in particular, due to the availability of liquid preparations. However, tolerance to H2RAs has been seen in children after 6 weeks of treatment, limiting their use in children with chronic symptoms.

Antacids: (ii) proton pump inhibitors (PPIs)

Key examples: omeprazole, lansoprazole

- *Preparations:* multiple unit pellet system 10 mg, 20 mg, 40 mg; capsules
- *Cautions:* no PPIs are licensed for < 1-year-olds, and lansoprazole is not licensed for use in children.
- *Pharmacokinetics:* maximal effect seen within 4 days of starting treatment (increase of gastric pH of ≥ 3 for a mean of 17 hours in a 24-hour period). Concomitant intake of food has no influence on the bioavailability.
- *Side-effects:*
  - *Common:* headache, abdominal pain, constipation, diarrhoea, nausea
  - *Uncommon:* liver enzyme derangement
- *Advice:* for healing of erosive oesophagitis and relief of GORD, PPIs are superior to H2RAs. Once-daily dosing at the lowest effective dose is recommended, although twice-daily split dosing can be considered in children with resistant symptoms. By decreasing gastric acid acidity and causing hypochlorhydria, PPIs may increase the risk of gastrointestinal infections and rarely increase the risk of bacterial enterocolitis.[2]

Compound alginate preparations

- Although these agents can be useful for immediate relief of dyspepsia, there is no evidence of benefit in children with established GORD.
- Alginate therapy (e.g. Gaviscon®) can, however, be a useful thickening agent to reduce regurgitation in children. Preparations containing aluminium should not be used in neonates or infants.

Antispasmodics and other drugs altering gut motility

- Antispasmodics can be useful in the management of chronic abdominal pain, particularly in those suffering from irritable bowel syndrome. However, there is very limited evidence for their use. They could be used as part of a treatment plan that includes patient education, reassurance where appropriate and consideration of dietary modifications.
- There is little difference in efficacy between different antispasmodics, but side-effect profiles do vary. Antimuscarinics are contraindicated in paralytic ileus.

Antimuscarinics

Hyoscine butylbromide

- *Preparations:* tablets (10 mg)
- *Pharmacokinetics:* only partially absorbed orally, with peak plasma concentrations seen at 2 hours following ingestion. Acts principally on muscarinic receptors and nicotinic receptors on gastric smooth muscle.
- *Side-effects: uncommon:* constipation, transient bradycardia, dry mouth, dyshidrosis
- *Advice:* hyoscine butylbromide is poorly selective and is more likely to cause antimuscarinic adverse effects than alternatives such as mebeverine. It should, therefore, be considered as second-line treatment for children requiring longer term-treatment.

Mebeverine hydrochloride

- *Preparations:* tablets (135 mg), oral suspension (50 mg/5 mL)
- *Pharmacokinetics:* completely absorbed following oral administration and acts on muscarinic receptors on gastric smooth muscle. It is completely metabolised and excreted into the urine.
- *Side-effects:* similar to hyoscine butylbromide.
- *Advice:* it has been reported that there is a particular risk of adverse effects in children with Down's syndrome.

Motility stimulants

- Motility stimulants can be a useful adjunct in the management of children with delayed gastric emptying or slow intestinal transit, but the evidence is very limited for use.
- **Domperidone is no longer licensed in the management of GORD, and Medicines and Healthcare products Regulatory Agency (MHRA) advice cautions its use in children due to the risk of cardiac side-effects.**

Erythromycin

- *Preparations:* tablets (250 mg), suspension (125 mg/5 mL)
- *Pharmacokinetics:* peak plasma concentrations are achieved within 1 hour of dosing, and it has a half-life of around 2 hours. Its prokinetic properties are achieved through stimulation of the gastric antral and duodenal motilin receptors.
- *Side-effects:*
  - *Common:* nausea, vomiting, abdominal discomfort and diarrhoea
  - *Uncommon:* hepatotoxicity, cholestatic jaundice, rash, QT interval prolongation
    Note: P450 system inhibitor
- *Advice:* low dose can stimulate motility, but should be on the advice of a paediatric gastroenterologist. Note potential impact on antimicrobial resistance when considering risk/benefit.

Antisecretory drugs and mucosal protection

H2 receptor antagonists

See 'Antacids: (i) H2 receptor antagonists (H2RAs)'.

Chelates and complexes

- These can be used in children with refractory symptoms of GORD, for stress ulcer prophylaxis, reflux oesophagitis and mucositis. There is very limited evidence for the use of chelates such as sucralfate.

Sucralfate

- *Preparations:* suspension (1 g/5 mL)
- *Pharmacokinetics:* very small amounts are absorbed and excreted through the urine. The active ingredient, antepsin, exerts a generalised cytoprotective effect by preventing gastrointestinal mucosal injury.
- *Side-effects:*
  - *Common:* constipation
  - *Uncommon:* bezoar formation
- *Advice:* from available literature,[3,4] a dose of 0.5 – 1 g four times a day is recommended. It should be used in caution in children with delayed gastric emptying, following reports of bezoar formation, and in those under 14 years of age. There is a risk of aluminium toxicity with long term use.

Proton pump inhibitors

See 'Antacids: (ii) proton pump inhibitors'.

Acute diarrhoea

Anti-motility drugs

- Anti-motility drugs only have a role in uncomplicated diarrhoea in children over 12 years of age and should be used in conjunction with supportive measures. They should be used with caution in other situations, because of the risk of intestinal obstruction.

Loperamide hydrochloride

- *Preparations:* tablets (2 mg), suspension (1 mg/5 mL)
- *Pharmacokinetics:* absorbed readily in the gut; systemic bioavailability is only approximately 0.3% due to significant first-pass metabolism. It has a half-life of about 11 hours. It binds to the opioid receptor in the intestinal wall, reducing propulsive peristalsis and increasing intestinal transit time.
- *Side-effects: common:* constipation, flatulence, headache and nausea

Enkephalinase inhibitors

- Enkephalinase inhibitors should only be used in those children in which supportive measures are insufficient. However, there is currently insufficient evidence to demonstrate improved recovery rates with their use.

Racecadotril

- *Preparations:* sachets (10 mg)
- *Pharmacokinetics:* it is a prodrug of thiorphan, which reduces intestinal secretions by inhibiting the breakdown of endogenous opioids. It does not affect the duration of intestinal transit.
- *Side-effects:*
  - *Common:* headache
  - *Uncommon:* rash
- *Advice:* licensed in uncomplicated diarrhoea in children over 3 months of age as an adjunct to supportive measures. **Avoid in renal or hepatic impairment.**

Chronic bowel disorders

Aminosalicylates

- Aminosalicylates are used as first line management for induction and maintenance of remission in children with inflammatory bowel disease (ulcerative colitis). They are locally active and generally well tolerated.

Key examples: sulfasalazine, mesalazine, balsalazide

- *Preparations:* tablets, suspension (sulfasalazine only), granules, suppositories, enemas, foam enemas

- *Pharmacokinetics:* sulfasalazine is broken down by colonic bacteria to split the drug into sulfapyridine and mesalazine. Over 90% of the drug when taken enterally will reach the colon, with the drug and its metabolites acting on arachidonic acid cascade resulting in immunomodulatory effects. Sulfapyridine is responsible for many of the side-effects of sulfasalazine; consequently mesalazine is often better tolerated. Balsalazide consists of mesalazine linked to a carrier molecule, which is broken down into 5-aminosalicylic acid in the colon.
- *Side-effects:*
  - *Common:* nausea, headache, rash, anorexia
  - *Uncommon:* renal impairment, pancreatitis, liver impairment
- *Advice:* there is no evidence for improved efficacy between preparations; however, in those children with joint involvement secondary to inflammatory bowel disease, sulfasalazine has been demonstrated to have additional benefit. Sulfasalazine is also available as a suspension, which is particularly useful in smaller children or those unable to take tablets. Efficacy of mesalazine is the same taken once daily rather than split, which can aid compliance with medications.
- **Renal function should be monitored before starting an oral aminosalicylate, at 3 months of treatment, and then annually during treatment.**

Corticosteroids

- Corticosteroids should be used for induction of remission in children with moderate to severe active luminal Crohn's disease, where exclusive enteral nutrition is not an option or not tolerated, or for moderate to severely active ulcerative colitis. In severe inflammatory bowel disease, intravenous steroid therapy is usually required. Steroids should not be used as therapy to maintain remission.[5,6]

Key examples: budesonide, prednisolone, hydrocortisone

- *Preparations:*
  Prednisolone: tablets (1 mg, 5 mg, 25 mg)
  Budesonide: tablets (3 mg)
  Hydrocortisone: liquid, rectal foam (125 mg)
- *Pharmacokinetics:*
  Prednisolone: peak concentrations by 1–2 hours after oral dose. Half-life is between 2.5 and 3 hours. It is mainly (>90%) renally excreted.
  Budesonide: peak concentration by 5 hours. Maximum release occurs in the terminal ileum and caecum. It is mainly (>90%) metabolised in the liver.
  Hydrocortisone: half-life 2.4–3.5 hours. It is mainly metabolised in the liver.

- *Side-effects:*
  - *Common:* Cushingoid appearance, dyspepsia, hypertension, hirsutism, weight gain, increased appetite, insulin resistance, increased susceptibility to infection and reactivation of latent infection (e.g. tuberculosis)
  - *Uncommon:* pancreatitis, muscle weakness, osteoporosis, psychosis. (Budesonide has reduced suppression and systemic side-effects compared with systemic corticosteroids.)
- *Advice:* hydrocortisone or prednisolone can be used for the induction of remission in moderate to severe inflammatory bowel disease.
- In children with only terminal ileum involvement suspected, budesonide has been shown to have similar localised efficacy at doses clinically equivalent to those of systemically acting corticosteroids, with significantly less hypothalamic–pituitary–adrenal axis suppression, and has a lower impact on inflammatory markers.

Drugs affecting the immune response

- Immunomodulators are commonly required to maintain remission in children with inflammatory bowel disease. There is some evidence that it is appropriate to start early in severe cases or those with ileal or perianal disease. Generally, immunomodulation is started if initial treatments are unsuccessful or improvement in symptoms is not sustained.

Thiopurines

Key examples: azathioprine, 6-mercaptopurine (6-MP)

- Mercaptopurine and its prodrug, azathioprine, are used as first line systemic immunomodulatory therapy in the maintenance of remission in children with inflammatory bowel disease.
- *Preparations:*
  Azathioprine: tablets (25 mg, 50 mg), suspension (various)
  6-Mercaptopurine: tablets (10 mg, 50 mg), suspension (20 mg/mL)
- *Pharmacokinetics:* azathioprine is broken down into 6-mercaptopurine (6-MP). 6-MP is a purine antagonist that requires cellular uptake and intracellular anabolism to form thioguanine nucleotides (TGNs). TGNs and other metabolites inhibit *de novo* purine synthesis and purine nucleotide interconversions, resulting in immunosuppressive effects.
- *Side-effects:*
  - *Common:* depression of bone marrow function, leucopenia, thrombocytopenia, flu-like symptoms, pancreatitis, nausea
  - *Uncommon:* pneumonitis, red cell aplasia, lymphoma
- *Advice:* those with thiopurine methyltransferase (TPMT) deficiency develop very high cytotoxic TGN concentrations, increasing the risks of

bone marrow toxicity. All patients prior to starting thiopurines should have TPMP activity tested and the dose adjusted accordingly. Regular monitoring of blood counts and liver tests is recommended as per local protocols. Children who do not tolerate azathioprine may tolerate 6-MP.

Folic acid antagonists

Methotrexate

- *Preparations:* tablets (2.5 mg, 10 mg), injection (10 mg/mL, 25 mg/mL)
  Note: Never dispense different strength preparations to the same patient.
- *Pharmacokinetics:* the major site of action of folate antagonists is the enzyme dihydrofolate reductase, inhibiting DNA, RNA and protein synthesis. Methotrexate's main effect is during the S phase of cell division. It is rapidly absorbed from the gastrointestinal tract, with the majority excreted via the urine within 24 hours.
- *Side-effects:*
  - *Common:* nausea, vomiting, mouth ulcers, bone marrow suppression – especially leucopenia and thrombocytopenia – hepatitis, skin rashes
  - *Uncommon:* pneumonitis, chronic fibrosis
- *Advice:* folic acid should be taken 3–4 days after each dose of methotrexate. **Methotrexate is teratogenic**, therefore it is essential that parents of teenage children (both male and female) and the children themselves are aware of the need to use a reliable form of contraception during treatment and for at least 3 months afterwards. Breastfeeding should also be avoided.
- *Monitoring:* baseline full blood count, liver function tests, urea and electrolytes and creatinine prior to initiation of therapy. These should be repeated every 2 weeks for the first month of treatment, then monthly for 6–12 months; then may change to every 2–3 months provided there are no problems.

Calcineurin inhibitors

Ciclosporin

- *Preparations:* tablets (10 mg, 25 mg, 50 mg, 100 mg), suspension (100 mg/mL)
- *Pharmacokinetics:* peak blood concentrations are reached within 1–2 hours, with a 20–50% oral bioavailability. It is metabolised in the liver via cytochrome P450 pathways – therefore to be used with caution with other drugs broken down by the same system.
- *Side-effects:*
  - *Common:* nausea, anorexia, abdominal pain, gingival hyperplasia, increased susceptibility to infections, leucopenia, tremor, headache,

hyperlipidaemia, hypertension, abnormal liver function, hirsutism, myalgia
- *Uncommon:* thrombocytopenia, pancreatitis, insomnia, convulsions, muscle weakness, nephrotoxicity
- *Monitoring:* trough ciclosporin levels should be measured weekly and dosages adjusted until the ciclosporin levels are stable. Full blood count, urea and electrolytes and creatinine, liver function tests, blood pressure and urinalysis should be completed every 2 weeks for 3 months; thereafter monthly. Lipids should be monitored every 6 months. Liaise with local clinical biochemist for laboratory normal ranges.

Cytokine modulators

Key examples: infliximab, adalimumab

- *Preparations:* infliximab (100 mg vials for infusion); adalimumab (40 mg prefilled pen/vials for subcutaneous injections)
- *Pharmacokinetics:* infliximab is a chimeric human–murine monoclonal antibody that binds with high affinity to both soluble and transmembrane forms of tumour necrosis factor alpha (TNFα) and is given as an intravenous infusion. Adalimumab is a fully human monoclonal antibody that also binds specifically to TNFα and is given as a subcutaneous injection. Both act by blocking TNF's interaction with the p55 and p75 cell surface TNF receptors.
- *Side-effects:*
  - *Common:* increased susceptibility to infection (viral, bacterial, mycobacterial), immediate/anaphylactic reactions, delayed hypersensitivity reactions, neutropenia, leucopenia, insomnia, headache, conjunctivitis, palpitations, abdominal pain, nausea, pustular psoriasis, dermatitis, arthralgia
  - *Uncommon:* increased risk of malignancy (lymphomas, including hepatosplenic T-cell lymphoma, leukaemia, melanoma), thrombocytopenia, agranulocytosis, lupus-like syndrome, serum sickness-like reaction, transverse myelitis
- *Advice:* children should be evaluated for tuberculosis, hepatitis viruses and for previous varicella-zoster infections prior to commencement of biological therapy. It is important that children and their families are fully counselled prior to the use of biological therapies.

Constipation and laxatives

- Prior to the prescribing of laxatives to children, it is important to identify whether the child is constipated or has slow transit, and that there is not an underlying cause. NICE guidance for the diagnosis and management of idiopathic childhood constipation in primary and secondary care[7] provides a useful framework for health professionals looking after these children. First line treatment (see Box 1) is usually with an osmotic laxative (e.g. macrogols). If that is unsuccessful after 2 weeks, a stimulant (e.g. senna) should be considered. Refractory constipation should be managed by a health professional with specialist training.

Box 1 Stepwise approach to management of constipation in children

Step 1: Is diet and behavioural intervention needed?
Idiopathic constipation should *not be treated with lifestyle interventions alone*. Positive reinforcement of behavioural interventions and regular scheduled toileting helps to establish regular and effective bowel habit. Dietary modifications should ensure a balanced diet and sufficient fluids are consumed.

Step 2: Is faecal impaction present?
Consider disimpaction with macrogol 3350 (e.g. MOVICOL® Paediatric Plain) followed by maintenance therapy.

Step 3: Is maintenance therapy required?
Macrogol 3350 is the first line maintenance therapy and should be adjusted to symptoms and response. It is important that families are shown a Bristol stool chart and encouraged to vary the dose, aiming for type 4 stools. Regular reassessment is essential.

Step 4: Is a stimulant laxative required?
If a macrogol alone is insufficient for regular soft stooling, consider starting a stimulant laxative. Senna or docusate sodium should be used as first line stimulants. If there are frequent small stools, sodium picosulfate is a useful second line therapy.

Bulk-forming laxatives

- Bulk-forming laxatives are used to relieve constipation by increasing faecal mass and thereby stimulating intestinal peristalsis. They are most useful in children deficient in dietary fibre. The most commonly prescribed is ispaghula husk.

Ispaghula husk

- *Preparations:* sachets (3.5 g)
- *Pharmacokinetics:* ispaghula husk is capable of absorbing up to 40 times its own weight of water, acting as a simple bulking agent. In addition, colonic bacteria are believed to use the hydrated material as a metabolic substrate, further increasing faecal bulk.

- *Side-effects: uncommon:* hypersensitivity
- *Advice:* it must be given with water (at least 150 mL) due to risk of causing intestinal obstruction. It also contains aspartame, and therefore should not be given to children with phenylketonuria.

Stimulant laxatives

- Stimulant laxatives increase intestinal motility and, consequently, decrease intestinal transit times, but can cause abdominal cramping if stool remains hard. Consequently, they are often coadministered with osmotic laxatives to soften the stool. Prolonged use can lead to electrolyte imbalance, particularly hypokalaemia. First line treatment in children is usually with senna.

Bisacodyl

Preparations: tablets (5 mg); suppositories (5 mg, 10 mg), suspension (5 mg/5 mL)

Pharmacokinetics: bisacodyl is rapidly hydrolysed to the active principle bis-(p-hydroxyphenyl)-pyridyl-2-methane (BHPM), with maximum laxative effect occurring between 6–12 hours post administration.

Side-effects:
- *Common:* nausea, vomiting
- *Uncommon:* hypersensitivity, colitis, dizziness

Advice: it should not be used in children suspected of having an ileus, intestinal obstruction or acute inflammatory conditions.

Docusate sodium

- *Preparations:* tablets (100 mg), suspension (paediatric: 12.5 mg/5 mL), enema (120 mg in 10 g dose)
- *Pharmacokinetics:* docusate has both softening and stimulant action – it lowers the surface tension of faeces, allowing the softening of faeces by water and salts.
- *Side-effects: common:* nausea, diarrhoea, abdominal cramps

Glycerol

- *Preparations:* suppositories (1 g, 2 g, 4 g)
- *Pharmacokinetics:* glycerol by the rectal route promotes peristalsis and evacuation of the lower bowel by virtue of its irritant action.
- *Side-effects: uncommon:* local irritation, abdominal cramps
- *Advice:* glycerol can play a useful role as a short-term stimulant and lubricant for childhood constipation, but should only be used in conjunction with longer term management with other agents.

Senna

- *Preparations:* tablets (7.5 mg), suspension (7.5 mg/5 mL)
- *Pharmacokinetics:* senna is broken down by colonic bacteria, releasing anthraquinones which exert a laxative action usually 6–12 hours after administration.
- *Side-effects: common:* abdominal cramping
- *Advice:* senna is best given in the evening before bed, given its duration of action. It is generally well tolerated, but adverse effects are seen particularly in children who still have hard stool.

Sodium picosulfate, sodium picosulfate with magnesium citrate

- *Preparations:* suspension (5 mg/5 mL)
- *Pharmacokinetics:* sodium picosulfate is broken down into the active compound BHPM in the colon following bacterial cleavage. It stimulates the mucosa of both the large intestine and the rectum. The onset of action of the preparation is usually between 6 and 12 hours. Preparations containing magnesium citrate can also act as an osmotic laxative by retaining moisture in the colon.
- *Side-effects:*
  - *Common:* headache, nausea
  - *Uncommon:* hypersensitivity, vomiting, rash
- *Advice:* sodium picosulfate is a particularly good stimulant of the distal colon and rectum. Preparations with magnesium citrate are used for bowel preparation prior to procedures.

Faecal softeners

Arachis oil

- *Preparations:* enema
- *Pharmacokinetics:* localised lubricant and softener made from peanut oil
- *Advice:* contraindicated in those with peanut or soya allergy. Rarely used in clinical practice.

Osmotic laxatives

Lactulose

- *Preparations:* suspension (10 g/15 mL)
- *Pharmacokinetics:* largely non-absorbed disaccharide in the small bowel, it is broken down by colonic bacteria causing an increase of the osmotic gradient in the colon. This causes stimulation of peristalsis and an increase of the water content of the faeces.

- *Side-effects: common:* nausea, vomiting, flatulence, cramps, abdominal discomfort
- *Advice:* useful stool softener in mild constipation or in children who do not tolerate macrogol laxatives. **Contraindicated in galactosaemia.**

Macrogols

- *Example:* MOVICOL Paediatric Plain® (macrogol 3350)
- *Pharmacokinetics:* macrogols are not absorbed and act by increasing stool volume through their osmotic effect, thereby softening stool and increasing colonic peristalsis.
- *Side-effects: common:* abdominal distension and pain, nausea, flatulence
- *Advice:* recommended by NICE as first line laxative in children. Can be used for disimpaction and/or maintenance therapy. Preparations of other macrogols (e.g. KLEAN-PREP 3350®) can be used as bowel cleansing preparations prior to procedures or for constipation refractory to other therapies.

Phosphates

- *Example:* phosphate enemas, Fleet® ready-to-use enemas
- *Preparations:* enemas (118 mL, 128 mL)
- *Pharmacokinetics:* promotes distal colonic peristalsis and bowel movement through fluid accumulation and subsequent bowel distension
- *Side-effects: uncommon:* hypersensitivity, electrolyte imbalance, nausea, vomiting, abdominal pain, abdominal distension
- *Advice:* useful in stool clearance of distal colonic tracts (descending, sigmoid and rectum), but rarely required as maintenance therapy.

Drugs affecting intestinal secretions

Drugs affecting biliary composition and flow

Ursodeoxycholic acid

- *Preparations:* tablets (150 mg, 300 mg), suspension (250 mg/5 mL)
- *Pharmacokinetics:* ursodeoxycholic acid is rapidly and completely absorbed, causing a reduction in cholesterol in biliary fluid primarily by dispersing the cholesterol and forming a liquid-crystal phase.
- *Side-effects: uncommon:* diarrhoea, urticaria, gallstones
- *Advice:* ursodeoxycholic acid should be used in children with cholestatic conditions, on long term parental nutrition, post liver surgery or in those that have an inborn error of bile acid synthesis. Close monitoring of liver function tests is required to ensure a correct dose of medication.

Bile acid sequestrants

Colestyramine

- *Preparations:* powder (4 g sachets)
- *Pharmacokinetics:* prevents reabsorption of bile from the enterohepatic circulation through combining with the bile acids in the intestine to form an insoluble complex that is excreted in the faeces.
- *Side-effects: uncommon:* intestinal obstruction, hyperchloraemic acidosis, anorexia, nausea, vomiting
- *Advice:* useful postoperatively in children following ileal surgery or to relieve pruritus in children with partial biliary obstruction. It should be noted that it reduces absorption of fat-soluble vitamins (vitamins A, D, K and folic acid supplements), which may require supplementation if treatment is prolonged.

Conclusions

This chapter presents an overview of the key knowledge that should underpin prescribing in paediatric gastroenterology. To optimise the medication regimens of patients with complex gastroenterological conditions requires regular input from specialist multidisciplinary teams and close liaison with the community-based healthcare professionals caring for such patients in non-specialist settings.

References

1   Vandenplas Y *et al.* Gastroesophageal reflux clinical practice guidelines: joint recommendations of the North American Society for Pediatric Gastroenterology, Hepatology and Nutrition (NASPGHAN) and the European Society for Pediatric Gastroenterology, Hepatology and Nutrition (ESPGHAN). *JPGN* 2009; 49(4): 498–547.
2   Asseri M *et al.* Gastric acid suppression by proton pump inhibitors as a risk factor for *clostridium difficile*-associated diarrhea in hospitalized patients. *Am J Gastroentrol* 2008; 103: 2308–2313.
3   Simon B *et al.* Sucralfate gel versus placebo in patients with non-erosive gastro-oesophageal reflux disease. *Aliment Pharmacol Ther* 1996; 10: 441–446.
4   Arguelles-Martin F *et al.* Sucralfate versus cimetidine in the treatment of reflux esophagitis in children. *Am J Med* 1989; 86: 73–76.
5   Turner D *et al.* Management of pediatric ulcerative colitis: joint ECCO and ESPGHAN evidence-based consensus guidelines. *JPGN* 2012; 55(3): 340–361.
6   Ruemmele FM *et al.* Consensus guidelines of ECCO/ESPGHAN on the medical management of pediatric Crohn's disease. *J Crohns Colitis* 2014; 8(10): 1179–1207.
7   NICE. *Constipation in Children and Young People: Diagnosis and management.* NICE, 2010. www.nice.org.uk/guidance/CG099

39

Cardiovascular system

K Leonard and R Tulloh

Introduction

Prescribing in paediatric cardiology differs significantly from prescribing for adults. In particular, the dose is dependent on the patient's weight, a test dose is recommended for certain medicines, close monitoring of renal function is required, and a number of medicines must only be initiated after advice from a consultant paediatric cardiologist.[1,2]

The learning objectives of this chapter are:

➤ to learn which medications are used for heart failure, arrhythmias, pulmonary hypertension and Kawasaki disease
➤ to understand the key indications, pharmacokinetics, pharmacodynamics, side-effects and toxicity of common medications
➤ to learn how to adjust prescription in renal and hepatic impairment
➤ to know how to correctly monitor relevant medications.

Heart failure

Potassium sparing diuretics

- *Examples:* amiloride, spironolactone
- Amiloride inhibits sodium proton exchange (involved in sodium reabsorption in distal tubules and collecting tubules). Spironolactone inhibits the effect of aldosterone by competing for intracellular aldosterone receptors in the distal tubule cells. This leads to increased water and sodium secretion and decreased potassium excretion.
- *Contraindications:* hyperkalaemia, anuria, Addison's disease. Avoid in severe renal impairment.
- *Pharmacokinetics:* amiloride is readily absorbed, not metabolised and has a duration of 6–24 hours. Spironolactone is 90% protein bound, undergoes hepatic transformation to canrenone and has a duration of action of 3–5 days. Both are excreted in urine.

- *Side-effects:* dry mouth, jaundice, electrolyte disturbances and gynaeco-mastia
- *Key points:*
  - Monitor renal function closely.
  - Do not give concurrent potassium supplements.

Loop diuretics

- *Examples:* bumetanide, furosemide
- These inhibit the reabsorption of sodium, potassium and chloride from the ascending limb of the loop of Henle.
- *Contraindications:* severe hypokalaemia, severe hyponatraemia, anuria, renal failure due to nephrotoxics. Avoid in hepatic impairment.
- *Pharmacokinetics:* bumetanide is 97% protein bound, has a half-life of 60–90 minutes and undergoes hepatic metabolism. Furosemide has a half-life of 1.5 hours. Both have a duration of action of 4–5 hours and are metabolised by renal excretion.
- *Side-effects:* postural hypotension, acute urinary retention, hepatic encephalopathy, tinnitus and deafness
- *Key point:*
  - Meticulously monitor electrolytes.

Angiotensin-converting enzyme inhibitors

- *Examples:* captopril, enalapril, lisinopril
- These inhibit angiotensin-converting enzyme (ACE) and hence reduce conversion of angiotensin I to angiotensin II. This leads to arteriolar and venous dilation, reduction of aldosterone secretion and reduction of cardiac remodelling.
- *Contraindications:* hypersensitivity to ACE inhibitors (includes angioedema), bilateral renovascular disease, suspected renovascular disease. Monitor liver function tests closely if using in hepatic impairment.
- *Pharmacokinetics:* captopril has a bioavailability of 65% and a half-life of 2 hours. Enalapril is 55% bound in plasma and has an oral availability of 95%. The oral prodrug is converted in the liver by hydrolysis to enalaprilat. The half-life of enalaprilat is 11 hours. Lisinopril has a bioavailability of 25%, a half-life of 12 hours and is not metabolised. All undergo renal excretion.
- *Side-effects:* hypotension, renal impairment, dry cough, bronchospasm, dyspnoea, blurred vision
- *Key points:*
  - Toxicity leads to severe hypotension.
  - Monitor blood pressure, renal function, liver function, full blood count.

- Must initiate under specialist supervision with a test dose (refer to local guidelines).
- In practice, the three times daily dose is difficult for older children and so conversion often takes place to lisinopril (once daily) at a few years old.

Beta-adrenoceptor blocking drugs

- *Examples:* carvedilol, propranolol, atenolol, sotalol
- These block the beta adrenoceptors in the heart, peripheral vasculature, bronchi, pancreas and liver. Vasodilation results and this reduces the workload of the ischaemic myocardium, restores excitation–contraction coupling, reduces cardiac hypertrophy and fibrosis, and reduces myocyte apoptosis.
- *Contraindications:* acute or decompensated heart failure (requiring inotropes), second/third degree heart block, asthma, bradycardia, hypotension, sick sinus syndrome and phaeochromocytoma. Sotalol is contraindicated if the patient has long QT syndrome. Avoid beta blockers in hepatic impairment. A dose reduction is required in renal impairment.
- *Pharmacokinetics:* carvedilol – half-life 6–8 hours, plasma protein binding 98%, bioavailability 25–35%, extensively metabolised in the liver, excreted in urine and faeces. Propranolol – bioavailability 26%, half-life 1–6 hours, 90% protein bound, extensive hepatic metabolism. Atenolol – bioavailability 40–50%, 10% protein bound, water soluble, half-life 6–7 hours, excreted only by the kidney. Sotalol – bioavailability 95%, half-life 12 hours, 5% protein bound, not metabolised, not lipid insoluble, excreted by kidneys.
- *Side-effects:* postural hypotension, coldness of the extremities, bradycardia, fatigue, sleep disturbances, dizziness. Sotalol may prolong the QT interval and can cause torsades de pointes (rare).
- *Key points:*
  - **Toxicity** leads to light-headedness, dizziness, syncope, coma or convulsions. Manage in hospital with expert advice (maintain airway, atropine, glucagon +/– temporary pacing).
  - Monitor renal function when titrating the dose.
  - Seek advice when discontinuing the drug, as this needs to be done gradually over several weeks.
  - When prescribing sotalol, particular care is required to avoid hypokalaemia (life-threatening arrhythmias).

Cardiac glycoside

- *Example:* digoxin
- Digoxin partially inhibits the sodium pump (Na–K–ATPase pump), leading to increased intracellular sodium, reduced sodium/calcium

exchange, and hence increased intracellular calcium. This increases the force of myocardial contraction. Digoxin has cardio-selective parasympathomimetic effects. It decreases the automaticity of the sinoatrial node and reduces conductivity within the atrioventricular node.

- *Contraindications:* intermittent complete/second degree heart block, Wolff–Parkinson–White syndrome, ventricular tachycardia/fibrillation and hypertrophic cardiomyopathy. Reduce the dose in renal impairment.
- *Pharmacokinetics:* oral bioavailability 70%, 25% bound in plasma, distributed to tissues (including central nervous system), half-life 1.5 days, not extensively metabolised, excreted via the kidneys.
- *Side-effects:* light flashes, blurred/yellow vision, arrhythmias and conduction disturbances
- *Key points:*
  - **Toxicity** leads to bradycardia and arrhythmias. Management involves discontinuation of digoxin, potassium supplementation (if hypokalaemia), atropine/pacing (if sinus bradycardia/atrioventricular block). In life-threatening overdose, give digoxin-specific antibody fragments and discuss with national poisons information service.
  - Monitor digoxin levels (0.8–2 µg/L). Take the blood test 6 hours post dose.

Angiotensin-II receptor blockers

- *Example:* losartan
- Losartan is an angiotensin-II receptor blocker. It reduces vasoconstriction and aldosterone secretion.
- *Contraindications:* aortic/mitral valve stenosis, hypertrophic cardiomyopathy, history of angioedema. Use with caution in renal artery stenosis. Avoid in hepatic impairment and in severe renal impairment.
- *Pharmacokinetics:* bioavailability 33%, 99% protein bound, active metabolite's half-life 3–4 hours, metabolised in liver, excreted in urine (35%) and faeces (60%)
- *Side-effects:* hypotension, hyperkalaemia and angioedema
- *Key points:*
  - **Toxicity** leads to hypotension and tachycardia.
  - Monitor renal function, full blood count and blood pressure.

Arrhythmias

Verapamil is no longer used in children routinely, because it can cause complete collapse. Adenosine is the treatment of choice for supraventricular tachycardia.

Adenosine

- Adenosine acts via the A1 receptor and opens the potassium channel, increasing inward potassium flux, and hence blocks conduction, primarily at the atrioventricular node.
- *Contraindications:* heart block, pre-existing angina, heart failure and long QT syndrome. It can exacerbate asthma.
- *Pharmacokinetics:* adenosine has a very short half-life of a few seconds.
- *Key points:*
  - Adenosine should be administered as a rapid intravenous injection into a proximal large peripheral vein, followed immediately by a flush of normal saline.
  - When administered, adenosine can cause asystole: hence it is disconcerting to patients and may cause angina in addition. The heart rate usually recovers rapidly, but full resuscitation facilities need to be available.

Flecainide

- Flecainide inhibits His–Purkinje conduction and fast sodium channels (causing depression of the upstroke of the cardiac action potential).
- *Contraindications:* heart failure, chronic atrial fibrillation, haemodynamically significant valvar heart disease, sinus node dysfunction, conduction defects. Reduce the dose in severe hepatic impairment. In renal impairment, reduce the dose and monitor plasma flecainide concentration.
- *Pharmacokinetics:* bioavailability 95%, 40% protein bound, peak plasma levels at 2–4 hours, half-life 20 hours, two-thirds metabolised by the liver, one-third excreted unchanged by the kidneys
- *Side-effects:* oedema, dyspnoea, dizziness, fatigue and visual disturbances
- *Key point:*
  - An effective plasma flecainide concentration is 200–800 µg/L. Take the blood sample immediately before next dose.

Beta-adrenoceptor blocking drugs *(see heart failure section)*

Amiodarone

- Amiodarone prolongs phase three of the cardiac action potential, acting on sodium and potassium channels to increase the refractory period. Hence it slows intra-cardiac conduction of the action potential.
- *Contraindications:* bradycardia, sinoatrial heart block, sinus node disease, thyroid dysfunction and iodine sensitivity
- *Pharmacokinetics:* half-life 25–110 days; 30–50% gastrointestinal absorption; lipid-soluble with extensive distribution in body; hepatic

metabolism to the active metabolite desethyl-amiodarone; excretion by skin, biliary tract and lacrimal glands
- *Side-effects:* pulmonary fibrosis, peripheral neuropathy, ataxia, hypothyroidism, hyperthyroidism, photosensitivity, corneal micro deposits and hepatotoxicity
- *Key points:*
  - Initiate in hospital or under specialist supervision.
  - The therapeutic blood level is 1.0–2.5 µg/mL.
  - Monitor thyroid, pulmonary and liver function and perform regular eye examinations.

Pulmonary hypertension

Management of pulmonary hypertension is initially by maintenance of good airway mechanics: maintaining a low CO_2, high O_2, high pH and good cardiac function, often with intravenous inotropic support such as milrinone. If there is chest infection, this must be treated first. Only after this has been undertaken would acute management of pulmonary hypertension include pharmacological therapy.

Endothelin receptor antagonists

- *Example:* ambrisentan
- Endothelin 1 stimulates the endothelin receptors ET-A and ET-B on the vascular smooth muscle cell. ET-A is known to cause vasoconstriction, and ambrisentan antagonises ET-A receptors.[3]
- *Contraindications:* idiopathic pulmonary fibrosis, moderate-severe hepatic impairment, pulmonary venous hypertension
- *Pharmacokinetics:* bioavailability unknown, 99% protein bound, peak concentration at 2 hours, half-life 15 hours, insoluble in water, eliminated by non-renal pathways
- *Side-effects:* peripheral oedema, anaemia, nasal congestion and liver dysfunction
- *Key points:*
  - Toxicity leads to severe hypotension.
  - Monitor haemoglobin levels and liver function tests.
- *Example:* bosentan (newer version macitentan, not yet licensed in children)
- Bosentan competitively antagonises ET-A and ET-B receptors. This is thought to be helpful, since the ET-B receptors are part of the negative feedback loop on the endothelial cell. Antagonism of both might help with reduction of downregulation.
- *Contraindications:* acute porphyria, liver dysfunction

- *Pharmacokinetics:* bioavailability 50%, 98% protein bound, hepatic metabolism, half-life 5 hours
- *Side-effects:* flushing, hypotension, palpitations, oedema, syncope, anaemia, liver failure/cirrhosis (rare)
- *Key point:*
  - Monitor liver function tests and haemoglobin levels.

Calcium channel blockers

- *Example:* amlodipine
- Amlodipine interferes with the inward displacement of calcium ions through the slow channels of active cell membranes. Amlodipine, a dihydropyridine, relaxes vascular smooth muscle and dilates coronary and peripheral arteries.
- *Contraindications:* cardiogenic shock, significant aortic stenosis. A dose reduction is required in hepatic impairment.
- *Pharmacokinetics:* bioavailability 64–90%, peak blood levels at 6–12 hours, extensive hepatic metabolism to inactive metabolites, half-life 35–48 hours, excreted by kidneys, steady state in 7–8 days.
- *Side-effects:* flushing, oedema, palpitations, sleep disturbance and fatigue

Eicosanoids

- *Examples:* epoprostenol, iloprost
- Epoprostenol inhibits platelet activation and is a potent vasodilator. Iloprost is a synthetic analogue of prostacyclin. It dilates systemic and pulmonary arterial vascular beds and affects platelet aggregation.[4]
- *Contraindications:* left ventricular dysfunction, pulmonary veno-occlusive disease, severe coronary heart disease, arrhythmias, valvar defects and disease of the myocardium. In liver cirrhosis, halve the dose of iloprost.
- *Pharmacokinetics:* epoprostenol – half-life 42 seconds, converted into 6-oxo-prostaglandin F_1 alpha, which is a much weaker vasodilator. Can be inhaled or administered intravenously. Iloprost – half-life 30 minutes, 60% protein bound, metabolised via β-oxidation of the carboxyl side chain.
- *Side-effects:* systemic hypotension, haemorrhage, bradycardia, tachycardia, flushing, sepsis, jaw pain
- *Key points:*
  - Epoprostenol is given via a continuous 24-hour intravenous infusion
  - With regards to iloprost, monitor vital signs and do not initiate if systolic blood pressure is less than 85 mmHg.

Additional treatments

Magnesium sulfate

- Magnesium sulfate is a cofactor for enzymatic reactions and plays an important role in neurochemical transmission and muscular excitability. It also causes peripheral vasodilation.
- *Contraindications:* heart block, myocardial damage. Avoid in renal impairment.
- *Pharmacokinetics:* renal excretion
- *Side-effects:* thirst, hypotension, arrhythmias, coma, respiratory depression
- *Key points:*
  - **Signs of overdose:** Rapid hypotension, respiratory paralysis, loss of patellar reflexes, weakness, sensation of warmth, flushing, drowsiness, double vision, slurred speech. Treat with artificial ventilation (if required) and intravenous calcium.
  - Monitor patellar reflexes and respiratory rate.

Nitric oxide

- Nitric oxide acts on guanylate cyclase, resulting in smooth muscle relaxation.[5] Nitric oxide is a potent and selective pulmonary vasodilator, because it is given by inhalation.
- *Contraindications:* neonates who are known to be dependent on right-to-left shunting of blood
- *Pharmacokinetics:* good bioavailability, metabolised via pulmonary capillary bed, half-life 2–6 seconds, excreted via the kidneys
- *Key points:*
  - **Toxicity:** signs of met-haemoglobinaemia include dyspnoea, tachypnoea, central cyanosis and brown discolouration of blood. Treat with 100% oxygen, methylene blue, exchange transfusion and hyperbaric oxygen.
  - Met-haemoglobin concentration should be measured regularly.

Sildenafil

- Sildenafil is a phosphodiesterase type-5 inhibitor. Inhibition augments the vasodilatory effects of nitric oxide and promotes relaxation of vascular smooth muscle.
- *Contraindications:* recent stroke, non-arteritic anterior ischaemic optic neuropathy, hereditary degenerative retinal disorders, sickle cell anaemia, pulmonary veno-occlusive disease. Reduce dose in mild to moderate renal and hepatic impairment. Avoid use in severe hepatic impairment.
- *Pharmacokinetics:* bioavailability 40%, hepatic metabolism, half-life 3–4 hours, faecal (80%) and renal (13%) excretion
- *Side-effects:* gastritis, haemorrhoids, dry mouth, flushing, night sweats, alopecia
- *Key point:*
  - Discontinue if sudden visual or hearing loss.

Kawasaki disease

Aspirin

- Aspirin irreversibly acetylates cyclooxygenase. It prevents the production of pro-aggregatory thromboxane A_2 and in high doses inhibits prostacyclin formation in the vascular endothelium. Aspirin inhibits the inflammatory process in the coronary arteries in Kawasaki disease at a high dose (30–50 mg/kg/day in four divided doses). The resultant endothelial dysfunction can lead to *in situ* platelet aggregation, hence low-dose (3–5 mg/kg/day) aspirin is used for at least 6 weeks (or longer if the coronary arteries are abnormal) to mitigate this effect.
- *Contraindications:* active peptic ulceration, haemophilia or other bleeding disorders. Avoid in severe hepatic and renal impairment.
- *Pharmacokinetics:* bioavailability 80–100%; 85% protein bound; hepatic metabolism; half-life 2–3 hours; excreted in urine, sweat, saliva, faeces
- *Side-effects:* dyspepsia, vomiting, bronchospasm, gastrointestinal haemorrhage
- *Key point:*
  - Aspirin use is associated with Reye's syndrome. Discontinue in high fever.

Human immunoglobulin

- Human immunoglobulin is thought to involve the inhibitory Fc receptor.
- *Contraindications:* patients with selective immunoglobulin A (IgA) deficiency who have known antibody against IgA
- *Pharmacokinetics:* there is considerable variability between patients.
- *Side-effects:* chills, fever, dizziness, arthralgia, myalgia, muscle spasms, anaphylaxis (rare)
- *Key point:*
  - Monitor renal function and discontinue the drug if there is deterioration.

Infliximab

- Infliximab is a monoclonal antibody that inhibits tumour necrosis factor alpha (a proinflammatory cytokine).
- *Contraindications:* severe infections and heart failure
- *Pharmacokinetics:* 92% bioavailability, metabolised via the reticulo-endothelial system, half-life 9.5 days
- *Side-effects:* infections, blood disorders, hypersensitivity reactions, fever and headache
- *Key points:*
  - **Hypersensitivity reactions:** fever, chest pain, hypotension or hypertension, dyspnoea, transient visual loss, urticaria, angioedema,

anaphylaxis. Treat with resuscitation (if required). Give prophylactic antipyretics, antihistamines and hydrocortisone.

- Administer only under specialist supervision with adequate resuscitation equipment accessible.

General considerations

Note that the protein binding of drugs can affect their pharmacodynamics. It is the unbound component that is pharmacologically active. For drugs that are heavily protein bound (such as warfarin, 97%), then only the unbound component is causing the pharmacological effect.[6] This only matters if there is a change in the protein (such as albumin) concentration in the blood, leading to a recalculation of the dose required.

Conclusions

Drugs used in paediatric cardiology differ in their indications and pharmacodynamics when compared with those used in adults. However, most of the half-lives described above have been extrapolated from the adult literature, given the frequent paucity of paediatric pharmacokinetic data. When prescribing a drug or formulation with which you are unfamiliar, it is important to seek early advice from senior or specialist colleagues, pharmacists or specialist information sites.

References

1 The Paediatric Formulary Committee, BNF for Children. London: BMJ Group, the Royal Pharmaceutical Society of Great Britain and RCPCH Publications Ltd, 2017.

2 Opie LH. *Drugs for the Heart*, 4th edn. Philadelphia, USA: W.B. Saunders Company, 1995.

3 Gilead Sciences. Highlights of prescribing information for LETAIRIS® (ambrisentan). Foster City, USA: Gilead Sciences, 2015. www.gilead.com/~/media/Files/pdfs/medicines/cardiovascular/letairis/letairis_pi.pdf

4 Actelion Pharmaceuticals US, Inc. Highlights of prescribing information for VENTAVIS® (iloprost) inhalation solution. South San Francisco, USA: Actelion Pharmaceuticals US, Inc, 2017. www.4ventavis.com/pdf/Ventavis_PI.pdf

5 Bayer HealthCare Pharmaceuticals Inc. Highlights of prescribing information for ADEMPAS (riociguat) tablets. Whippany, USA: Bayer HealthCare Pharmaceuticals Inc, 2013. http://labeling.bayerhealthcare.com/html/products/pi/Adempas_PI.pdf

6 Katzung B *et al. Basic and Clinical Pharmacology*, 12th edn. London: McGraw-Hill, 2012.

40

Respiratory system

W Lenney

Introduction

The respiratory system accounts for high levels of prescribing in children.[1] It has been calculated that 30% of outpatient visits, 25% of inpatient stays and 20% of primary care visits in Europe occur because of children with respiratory problems, predominantly in the autumn and winter months. The commonest symptoms are chronic cough, wheezing and breathlessness, often associated with upper or lower respiratory tract infections or asthma. Medicines used to treat these symptoms will be highlighted in this chapter. Most respiratory infections are viral in nature, so antibiotics have little to offer. Some medicines used in cystic fibrosis will also be discussed, but the treatment of rare diseases such as idiopathic pulmonary fibrosis, pulmonary haemosiderosis, surfactant or immune deficiencies and sarcoidosis are beyond the scope of this text.[2]

The main learning objectives are:

➢ to know how to treat each symptom with an appropriate medicine and not overuse antibiotics
➢ to be aware of the main side-effects of each medicine
➢ when a treatment is started but has little benefit, to be prepared to stop it
➢ to understand and be able to teach inhaler technique to all children and their families for any inhaler that is prescribed.

Short acting β_2-adrenergic agonists (SABAs) – salbutamol/terbutaline

SABAs are sympathomimetic amines comprising a benzene ring attached to an amine group via carbon atoms. They were discovered by making large substitutions on the amine group to increase β activity and reduce α activity, conferring bronchial selectivity and less cardiotoxicity. Within the respiratory system, B$_2$ receptors are present from the throat to the alveoli. SABAs bind to β$_2$ receptors, stimulate adenylate cyclase and encourage the formation of cyclic AMP. Stimulation of β$_2$ receptors causes relaxation of smooth muscle (thereby inducing bronchodilation), reduction in oedema and increased mucociliary clearance. Following inhalation, the onset of action is within 5 minutes, maximal effect occurring within 20 minutes, and the half-life is approximately 90 minutes.

Use SABAs as required but not as regular inhaled therapy. The usual dosage range for salbutamol is 2–8 puffs 4 hourly in all ages (where 1 puff equates to a dose of 100 µg). Note that SABAs are less effective in children under 18 months old.

Inhalation technique must be well taught and rechecked at each future consultation.

Main side-effects: fine tremor, tachycardia, headache

Long acting β$_2$-agonists (LABAs) – formoterol and salmeterol

These hydrophobic compounds have much greater affinity for the β$_2$ receptor, hence one reason for their longer action of up to 9–12 hours in duration. Salmeterol also shows intense binding of its very long sidearm to an area of the receptor known as the exosite, conferring on it a unique mode of action. This binding allows the other end of the molecule to interact freely with the active site, thereby reducing desensitisation and tachyphylaxis, the development of early tolerance to the long action of LABAs. Unlike SABAs, LABAs should not be used on an as-required basis and should only be prescribed alongside inhaled corticosteroids, usually twice daily, either as a separate inhaler or as combination therapy for improved adherence and patient preference purposes (see below).

Main side-effects: similar to SABAs

Corticosteroids: inhaled and systemic

At the cellular level, corticosteroids attach themselves to specific cytoplasmic glucocorticoid receptors and then enter the cell nucleus, where they bind with genes involved in inflammatory changes. Through effects on gene transcription and its regulation, they activate genes responsible for reducing inflammation and suppress genes that enhance inflammation. They have no effect on the leukotriene driven inflammatory pathway.

Inhaled corticosteroids (ICS) are the gold standard for use in all but the very mildest forms of allergic asthma and are particularly helpful in children of school age. They are less effective for viral induced wheeze; viral infection is the commonest reason for symptoms such as wheezing in the pre-school-age group. ICS are overused in these children, especially in those under 3 years old. Montelukast is now often the first treatment of choice in this very young age group. It is imperative to demonstrate good inhalation technique to all patients if they are to obtain maximum benefit from inhaled medicines. This takes time, and reports frequently comment that insufficient time is dedicated to such teaching and training. (See paragraph on inhalers and nebulisers.)

At recommended international asthma management guideline dosages, ICS efficacy is very high and side-effects are rare. There is still a fear of the word 'steroid' in many European communities, and much of this is inappropriately related to concerns about anabolic steroids.

There is little to choose between the various ICS brands available in relation to efficacy, but some are more potent than others – i.e. they attach themselves more readily and remain more firmly attached to the steroid receptor. Similarly, there are some differences in the side-effect profile, particularly in relation to oral absorption and first-pass metabolism through the liver. Dosage recommendations in guidelines take account of these differences.

At each consultation it is important to assess any ICS side-effects in each child: monitor height and weight (and plot these on a growth chart), check the mouth for evidence of candidiasis and, although a very rare issue, ask about dizzy spells or other signs/symptoms of low blood sugar levels, which may indicate adrenal suppression.

Main side-effects: rare when used at recommended guideline doses; high dosages may slow growth

Oral corticosteroids

Use in asthma: Prednisolone is used in short courses to regain asthma control. Guidelines recommend 1–2 mg/kg for 1–3 or 5 days. Evidence for the best dosage is lacking, and 0.5 mg/kg is also used in some centres. In more severe asthma, longer courses of prednisolone are needed. The dose does not need to be tapered if the course duration is less than 14 days. Prednisolone is available as tablets, enteric coated tablets and dissolvable/soluble formulations. Most children are offered soluble preparations, which are more expensive. The most appropriate dosage form for each child should be determined. Some children with very severe asthma may need low dose prednisolone on a regular daily basis but, if so, they should be under the care of a respiratory paediatrician.

Use in acute viral croup: Almost all the clinical studies undertaken to assess corticosteroid treatment in the management of acute viral croup used dexamethasone, hence the present recommendation for dexamethasone rather than prednisolone. Prednisolone, however, is likely to be equally effective.

Main side-effects: mild behavioural change even with short courses; weight gain and increased appetite with prolonged use

Combination therapy

The use of combination therapy has been increasing over the last 15 years in children 5 years and older whose asthma is not well controlled on ICS alone. The main therapies have been Seretide® (salmeterol and fluticasone) and Symbicort® (formoterol and budesonide), both licensed for regular twice-daily use. The efficacy and side-effect profiles are the same. Seretide® is available in metered dose and dry powder formulations, Symbicort® only as dry powder. The clinical difference in usage rests on the rapid onset of action of formoterol, being similar to that of salbutamol and terbutaline (within 5 minutes), whereas salmeterol has a slow onset (up to 20 minutes). To improve control when using regular twice-daily Symbicort®, an additional two or three inhalations can be given each day, whereas if control needs improving when using Seretide®, it should be in the form of additional salbutamol or terbutaline inhalations. A number of other twice-daily combination products are now available, as is once-daily therapy using a combination of vilanterol and fluticasone furoate (which, at the time of writing, is only licensed for children 12 years and above).

Main side-effects: as for ICS plus LABAs

Other treatments for asthma and wheezing

Montelukast

Leukotrienes are produced as part of the inflammatory process. They are not suppressed by corticosteroids. Cysteinyl leukotrienes increase mucus production, encourage eosinophil recruitment and cause bronchoconstriction. Montelukast, a leukotriene receptor antagonist, is licensed for use in viral induced wheezing and asthma in all age groups from 6 months upwards. It is given as granules to those under 2 years of age, which helps administration at this very young age, and as a once-daily chewable tablet from 2–14 years of age. It is thought that adherence is higher because of its ease of administration, and it is recommended as first line treatment in the pre-school-age group. It works rapidly, so response should be seen within the first few days of use. If there is no response after 14 days, consider stopping.

Main side-effects: sleep disturbance, abdominal pain

Omalizumab

Omalizumab is a humanised monoclonal antibody which binds to free immunoglobulin E (IgE) and inhibits mast cell degranulation. Severity of asthma is related to degree of atopy and IgE levels. Omalizumab is used in children aged 6 years and older with asthma that is uncontrollable on conventional treatment. Fortnightly or monthly subcutaneous injections are administered – the dose depends on body weight and total IgE blood level. Omalizumab is very expensive, and treatment should be under the supervision of a tertiary respiratory paediatric service.

Main side-effects: headache, abdominal pain (rare)

Sodium cromoglicate and nedocromil sodium

These medications are now rarely used in children with asthma. There is very little evidence to support their use.

Respiratory medicines used in cystic fibrosis (CF)

Respiratory disease in CF is characterised by airway obstruction, mucus retention and repeated infections with both viruses and bacteria. These lead to deterioration in lung function, with 90% of deaths from CF being due to respiratory causes.

Mucolytics: hypertonic saline and DNase

Airway surface liquid is abnormal in CF. The mucus is tenacious and difficult to expectorate. Nebulised hypertonic saline, prior to physiotherapy, enhances mucociliary clearance, with a concentration of 7% having the most supportive evidence from clinical studies. Side-effects are rare providing the child can tolerate the salty taste.

In CF, extracellular DNA accumulates in the airways in response to infection, which increases sputum viscoelasticity. The administration of once-daily nebulised phosphorylated glycosylated recombinant human deoxyribonuclease (rhDNase) 1 hour before physiotherapy helps to break up mucus strands, reduces respiratory symptoms, may improve lung function, and can lower the frequency of infective exacerbations.

Main side-effects: pharyngitis, vocal changes

Ivacaftor

Genetic mutations in the cystic fibrosis transmembrane conductance regulator (CFTR) result in reduced protein transfer to the apical surface of airway epithelial cells. The combination of the $\Delta F508$ and the G551D mutation is found in approximately 5% of patients with CF and is a class 3 'gating' defect. Ivacaftor administered as one tablet twice daily in such patients has enabled an abnormal sweat test result to return to within the normal range, halted deterioration in pulmonary progression, and in some patients improved their lung function levels. This is the first medicine used in CF that works at a cellular level to normalise the function of the mutant gene. The major issue is its cost, at approximately £120,000 per patient per year.

Main side-effects: abdominal pain, diarrhoea, headache

Antibiotics

A wide range of oral, nebulised and intravenous antibiotics are regularly used in CF. Colomycin and tobramycin are worthy of mention because of their wide bactericidal spectrum, their modes of action and their frequent use in nebulised and intravenous formulations.

Colomycin

Colomycin, a cyclical polypeptide, is derived from a polymixin bacillus. Its main action is to damage the bacterial cell membrane, which proves lethal to bacteria with a hydrophobic outer cell wall. Absorption is variable following nebulised therapy, but some systemic absorption can occur. There is no absorption from the gastrointestinal tract. The half-life of intravenous colomycin is 1.5 hours, and colomycin is eliminated by the kidneys.

Main side-effects: neurotoxicity and nephrotoxicity when given parenterally; sore throat when given by inhalation

Tobramycin

Tobramycin is a rapidly bactericidal aminoglycoside that shows concentration dependent killing. Between-patient variation is less in high-dose once-daily usage. Its elimination half-life is 2–3 hours, but this is increased in high-dose once-daily regimens. The best predictor of efficacy is area under the curve (AUC) over 24 hours: mean inhibitory concentration (MIC). Note that all aminoglycosides are nephrotoxic. Hearing tests are recommended following every 10 courses of intravenous aminoglycosides.

Main side-effects: bronchospasm, nephrotoxicity

Ciprofloxacin

Ciprofloxacin is the only oral antibiotic that is clinically effective against *Pseudomonas aeruginosa*. It has been used as first line eradication therapy when *Pseudomonas* is first grown in CF patients. Its value has been questioned, however, and a large study in the UK will determine whether oral ciprofloxacin monotherapy or intravenous tobramycin and ceftazidime dual therapy is more effective.

Main side-effects: nausea, diarrhoea, joint pains

Inhalers and nebulisers

National standards of care now state that every consultation requires demonstration by the patient and family that all children are able to use their inhalers effectively. This is because efficacy will be severely compromised if the technique is inadequate. There remains a reticence to teach and train inhaler technique to all patients from the first visit onwards. This is worrying when most reports from around the world show that control of asthma is poor. Thus the published benefit–risk balance for inhaled versus oral medication usage is meaningless without education and regular checking of technique at every consultation. Inhaled therapies need to be carefully evaluated, particularly in children, to ensure the appropriate inhalation device is chosen for each child so that maximal (or indeed any) benefit is obtained from the prescribed medication.[3]

Conclusions

The burden of respiratory disease in children remains significant, and therefore high quality prescribing in this area is essential. After treatment initiation, patients' medications should be reviewed regularly and stopped where appropriate. The importance of patient/parent education as a key component of respiratory pharmacotherapy should not be underestimated, particularly for inhaler technique in the context of asthma.

References

1 Zar HJ, Ferkol TW. The global burden of respiratory disease-impact on child health. *Pediatr Pulmonol* 2014; 49(5): 430–434.

2 Lenney W *et al*. Medicines used in respiratory diseases only seen in children. *Eur Respir J* 2009; 34(3): 531–551.

3 van Aalderen WM *et al*. How to match the optimal currently available inhaler device to an individual child with asthma or recurrent wheeze. *NPJ Prim Care Respir Med* 2015; 25: 14088.

41

Antiepileptic drug therapy

M Anderson

Introduction

The goal of the pharmacological treatment of epilepsy is complete seizure control with an absence of significant adverse effects. This chapter provides an overview of the principles to consider when treating paediatric epilepsy with antiepileptic drugs (AEDs) and of the individual drugs currently available for use in the UK.

The learning objectives of this chapter are:

➤ to understand the key principles of AED therapy
➤ to know the first and second line treatment options for different seizure/epilepsy syndrome types
➤ to recognise common adverse drug reactions associated with AEDs used in children.

Principles of AED therapy

Certain AEDs are considered to be 'first line' for the different seizure types and epilepsy syndromes; others are considered 'second line' in comparison, either because of reduced efficacy or, more often, a poorer adverse effect profile. However, it is well recognised that there is significant difficulty in categorising seizure types and epilepsy syndromes, and sometimes the most effective AED for a child may have to be found by trial and error. Seizure types and syndromes with their associated first and second line drugs are listed in Table 1.

Initially, the appropriate first line AED is introduced at a low dose and increased to achieve a therapeutic dose at the lower end of the dosage range. A slow introduction over several weeks reduces the incidence of unwanted adverse effects, although the AEDs levetiracetam and gabapentin are well tolerated and can be increased rapidly. If the seizures do not respond, the dose should be increased until the maximum dose is reached or adverse effects occur. In the event of inefficacy at maximum dose or of

Table 1 AEDs by seizure/epilepsy syndrome type		
Seizure type/epilepsy syndrome	First line AED(s)[*]	Second line AED(s)[*]
Generalised tonic–clonic	Sodium valproate Lamotrigine Carbamazepine (not in generalised genetic epilepsy)	**Levetiracetam Clobazam Topiramate**
Tonic or atonic	Sodium valproate	**Lamotrigine**
Absence	Ethosuximide Sodium valproate Lamotrigine	**Clobazam Clonazepam Levetiracetam Topiramate Zonisamide**
Myoclonic	Levetiracetam Sodium valproate Topiramate	**Clobazam Clonazepam Zonisamide**
Focal	Carbamazepine/Oxcarbazepine Levetiracetam Lamotrigine	**Topiramate Gabapentin Sodium valproate Phenobarbital Phenytoin Lacosamide Tiagabine Zonisamide**
Childhood absence epilepsy	Ethosuximide Sodium valproate	**Lamotrigine Clobazam Clonazepam Topiramate**
Juvenile absence epilepsy	Ethosuximide Sodium valproate Lamotrigine	**Clobazam Clonazepam Levetiracetam Topiramate Zonisamide**
Juvenile myoclonic epilepsy	Lamotrigine Levetiracetam Sodium valproate	**Clobazam Clonazepam Topiramate**
Genetic generalised epilepsy	Sodium valproate Lamotrigine	**Levetiracetam Topiramate Clobazam**
Infantile spasms	Vigabatrin Steroids (prednisolone or depot tetracosactide)	**Sodium valproate**

Table 1 (*Continued*)		
Seizure type/epilepsy syndrome	**First line AED(s)***	**Second line AED(s)***
Benign epilepsy with centrotemporal spikes	Carbamazepine/Oxcarbazepine Lamotrigine Levetiracetam Sodium valproate	**Clobazam Gabapentin Topiramate**
Severe myoclonic epilepsy of infancy (Dravet syndrome)	Sodium valproate	**Clobazam Stiripentol**
Lennox–Gastaut syndrome	Sodium valproate	**Clobazam Levetiracetam Topiramate Rufinamide**

*Not all AEDs listed have a licence for the indication.

treatment-limiting adverse effects, an alternative first line AED or a second line AED should be selected and introduced in the same fashion.

There is a risk of precipitating seizures if AEDs are suddenly withdrawn. To avoid this, the new AED should be introduced alongside the old AED for a period of time prior to gradual withdrawal of the old AED. For the same reason, AED therapy should not be interrupted, where possible, for reasons such as intercurrent illness or operations. If necessary, intravenous antiepileptic medication can be given to a child who is nil by mouth or unable to take medication by mouth. If AED therapy is no longer deemed necessary, for example when a child has been seizure free for greater than 2 years for an epilepsy known to be age limited, gradual dose reduction should be undertaken over a period of several weeks.

Sometimes two AEDs administered concurrently are required to control seizures. The relative disadvantages of using more than two AEDs may outweigh the benefits. It is vital to consider drug interactions whenever more than one drug is being used.

Therapeutic drug monitoring (TDM) is available for a number of AEDs. It is vital that it is interpreted in the clinical context, as the pharmacokinetic/pharmacodynamic inter-individual variability is significant. It may be acceptable for the drug concentration to be below the target range if seizures are well controlled, or above the range if this is required for seizure control and there are no adverse effects, giving rise to the concept of individual therapeutic concentrations rather than target ranges. TDM is generally useful in the following situations:

- To guide and monitor dosing when using phenytoin or phenobarbital
- To evaluate loss of seizure control for causes such as non-compliance
- To evaluate toxicity

Reference ranges for therapeutic drug concentrations, where quoted in this chapter, are generally internationally accepted,[1] but guidance may vary and readers are advised to comply with local policies.

A number of AEDs are strongly associated with Stevens–Johnson syndrome or toxic epidermal necrolysis (TEN): lamotrigine, carbamazepine, phenytoin and phenobarbital. These drugs may also cause benign rashes, which are unfortunately indistinguishable from the early stages of the more serious skin manifestations. If a child develops a rash with benign characteristics (no systemic features, non-confluent), the drug should be stopped or dose increases should be halted, and close monitoring is advisable. If the rash settles, cautious reintroduction can be considered, but recurrence of the rash indicates that the drug should not be restarted. If a child develops a rash with serious characteristics (confluent, involvement of mucous membranes, systemic features), the drug should be stopped and admission to hospital is advised; the drug should not be restarted.

AEDs

Carbamazepine and oxcarbazepine

- *Use and efficacy:*
  - Carbamazepine: first line drug for focal seizures with or without secondary generalisation. Also effective for primary generalised tonic–clonic seizures, but should be avoided in genetic (idiopathic) generalised epilepsy due to lack of efficacy. Exaggerates absence, myoclonic and atonic seizures and is contraindicated in epilepsies with these seizure types.
  - Oxcarbazepine: very similar antiepileptic efficacy to carbamazepine; may be useful in patients in whom carbamazepine has been effective but not tolerated due to adverse effects.
- *Adverse effects:*
  - Carbamazepine: commonly causes sedation and dizziness – usually dose dependent and reversible and can be avoided by slow upward dose adjustments; rarely, can cause agranulocytosis or aplastic anaemia (patients should be warned to watch for signs of unusual bruising or bleeding and severe infection). Stevens–Johnson syndrome – strongly associated with the HLA-B*1502 allele present in Southeast Asian populations – should be tested for prior to initiation of carbamazepine in patients from these populations.[2]
  - Oxcarbazepine: similar adverse effects to carbamazepine, except lower rate of Stevens–Johnson syndrome – approximately 25% of patients presenting with a skin rash with carbamazepine will also have a rash with oxcarbazepine.

- Carbamazepine concentrations in blood can be measured but are not needed routinely. Reference range is 4–12 mg/L, but this must be interpreted in relation to clinical control.
- *Metabolism and elimination:*
  - Carbamazepine: hepatic metabolism, mainly by CYP3A4, to a pharmacologically active epoxide metabolite, which is in turn inactivated in the liver; undergoes autoinduction, increasing clearance over the first few weeks of therapy, which may lead to a need for dose adjustment; elimination half-life after a single dose is 3–32 hours; during repeated therapeutic dosing elimination half-life falls to 10–13 hours.
  - Oxcarbazepine: hepatic metabolism to primary active metabolite 10-hydroxycarbazepine – oxcarbazepine is essentially a prodrug; elimination half-life for 10-hydroxycarbazepine is 8–15 hours.
- *Important drug interactions:*
  - A wide range of medications induce CYP3A4, increasing the clearance of carbamazepine.
  - Carbamazepine and oxcarbazepine enhance the metabolism of oral contraceptives, leading to a reduction in effectiveness.

Ethosuximide

- *Use and efficacy:*
  - First line drug for typical childhood absence seizures; may also be useful for atypical absence, myoclonic and atonic seizures
  - Ineffective for generalised tonic–clonic seizures and may exacerbate these
- *Adverse effects:*
  - Unusual: may cause mild gastrointestinal side-effects such as abdominal pain and nausea; severe side-effects are very rare
- *Metabolism and elimination:*
  - Hepatic metabolism to inactive metabolites primarily by CYP3A; elimination half-life is 30–40 hours
- *Important drug interactions:*
  - Combination therapy of ethosuximide and valproate can lead to seizure control in patients in whom monotherapy with either drug is not successful
  - Does not enhance metabolism of oral contraceptives

Gabapentin

- *Use and efficacy:*
  - Second line drug for focal seizures, with limited role due to lack of efficacy compared with other AEDs

- May exacerbate absence, myoclonic and generalised tonic–clonic seizures
- *Adverse effects:*
  - Unusual – may cause mild central nervous system (CNS) side-effects such as sedation and dizziness; severe side-effects are very rare
- *Metabolism and elimination:*
  - Not metabolised; gabapentin is excreted unchanged in urine; elimination half-life is 5–9 hours
- *Important drug interactions:*
  - Does not enhance metabolism of oral contraceptives

Lacosamide

- *Use and efficacy:*
  - Licensed for use as adjunctive therapy for adults with focal seizures; published case series in children suggest equivalent efficacy, but too little evidence to define the precise role of lacosamide
- *Adverse effects:*
  - Very limited data for children; common side-effects in adults include CNS effects and gastrointestinal effects
- *Metabolism and elimination:*
  - Hepatic metabolism by demethylation to inactive metabolites; elimination half-life is approximately 13 hours
- *Important drug interactions:*
  - Does not enhance metabolism of oral contraceptives

Lamotrigine

- *Use and efficacy:*
  - First line drug for focal and generalised seizures and Lennox–Gastaut syndrome
  - Second line drug for many other seizure types
  - Particularly effective in combination with valproate
  - Less effective than ethosuximide and valproate for absence seizures
- *Adverse effects:*
  - Commonly causes mild CNS and gastrointestinal side-effects
  - A benign rash is common, but lamotrigine may also cause Stevens–Johnson syndrome and toxic epidermal necrolysis with an increased risk in children under the age of 12 years and those taking valproate
- *Metabolism and elimination:*
  - Hepatic metabolism by glucuronidation to inactive metabolites; undergoes autoinduction, increasing clearance over the first few weeks of therapy, which may lead to a need for dose adjustment; elimination half-life is 15–35 hours

- *Important drug interactions:*
  - Administration with valproate is associated with significant increased efficacy of small doses of lamotrigine, but also the possibility of a significant increase in adverse effects; lamotrigine may also increase the risk of side-effects with carbamazepine.
  - Lamotrigine metabolism is accelerated by enzyme-inducing AEDs.
  - Oral contraceptives can increase the elimination of lamotrigine, leading to loss of seizure control; conversely, the pill-free week with the combined oral contraceptive pill may result in increased adverse effects; lamotrigine may enhance the metabolism of the progestogen-only pill, leading to contraceptive failure.

Levetiracetam

- *Use and efficacy:*
  - First or second line drug for genetic generalised epilepsies, in particular juvenile myoclonic epilepsy and focal seizures with or without generalisation
  - Dose can be rapidly titrated upwards
- *Adverse effects:*
  - Well tolerated, although behavioural symptoms (agitation, emotional lability, oppositional behaviour) are more common in children than adults
- *Metabolism and elimination:*
  - Minimal metabolism by hydrolysis in blood; remainder excreted unchanged in urine; elimination half-life 5–6 hours
- *Important drug interactions:*
  - Does not enhance metabolism of oral contraceptives

Perampanel

- *Use and efficacy:*
  - Licensed for use as adjunctive therapy for adults with focal seizures; very limited evidence in children
- *Adverse effects:*
  - Commonly causes CNS effects (sedation, dizziness)
- *Metabolism and elimination:*
  - Hepatic metabolism by CYP3A4 to inactive metabolites; elimination half-life is 66–90 hours
- *Important drug interactions:*
  - Does not enhance metabolism of oestrogen component of oral contraceptives, but can enhance metabolism of progesterone, leading to contraceptive failure of progestogen-only pill

Phenobarbital and primidone

- *Use and efficacy:*
  - Phenobarbital:
    - Effective in all seizure types except absence seizures; adverse sedative and cognitive defects limit usefulness as a first line drug
    - First line drug for neonatal seizures
    - Used intravenously as an alternative to phenytoin in status epilepticus
  - Primidone:
    - Prodrug of phenobarbital – limited use
- *Adverse effects:*
  - Commonly causes CNS effects, in particular sedation, and also paradoxical hyperactivity and irritability in young children; primidone may additionally cause transient initial adverse effects including drowsiness, dizziness and ataxia.
  - TDM is helpful in view of high degree of pharmacokinetic inter-individual variability; target plasma concentrations are 10–40 mg/L. In view of the long elimination half-life, steady state plasma levels are only reached 2–3 weeks after dose changes, unless a loading dose is administered, and blood samples can be obtained at any time of day.
- *Metabolism and elimination:*
  - Hepatic metabolism to inactive metabolites; undergoes autoinduction, increasing clearance over the first few weeks of therapy, which may lead to a need for dose adjustment; elimination half-life 60–70 hours (children < 5 years), 70–140 hours (older children), 40–200 hours (neonates).
- *Important drug interactions:*
  - Increases clearance of many drugs, including other AEDs
  - Enhances metabolism of oral contraceptives, leading to a reduction in effectiveness

Phenytoin and fosphenytoin

- *Use and efficacy:*
  - Very effective for focal and generalised seizures, but complicated pharmacokinetics and cognitive and cosmetic adverse effects limit use in children and young people
  - Intravenous drug of choice for benzodiazepine resistant status epilepticus; fosphenytoin is an injectable prodrug of phenytoin which is water-soluble and may be easier and quicker to administer intravenously than phenytoin

- *Adverse effects:*
  - Commonly causes CNS effects such as ataxia and decreased coordination; gingival hyperplasia and hirsutism are also common
  - May cause Stevens–Johnson syndrome and toxic epidermal necrolysis
  - Wide inter-individual pharmacokinetic variability and non-linear pharmacokinetics mean that plasma concentrations can increase disproportionately with dose increases. Dosing must be undertaken with guidance from TDM – target plasma concentrations are 10–20 mg/L. Intermittent monitoring even in the absence of dose alteration is advisable.
- *Metabolism and elimination:*
  - Hepatic metabolism by CYP2C9 and CYP2C19 to inactive metabolites; undergoes autoinduction, increasing clearance over the first few weeks of therapy, which may lead to a need for dose adjustment. Metabolism is saturable – clearance decreases with increasing dose, and elimination half-life increases with increasing plasma concentration. In young children, the half-life can be < 10 hours compared with 30–100 hours in adults.[3]
- *Important drug interactions:*
  - Increases clearance of many drugs, including other AEDs
  - Enhances metabolism of oral contraceptives, leading to a reduction in effectiveness

Rufinamide

- *Use and efficacy:*
  - Second line drug for Lennox–Gastaut syndrome
- *Adverse effects:*
  - Commonly causes CNS side-effects such as sedation and dizziness; a hypersensitivity syndrome (fever, rash, lymphadenopathy) has been reported
- *Metabolism and elimination:*
  - Hepatic metabolism by CYP-independent hydrolysis to inactive metabolites; elimination half-life in adults is 6–10 hours, but likely to be shorter in children
- *Important drug interactions:*
  - Enhances metabolism of oral contraceptives, leading to a reduction in effectiveness

Stiripentol

- *Use and efficacy:*
  - Licensed for the adjunctive treatment of severe myoclonic epilepsy of infancy (Dravet syndrome)

- *Adverse effects:*
  - Commonly causes anorexia and variable CNS effects (sedation or insomnia, irritability)
- *Metabolism and elimination:*
  - Hepatic metabolism by desmethylation and glucuronidation to inactive metabolites
- *Important drug interactions:*
  - Very limited data – stiripentol is a potent inhibitor of hepatic enzymes, and care must be exercised when using in combination with any drug that is metabolised by the liver

Tiagabine

- *Use and efficacy:*
  - Limited to focal seizures unresponsive to other AEDs; very limited experience in children
  - May precipitate absence seizures in genetic generalised epilepsies
- *Adverse effects:*
  - Commonly causes CNS side-effects including sedation, difficulty concentrating and behavioural problems
- *Metabolism and elimination:*
  - Hepatic metabolism by CYP3A4 to inactive metabolites; half-life 5–9 hours
- *Important drug interactions:*
  - Does not enhance metabolism of oral contraceptives

Topiramate

- *Use and efficacy:*
  - Second line drug in focal seizures and genetic generalised epilepsies as an adjunctive to other AEDs or as monotherapy in older children
- *Adverse effects:*
  - Commonly causes sedation, cognitive effects and changes in behaviour and mood; anorexia leading to weight loss is frequent
  - Renal stones and narrow angle (angle-closure) glaucoma may be precipitated
- *Metabolism and elimination:*
  - Metabolic pathway not fully elucidated – 40–50% of dose excreted unchanged in urine; half-life 10–20 hours
- *Important drug interactions:*
  - May enhance the valproate associated risk of hyperammonaemic encephalopathy
  - Enhances metabolism of oral contraceptives, leading to a reduction in effectiveness

Valproate

- *Use and efficacy:*
  - First line drug for all types of seizures and epilepsy syndromes
  - Slightly less effective than carbamazepine for focal seizures
- *Adverse effects:*
  - Commonly causes CNS side-effects, including sedation and tremor; hair loss, increased weight gain and thrombocytopenia are common dose-dependent side-effects
  - Fatal hepatotoxicity has been reported; this appears to be a particular risk in children aged under 2 years with other neurodevelopmental problems – some of these cases may be due to unrecognised Alpers syndrome; liver function tests and serum ammonia should be measured if symptoms suggestive of hepatotoxicity occur
  - Should be avoided in girls and young women due to risks of teratogenicity[4]
  - Valproate concentrations in blood can be measured, but are not needed routinely; target range is 50–100 mg/L, but this must be interpreted in relation to clinical control
- *Metabolism and elimination:*
  - Hepatic metabolism by multiple pathways to active and inactive metabolites; half-life 7–15 hours
- *Important drug interactions:*
  - Many interactions with drugs, including other AEDs:
    - Use of valproate and lamotrigine together may result in better seizure control than expected from using either alone, but entail a concomitant risk of increased adverse effects.
    - Use of valproate and ethosuximide together may result in better control of absence seizures than expected from using either alone.
    - Topiramate may enhance the risk of valproate associated adverse effects.
  - Does not enhance metabolism of oral contraceptives

Vigabatrin

- *Use and efficacy:*
  - First line drug for the treatment of infantile spasms, particularly in patients with tuberous sclerosis
  - Also used for focal seizures with or without secondary generalisation when other AEDs are ineffective
- *Adverse effects:*
  - Commonly causes CNS side-effects, including sedation and impaired cognition

- Irreversible visual field defects may occur after 6 months of treatment – patients and families require particularly careful counselling about this side-effect
- *Metabolism and elimination:*
  - Excreted unchanged in urine; half-life 5–8 hours
- *Important drug interactions:*
  - Does not enhance metabolism of oral contraceptives

Zonisamide

- *Use and efficacy:*
  - Second line drug for focal seizures and progressive myoclonic epilepsy
  - Also used in refractory generalised epilepsies
- *Adverse effects:*
  - Commonly causes CNS side-effects, including sedation, cognitive slowing and behavioural effects; anorexia leading to weight loss is common
  - May predispose to renal stones
- *Metabolism and elimination:*
  - Hepatic metabolism by CYP3A4 to inactive metabolites; half-life 50–70 hours
- *Important drug interactions:*
  - Does not enhance metabolism of oral contraceptives

Clobazam and clonazepam

- *Use and efficacy:*
  - Clobazam and clonazepam are commonly used for adjunctive treatment of drug resistant focal and generalised seizures
  - Clobazam is particularly used for intermittent use for seizure clusters (e.g. catamenial seizures) and also for myoclonic and atonic seizures
  - Clonazepam is particularly used for progressive myoclonic epilepsy
- *Adverse effects:*
  - Major side-effect is sedation, which may be severe enough to limit therapy
  - Paradoxical agitation may occur in young children
- *Metabolism and elimination:*
  - Clobazam: hepatic metabolism to active metabolites; half-life 16 hours
  - Clonazepam: hepatic metabolism to active and inactive metabolites; half-life 22–33 hours
- *Important drug interactions:*
  - Benzodiazepines can potentiate the effects of CNS depressant drugs
  - Does not enhance metabolism of oral contraceptives

Drugs used in status epilepticus

Diazepam, lorazepam and midazolam

- *Use and efficacy:*
  - The benzodiazepines diazepam, lorazepam and midazolam are primarily used as first line drugs for the treatment of prolonged (>5 minutes) or repetitive serial seizures.
  - For home use and situations where intravenous access is not available, midazolam administered into the buccal cavity is the drug of choice; rectal diazepam may also be used, although this route is less acceptable to patient and caregiver.
  - For situations where intravenous access is available, lorazepam is the drug of choice due to its more prolonged duration of anticonvulsant action.
- *Adverse effects:*
  - The primary adverse effect of all three drugs of relevance to the emergency situation is that of respiratory depression, although a significant proportion of this may relate to the effect of the prolonged seizure rather than the drug; lorazepam may lead to a lower incidence of respiratory depression than midazolam or diazepam.[5]
- *Metabolism and elimination:*
  - Diazepam: hepatic metabolism by CYP2C19 and CYP3A4 to multiple active metabolites; rapid redistribution to lipid compartment leads to rapid initial fall in plasma concentrations, accounting for short duration of action despite long elimination half-life
  - Lorazepam: hepatic metabolism by glucuronidation to inactive metabolite; half-life 8–14 hours in children, approximately 40 hours in neonates
  - Midazolam: hepatic metabolism by CYP3A4 to active metabolite; half-life 1–3 hours in children, up to 12 hours in neonates (accounting for risk of accumulation with repeated doses in this age group)
- *Important drug interactions:*
  - None of relevance to the emergency situation

Paraldehyde

- *Use and efficacy:*
  - A second line drug for prolonged seizures, used per rectum; evidence of efficacy is limited, but drug is useful for some patients in whom benzodiazepines are deemed ineffective
- *Adverse effects:*
  - Very safe, with no associated respiratory depression; repeated administration may cause rectal irritation

- *Metabolism and elimination:*
  - Hepatic metabolism; half-life 3–9 hours
- *Important drug interactions:*
  - None of relevance to the emergency situation

Phenobarbital, phenytoin and fosphenytoin

See entries above.

Conclusions

This chapter gives an introduction to the core principles of AED therapy in children. It is important to follow national or local guidelines when treating seizures and epilepsy syndromes, and to be aware of common adverse drug reactions associated with AEDs and their management. When managing complex cases, seek early expert advice from a paediatric neurologist. Beyond the pharmacotherapy, epilepsy management should always be supported by a multidisciplinary team.

References

1 Patsalos PN *et al.* Antiepileptic drugs – best practice guidelines for therapeutic drug monitoring: A position paper by the subcommission on therapeutic drug monitoring, ILAE Commission on Therapeutic Strategies. *Epilepsia* 2008; 49: 1239–1276.
2 Amstutz U *et al.* Recommendations for HLA-B*15:02 and HLA-A*31:01 genetic testing to reduce the risk of carbamazepine-induced hypersensitivity reactions. *Epilepsia* 2014; 55: 496–506.
3 Cloyd J *et al.* Clinical pharmacology of phenytoin in the elderly. *Epilepsia* 2001; 42(Suppl 2): 11–12.
4 Medicines and Healthcare products Regulatory Agency (MHRA). Medicines related to valproate: risk of abnormal pregnancy outcomes. Drug Safety Update 2015. www.gov.uk/drug-safety-update/medicines-related-to-valproate-risk-of-abnormal-pregnancy-outcomes
5 Chiulli DA *et al.* The influence of diazepam or lorazepam on the frequency of endotracheal intubation in childhood status epilepticus. *J Emerg Med* 1991; 9: 13–17.

42

Prescribing in infection: antibacterials

D Gbesemete and S Faust

Introduction

Antimicrobials are among the most commonly prescribed drugs in paediatric practice, across primary and hospital care. This chapter focuses on how to optimise antibiotic prescribing for children and neonates. Prescription of antibiotics in an appropriate and effective manner not only ensures adequate treatment of infections, but also avoids the emergence of resistance (personal and community), adverse reactions and unnecessary use of resources.

The learning objectives of this chapter are:

➤ to know the key classes of antibacterial drugs, common indications and cautions when prescribing
➤ to understand the key principles of antimicrobial stewardship, including that agent choice should be based on knowledge of the suspected pathogen(s) and local epidemiology
➤ to understand that consideration should also be given to the drug's ability to reach the site of infection, such as considering bone penetration in osteomyelitis
➤ to be aware of age related or disease related factors that can alter compliance with antibiotic therapy
➤ to recognise common and serious adverse reactions to antimicrobials.

Antibiotic prescribing: general principles

When prescribing antibiotics for children, there are a variety of practical factors that should always be taken into account.

Taste

Children are much less likely to take medication that tastes unpleasant. A taste test may be performed prior to prescription or discharge from hospital. A general guide to palatability of common antibiotics is included in Table 1.[1]

Number of doses

Children and parents are more likely to adhere to regimens requiring fewer doses per day or a shorter overall course. A regimen of fewer doses per day also improves the feasibility of outpatient/ambulant intravenous (IV) antibiotic treatment.

Route

Consider the best route of administration based on infection severity, drug pharmacokinetics and pharmacodynamics, and the patient's ability to tolerate/absorb oral medication. Use IV antibiotics first in systemically unwell patients and in serious infections, e.g. meningitis, bone and joint infection, endocarditis, and in high risk groups, e.g. neonates and neutropenic or immunodeficient patients.

Some parenteral regimens may be suitable for course completion at home while the patient remains under hospital supervision; paediatric outpatient parenteral antimicrobial therapy (OPAT) services are increasingly available. Advantages include improved patient experience, reduced inpatient stay (with associated economic benefits) and reduced risk of nosocomial infections. Different antimicrobials are more, or less, suitable for OPAT use, and this is summarised in Table 1 and Table 3.[2]

Timing

Start antimicrobial treatment as soon as possible following collection of microbiological samples, then try to organise dose timings to improve compliance. Where possible, prescribe oral medication during the child's waking hours, and ambulatory/OPAT doses during working hours. This might mean choosing a broader-spectrum agent given two or three times per day rather than a four times daily narrow-spectrum regimen. The following points can aid pragmatic prescribing.

- If a first dose of ceftriaxone has been given overnight, it can be moved to daytime by giving the second dose early, at any time from 12 hours following the initial dose.

  A regimen of 80 mg/kg with the first two doses being given at a 12-hourly interval was previously widely and effectively used for paediatric meningococcal sepsis, without adverse effects.

- Make sure parents are aware of time windows to give antimicrobials, for example a three times per day routine might be explicitly described as 'at 08:00 before school, at 16:00 on coming home and at midnight before parents go to sleep'.

Duration

There is little evidence for antimicrobial treatment course duration, which is currently based mainly on experience and expert opinion. Some evidence suggests an increased risk of resistance developing with longer courses of lower doses, and a reduced risk with higher doses for shorter courses.[3,4] Shorter courses also improve compliance and reduced the risk of adverse effects.[4] However, course duration needs to be sufficient to fully treat the infection, and is an area requiring further research.

Antimicrobial stewardship

This is the process of responsible planning and management of antimicrobial use with the aims of optimising treatment and minimising risk of adverse effects to the individual, and minimising the development of resistance at the individual and community level. Public Health England 2015 guidelines for antimicrobial prescribing, *Start Smart – Then Focus*,[5] include points relevant to paediatrics (see Figure 1).[6]

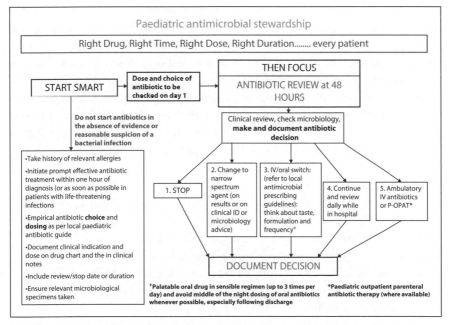

Figure 1 Principles of paediatric antimicrobial stewardship. Adapted for children from Public Health England's Start Smart – Then Focus[5]

Antibiotics

Beta-lactam antibiotics

- Large family of antibiotics (see Table 1)
- Characterised by presence of beta-lactam ring
  - Different ring structures and side chains confer differing activity
- Act by inhibition of cell wall synthesis
  - Mediated via penicillin-binding proteins[7]
- Therefore not effective against:
  - intracellular organisms
  - pathogens that lack a cell wall
  - organisms with impenetrable cell wall, i.e. mycobacteria[8]

Due to formularies frequently following formal drug licensing indications, many of which have inadequate evidence to guide them, many beta-lactams have a dose range for children or an option to double the dose in severe infection. Any patients requiring hospitalisation and IV antibiotics will typically be considered to have a severe infection and, if so, should be commenced on the highest formulary dose allowed for their weight/age. For example, we recommend that all patients commenced on ceftriaxone should start on 80 mg/kg IV (maximum 4 g once daily). Inadequate dosing can cause increased risk of treatment failure and resistance emerging, particularly when dealing with infections in difficult sites, e.g. central nervous system (CNS), bone and joint. Similarly, as most children presenting in primary care with infection have viral infections not requiring antibiotics, any child starting oral antibiotics in the community for a suspected bacterial infection should be given a high oral dose for the shortest possible course. The potential inadequacy of formulary oral beta-lactam age based oral dose recommendations was recognised for amoxicillin and ampicillin in April 2014;[9] the standard age band doses per kilogram of amoxicillin were subsequently doubled from those previously recommended, to the high dose alternative.[10] In primary or hospital care, all oral beta-lactam prescriptions should use the higher available dose recommendation with minimum course duration.

Resistance to beta-lactams

- Resistance to beta-lactams is increasingly significant globally, although uncommon in the UK.[11]
- Resistance can arise by beta-lactamase production.
- Beta-lactamase enzymes hydrolyse the beta-lactam ring.
  - Some beta-lactamases only cause resistance to penicillins.
  - Sensitivity is maintained to beta-lactamase resistant antibiotics, e.g. flucloxacillin.

- Other bacteria can produce extended spectrum beta-lactamase (ESBL).
  - Confers resistance to broader range of beta-lactams.
- Beta-lactamase inhibitors such as clavulanic acid and tazobactam have no specific antimicrobial activity themselves, but giving in combination with beta-lactam antibiotics can allow them to remain active against pathogens that would otherwise be resistant.[8]
- Another mechanism of resistance is a change in the penicillin-binding site seen with methicillin resistant *Staphylococcus aureus* (MRSA), which results in resistance to all members of the beta-lactam family of antibiotics.[8]

Macrolides

- Macrolides are bacteriostatic agents (Table 2)
- Bind to bacterial ribosomal RNA, blocking protein synthesis
- Similar spectrum of activity to beta-lactams
- Often used as an alternative in penicillin-allergic patients
- Widely distributed and achieve high tissue concentrations, particularly in bronchial tree and tonsils
- Concentrate in intracellular compartment – thus useful for intracellular infections, e.g. *M. pneumoniae*, Rickettsiae and Chlamydiae[7]
- Also active against some atypical mycobacteria
- Acquired resistance increasingly common in Staphylococci and group A Streptococci[7]

Glycopeptides

- Include vancomycin and teicoplanin (see Table 3)
- Inhibit peptidoglycan synthesis → inhibits bacterial cell wall synthesis
- Bactericidal and active against Gram positive organisms
- Often used when beta-lactams ineffective due to resistance (e.g. MRSA) or hypersensitivity
- Due to large molecular size, mostly inactive against Gram negative bacteria (except *Neisseria* spp.) as unable to penetrate outer membrane[8]
- Parenteral administration (as not absorbed via gastrointestinal tract)
  - Exception is oral vancomycin to treat *Clostridium difficile*-associated pseudomembranous colitis
- Do not cross intact blood–brain barrier
- Will cross in presence of meningeal inflammation[8]
- Vancomycin
  - Must be given by slow (> 1 hour) IV infusion

Table 1 Beta-lactam antibiotics – commonly used examples[1,2,7,8]

Class	Category	Parenteral drug	OPAT[a]	Enteral drug	Taste[b]	Active against	Excretion	Special notes
Penicillins	Natural penicillin	**Benzylpenicillin (penicillin G)**	Use ceftriaxone instead due to dose frequency.	**Phenoxymethylpenicillin (penicillin V)**	2	Gram positive – Streptococci, Gram negative – *Neisseria*	Rapid renal excretion	Inactivated by bacterial beta-lactamases (produced by most Staphylococci).
	Semi-synthetic (beta-lactamase resistant) penicillin	**Flucloxacillin**	Intermittent infusions not suitable due to frequency. Often successful use of ceftriaxone as alternative in UK. 24 hour infusion via elastomeric device is possible.	**Flucloxacillin**	4	Gram positive including Beta-lactamase producing Staphylococci.	Rapid renal excretion	
	Semi-synthetic (amino) penicillin	**Amoxicillin**	Use ceftriaxone instead due to dose frequency.	**Amoxicillin**	1	Gram positive – Streptococci, Gram negative – *Neisseria, Haemophilus, Listeria monocytogenes, Borrelia* (Lyme)	Renal	Inactivated by bacterial beta-lactamases. Risk of non-allergy mediated rash in EBV infection.
		Amoxicillin and clavulanic acid (co-amoxiclav)		**Co-amoxiclav**	1	As above plus beta-lactamase producing Gram positive		Contains clavulanic acid – beta-lactamase inhibitor.
	Semi-synthetic (ureido) penicillin	**Piperacillin/tazobactam (piptazobactam)**	Intermittent infusions not suitable due to frequency. 24 hour infusion via elastomeric device is possible.			Gram positive Enhanced Gram negative particularly *Pseudomonas* and *Klebsiella*	Renal	Contains tazobactam – beta-lactamase inhibitor.

Cephalosporins	First generation	Cefalexin [a]			Gram positive – Streptococci, Staphylococci	Renal	
	Second generation	Cefaclor [a] 1	Cefuroxime	Use ceftriaxone instead due to dose frequency.	Gram negative – Neisseria haemophilus, Enterobacteria (parenteral agents)		
	Third generation		Cefotaxime	Intermittent infusions not suitable due to frequency. 24 hour infusion via elastomeric device is possible.	Ceftazidime – Pseudomonas		Antipseudomonal activity.
			Ceftazidime				
			Ceftriaxone	Suitable for daily infusion.		50–60% renal 40–50% biliary long half-life	Only use 80 mg/Kg IV. Second dose can be given any time from 12 hours following the initial dose. Do not use in neonates if IV calcium used concomitantly.[c]
Carbapenems			Meropenem	Not advised, as concerns about stability.	Gram positive and Gram negative	Renal	Not to be used first line due to increase in resistance.

[a] Suitability for outpatient parenteral antibiotic therapy

[b] Taste – ranked 1–4, where 1 is the most palatable.

[c] In neonates (up to 28 days of age), ceftriaxone is contraindicated if:
- jaundice (> 50 µmol/L)
- hypoalbuminaemia (albumin < 25 g/L)
- acidosis (pH < 7.35)

Notes:

In patients of any age, ceftriaxone must not be mixed or administered *simultaneously* with any calcium-containing IV solutions (such as total parenteral nutrition or Hartmann's), even via different infusion lines or at different infusion sites.

In patients older than 28 days of age, ceftriaxone and calcium-containing solutions may be administered *sequentially* one after another through a different IV site or through the same IV site if thoroughly flushed with normal saline.

Table 2 Macrolides[7,8,12]

Drug	Route	Activity	Excretion	Adverse effects	Special notes
Erythromycin	Oral IV	Gram positive cocci Intracellular bacteria • Mycoplasmas • Chlamydiae • Rickettsiae • *Legionella pneumophila* • *Campylobacter jejuni*	Excreted in bile Some renal excretion	Nausea and vomiting	Poor taste and tolerability, Four times/day regimen so best avoided Good oral absorption Good tissue distribution
Clarithromycin	Oral IV	As erythromycin Improved activity against Gram positive bacteria and *Legionella pneumophila*		Reduced adverse effects	
Azithromycin	Oral	As erythromycin Improved activity against Gram negative bacteria			High tissue concentrations and post-antibiotic effect allow dose to be given once daily for just 3 consecutive days

- Minimises risk of red man syndrome (upper torso flushing, erythema and pruritis caused by rapid histamine release)
- More rarely, this can cause angio-oedema, anaphylactoid reactions and cardiovascular collapse
- Intramuscular (IM) injection causes pain and necrosis
- Can cause nephrotoxicity and ototoxicity
- Monitor plasma concentrations carefully (associated with risk of toxicity) (see chapter 35)
- Modify dose in renal failure (see chapter 47)
- Avoid using in combination with aminoglycosides or loop diuretics, to reduce risk of nephrotoxicity[7]
- High level acquired vancomycin resistance can occur
  - Arises following acquisition of resistance associated genes
- Notable problem in Enterococci (vancomycin resistant Enterococci; VRE)

- Transfer of resistance genes to Staphylococci also observed
    - Some strains of VRE remain sensitive to teicoplanin[7,8]
- Teicoplanin
    - Less active against some coagulase negative Staphylococci
    - Less risk of nephrotoxicity and ototoxicity
    - Toxicity is not dose dependent; no need for therapeutic drug monitoring
    - Can be safely given intramuscularly or by IV bolus
    - Added advantage of longer half-life, allowing once daily dosing[7]

Aminoglycosides

- Include gentamicin, amikacin, tobramycin (see Table 3)
- Bind to bacterial ribosomal subunit → inhibit protein synthesis
- Potent, broad spectrum, bactericidal agents
- Used for serious Gram negative infections
    - Particularly if reduction in host defences
- They are active against most aerobic Gram negative pathogens (except *Neisseria* spp)
- Not active against anaerobes and most Gram positive bacteria (except Staphylococci)
- Must be given parenterally
    - Poorly absorbed from gastrointestinal tract
- Do not penetrate well into tissues and bone or via the blood–brain barrier
    - Thus often used in first stages of bacterial sepsis then stopped once there is clinical stability
- Act synergistically with beta-lactams
    - Often used in combination with them, especially if infection blood surface associated, e.g. endocarditis
- Risk of nephrotoxicity and ototoxicity
    - Necessitates careful monitoring of plasma concentrations (see chapter 35)
    - Dose adjust in renal impairment (see chapter 47)
- Acquired resistance is relatively rare[7,8]

The key features of several other commonly used classes of antibiotic are summarised below in Table 4.

Anti-mycobacterial agents

- Mycobacteria are challenging organisms to treat:
    - Impermeable cell wall
    - Intracellular location
    - Extremely slow growth

Table 3 Glycopeptides and aminoglycosides[2,7,8]

Family	Mechanism	Drug	Route	OPAT[a]	Uses / Activity	Excretion	Special notes
Glycopeptides	Inhibition of cell wall formation	**Vancomycin**	IV slow infusion	Intermittent infusions not suitable due to frequency. 24 hour infusion via elastomeric device is possible.	**Gram positive** ● Staphylococci ● Streptococci ● Enterococci (unless vancomycin resistant) **Gram negative** ● *Neisseria*	Renal (glomerular)	Risk of nephrotoxicity and ototoxicity – levels required Caution and reduced dose in renal impairment Risk of red man syndrome with rapid IV infusion
		Teicoplanin	IV or IM	Once-daily infusion via silicone-free syringe			Reduced risk of adverse effects Potentially reduced activity against coagulase-negative staphylococci
Aminoglyco-sides	Inhibitors of protein synthesis	**Gentamicin**	IV or IM	Once-daily infusion via syringe	**Gram negative aerobes** ● E. coli ● Klebsiella ● Enterobacter ● Proteus ● Shigella ● Salmonella ● Serratia ● H. influenzae ● Pseudomonas (particularly tobramycin) **Gram positive** ● Staphylococci	Renal (glomerular)	Use in severe infections, often in association with a beta-lactam in the early stages of sepsis treatment on paediatric intensive care unit
		Tobramycin	IV	Once-daily infusion via syringe			Similar to gentamicin but improved activity against *Pseudomonas aeruginosa* Often used in CF patients with *Pseudomonas*
		Amikacin	IV				Active against many gentamicin-resistant Gram negative rods

[a] Suitability for outpatient parenteral antibiotic therapy

Table 4 Other antibiotics[7,8]

Mechanism	Family	Drug	Route	Activity	Excretion	Adverse effects	Special notes
Inhibitors of protein synthesis	Tetracyclines	**Doxycycline**	Oral	*Chlamydiae Rickettsiae* Mycoplasmas *Borrelia* (Lyme) Spectrum of activity broad but acquired resistance common	Renal Faecal	GI upset Brown staining teeth Interference with bone development Risk of hepatotoxicity	UK formulary advises do not use < 9 years or in pregnancy / breast feeding. However evidence from the USA suggests short course therapy with doxycycline is not associated with long lasting adverse effects
	Chloramphenicol	**Chloramphenicol**	Oral – well absorbed IV – if NBM	*H. influenzae* meningitis Broad spectrum of activity but not used if alternative available due to toxicity	Metabolised in liver, excreted renally	Bone marrow toxicity – usually dose dependant and reversible Rarely idiosyncratic and irreversible	Achieves good CNS penetration High rates of resistance
	Lincosamides	**Clindamycin**	Usually oral IV or IM	Gram positive bacteria – particularly *Staphylococcus aureus* Anaerobic bacteria	Metabolised in liver, excreted in faeces	Not active against *Clostridium difficile* so risk of pseudomembranous colitis	Good bone penetration – useful in osteomyelitis Poor cerebrospinal fluid (CSF) penetration even via inflamed meninges
	Oxazolidinones	**Linezolid**	Oral or IV	Gram positive bacteria including many multiresistant strains Resistance rare	Metabolised in liver	Bone marrow suppression and optic neuropathy following prolonged use	Reserve for use against multi-resistant pathogens

(continued)

Table 4 (Continued)

Mechanism	Family	Drug	Route	Activity	Excretion	Adverse effects	Special notes
Inhibitors of nucleic acid synthesis	Quinolones	**Ciprofloxacin**	Oral or IV	Gram positive • Staphylococci Gram negative bacteria • *Pseudomonas aeruginosa* Intracellular bacteria	Renal Some excreted in faeces	Avoid in patients with increased risk of seizures	Good oral absorption. Use IV only if unable to take orally
	Rifamycins	**Rifampicin**	Oral	Prophylaxis for contacts of *Haemophilus influenza* and *meningococcal meningitis*	Metabolised in liver Excreted in bile	Turns urine, sweat and saliva orange Rapid development of resistance if used as monotherapy	Well absorbed and distributed Crosses blood brain barrier Affinity for plastics – reported useful in adults for attempting treatment of infections associated with prostheses If used as anti-Staphylococcal agent never use as monotherapy
	Trimethoprim	**Trimethoprim**	Oral	Gram negative rods (not *Pseudomonas* spp.)	Renal excretion – more rapidly excreted in renal failure	Neutropenia Nausea and vomiting Adverse effects more common in HIV infection	Treatment and prophylaxis of urinary tract infections Often given in combination with sulfamethoxazole as co-trimoxazole – act synergistically
	Nitroimidazoles	**Metronidazole**	Oral or IV	Anaerobes	Renal excretion	Peripheral neuropathy in prolonged use or high doses – rare	Good oral absorption, distribution to tissues and CSF

- Long treatment courses are required[8]
- Manage patients under guidance of paediatric infectious disease or tuberculosis (TB) specialists
- Standard recommended regimen for *M. tuberculosis* infection is:
  - Four drug regimen for the first 2 months (see Table 5)
    - Usually isoniazid, rifampicin, pyrazinamide and ethambutol
  - Followed by isoniazid and rifampicin for a further 4 months
- In meningeal involvement, continue isoniazid and rifampicin for a total of 12 months
- If meningeal or pericardial involvement, commence a glucocorticoid at treatment outset and wean off after the first 2–3 weeks[13]
- Multiple agents in combination are necessary to kill both replicating and dormant bacilli and to reduce the risk of resistance developing
- Majority of organisms will be killed in the early intensive phase of treatment, leaving a minority of persistently dormant organisms to be killed by rifampicin in continuation phase
- Isoniazid is also continued in case any rifampicin resistant organisms begin to replicate[7]

Multiple drug resistant TB

- Multiple drug resistance is an increasing problem worldwide
- Resistance can quickly develop
  - Exacerbated by monotherapy or poor compliance
- Patients must be counselled regarding risks
- Directly observed therapy is not currently routinely recommended in the UK
- Considered in patients at high risk of poor adherence[13]
- Other agents or regimens will be necessary for drug resistant strains
  - Treatment regimens are guided by isolate sensitivity patterns whenever available

Allergies and adverse drug reactions

Adverse events while taking antimicrobials (particularly beta-lactams) are common. A large proportion of children are labelled as antibiotic allergic as a result. Many of these events will be unrelated to the antibiotic or will not be a hypersensitivity reaction. Only 6–24% of children with a suspected antibiotic allergy will have a positive result on drug provocation testing.[14] This can have significant implications, limiting the range of potentially

Table 5 Antimycobacterials[7,8]

Drug	Mechanism of action	Absorption and distribution	Excretion	Adverse effects
Isoniazid	Inhibition of mycolic acid synthesis (mycobacterial cell wall component) Rapidly bactericidal against replicating organisms Minimal effect on dormant organisms	Good GI absorption	Metabolised by acetylation	Potential neurotoxicity – prevented by concomitant pyridoxine (ask child or young person to report pins and needles) Hepatitis – rare and reversible in children Can cause high levels of anticonvulsants in slow acetylators
Rifampicin	Blocks mRNA synthesis Active against nearly dormant organisms	Good GI absorption Well distributed and crosses blood–brain barrier	Metabolised in liver, excreted in bile	Orange urine/saliva/sweat – non-harmful and an indicator of compliance If used as anti-Staphylococcal agent never use as monotherapy
Pyrazinamide	Inhibition of mycolic acid synthesis Active against slowly replicating bacilli in acidic environments	Good GI absorption Well distributed and crosses blood–brain barrier	Metabolised in liver, excreted in urine	Potential hepatotoxicity but usually well tolerated
Ethambutol	Inhibits arabinogalactan polymerisation (mycobacterial cell wall component)	Good GI absorption Well distributed and crosses blood–brain barrier if meninges inflamed	Renal excretion	Optic neuritis – monitor visual acuity, and discontinue if any change. Can be irreversible if treatment continued

life-saving antibiotics available to them. Drug provocation testing can be helpful in patients with mild symptoms of suspected drug allergy, particularly those who will require further antibiotic therapy.[14,15]

It is very important to recognise true IgE mediated hypersensitivity reactions, which can be life-threatening. In patients with true penicillin hypersensitivity, there can be cross-sensitivity to other beta-lactams: 3–9% of penicillin-allergic patients may also be allergic to cephalosporins.[7] Due to the relatively low risk, intensive care clinicians may choose to use a third generation cephalosporin for treating community acquired sepsis, which can be appropriate; however, it is important to carefully assess any potential reaction to guide appropriate future use/avoidance of antibiotics. Table 6 summarises the key features of important adverse drug reactions.

When antibiotic allergy is suspected:

- Characteristics typical of type I (IgE mediated) hypersensitivity reactions are: early onset after exposure (usually 1–4 hours; range up to 72 hours), angio-oedema, urticaria, diffuse erythema, bronchospasm, laryngeal oedema and anaphylaxis.
- In type I hypersensitivity and severe non-IgE mediated reactions, all penicillins are absolutely contraindicated; other beta-lactams should only be used if there is no alternative, and then under expert guidance.
- In patients with mild non-IgE mediated reactions (e.g. non-urticarial rash), avoid penicillins unless there is no alternative; use other beta-lactams with caution.[6]

When penicillin allergy is suspected:

- Erythromycin is commonly prescribed but is not ideal because it:
  - is unpalatable
  - requires four times daily dosing
  - has a poor adverse effect profile.
- Clarithromycin has good anti-Staphylococcal activity but is less palatable than amoxicillin.
- Azithromycin is more palatable and has a useful pharmacokinetic profile:
  - High and persistent tissue concentration
  - Once-daily dosing for 3 consecutive days achieves therapeutic levels (sustained for up to 10 days[12])
  - Three days is a sufficient treatment course
  - Effective prophylactic agent in certain patient groups
  - For prophylaxis, prescribe for 3 consecutive days per week

Table 6 Adverse drug reactions

Allergic response	Timing	Symptoms	Immunological mechanism	Prognosis
Maculopapular eruption	6–10 days after first exposure < 3 days after second exposure	Widespread red macules / papules Variable in size and distribution Can resemble urticaria	T-cell mediated	Lesions last 5–10 days
Fixed drug eruption	6–10 days after first exposure < 3 days after second exposure	Localised inflamed skin – always at same site	T-cell mediated	Will recur with repeated use of drug Will resolve days to weeks after drug cessation
Urticaria/angio-oedema	< 1 hour after exposure	Urticaria – erythematous swollen lesions with brightest erythema at periphery and paler in centre. Distribution of lesions will change over hours to days Angio-oedema – swelling, typically of face, hands, feet If severe, can affect airway	IgE mediated mast cell degranulation	May last for several days May rapidly evolve into airway compromise or anaphylaxis Potential for late phase reaction
Anaphylaxis	< 1 hour after exposure	Severe systemic reaction Urticaria/angio-oedema/erythema + hypotension and/or bronchospasm	IgE mediated mast cell degranulation	Immediately life-threatening
Drug reaction with eosinophilia and systemic symptoms (DRESS)	2–6 weeks after first exposure < 3 days after Second exposure	Widespread maculopapular rash or erythroderma Eosinophilia Fever Lymphadenopathy Liver/renal/bone marrow dysfunction	T-cell mediated	Can result in prolonged symptoms even after cessation of drug Mortality up to 10%

Erythema multiforme (EM)	1–2 weeks after first exposure <3 days after second exposure	Distinct circular lesions 1–2 cm diameter, flat or raised Darker in centre, paler peripherally, may be concentric rings – target lesions May be associated blistering of lesions and systemic symptoms	T-cell mediated	Risk of mortality increases with increasing body surface area involvement, age, biochemical and haemodynamic instability Mortality up to 90% in most severe cases SJS/TEN likely to require intensive care
Stevens–Johnson syndrome (SJS)		As EM, with blistering/skin oss 1–10% of body surface area Mucosal involvement		
Toxic epidermal necrolysis (TEN)		Blistering/skin loss > 30% Mucosal involvement		
SJS/TEN overlap		Blistering/skin loss 10-30% Mucosal involvement		
Acute generalised exanthematous pustulosis (AGEP)	3 – 5 days after exposure	Widespread pustules Fever Neutrophilia	T-cell mediated	Will resolve within days of drug cessation

Conclusions

High quality antimicrobial prescribing can benefit both children and communities, and the benefits of antimicrobial stewardship are broad. However, changing antibiotic prescribing practices among physicians requires insights into behaviour as well as science. For complex cases, have a low threshold to discuss with specialists in paediatric infectious diseases and microbiology.

References

1   Baguley D *et al*. Prescribing for children – taste and palatability affect adherence to antibiotics: a review. *Arch Dis Child* 2012; 97(3): 293–297.
2   Patel S *et al*. Good practice recommendations for paediatric outpatient parenteral antibiotic therapy (p-OPAT) in the UK: a consensus statement. *J Antimicrob Chemother* 2015; 70(2): 360–373.
3   Guillemot D *et al*. Low dosage and long treatment duration of beta-lactam: risk factors for carriage of penicillin-resistant Streptococcus pneumoniae. *Jama* 1998; 279(5): 365–370.
4   Kerrison C, Riordan FA. How long should we treat this infection for? *Arch Dis Child Educ Pract Ed* 2013; 98(4): 136–140.
5   Public Health England. *Start Smart – Then Focus. Antimicrobial Stewardship Toolkit for English Hospitals*. London, UK: Public Health England. 2015 www.gov.uk/government/uploads/system/uploads/attachment_data/file/417032/Start_Smart_Then_Focus_FINAL.PDF
6   University Hospital Southampton NHS Foundation Trust. First-line empirical antibiotic therapy for specific childhood infections. Paediatric microguide, 2015.
7   Finch RG *et al*. *Antibiotic and Chemotherapy, Anti-Infective Agents and Their Use in Therapy*, 8th edn. Philadelphia, USA: Churchill Livingstone, 2003.
8   Goering R *et al*. *Mims' Medical Microbiology*, 5th edn. London, UK: Saunders, 2013.
9   Saxena S *et al*. Oral penicillin prescribing for children in the UK: a comparison with BNF for Children age-band recommendations. *Br J Gen Pract* 2014; 64(621): e217–e222.
10 *British National Formulary*. April 2014 BNF e-newsletter. www.pharmpress.com/mailouts/bnf/apr14/BNF_enewsletter.html
11 Centers for Disease Control and Prevention. *Antibiotic Resistance Threats in the United States,* 2013. Centers for Disease Control and Prevention, 2013.
12 Foulds G, Johnson RB. Selection of dose regimens of azithromycin. *J Antimicrob Chemother* 1993; 31 Suppl E: 39–50.
13 NICE. Tuberculosis: Clinical diagnosis and management of tuberculosis, and measures for its prevention and control. Clinical guideline CG117. London, UK: NICE, March 2011. www.nice.org.uk/guidance/cg117
14 Marrs T *et al*. The diagnosis and management of antibiotic allergy in children: systematic review to inform a contemporary approach. *Arch Dis Child* 2014; 0: 1–6.
15 du Toit G *et al*. The RCPCH care pathway for children with drug allergies: an evidence and consensus based national approach. *Arch Dis Child* 2011; 96 Suppl 2: i15–i18.

Further recommended reading

Ardern-Jones MR, Friedmann PS. Skin manifestations of drug allergy. *Br J Clin Pharmacol* 2011; 71(5): 672–683.
Ashiru-Oredope D *et al*. Improving the quality of antibiotic prescribing in the NHS by developing a new antimicrobial stewardship programme: Start Smart – Then Focus. *J Antimicrob Chemother* 2012; 67 Suppl 1: i51–i63.

Dworzynski K *et al*. Diagnosis and management of drug allergy in adults, children and young people: summary of NICE guidance. *BMJ* 2014; 349: g4852.

Electronic Medicines Compendium. Summary of product characteristics, Rocephin 250mg powder for solution for injection, 1g powder for solution for injection or infusion, 2g powder for solution for injection/infusion vials. www.medicines.org.uk/emc/medicine/1729

Kim DH, Koh YI. Comparison of diagnostic criteria and determination of prognostic factors for drug reaction with eosinophilia and systemic symptoms syndrome. *Allergy Asthma Immunol Res* 2014; 6(3): 216–221.

Kostopoulos TC *et al*. Acute generalized exanthematous pustulosis: atypical presentations and outcomes. *J Eur Acad Dermatol Venereol* 2015; 29(2): 209–214.

Todd SR *et al*. No visible dental staining in children treated with doxycycline for suspected Rocky Mountain spotted fever. *J Pediatr* 2015; 166(5): 1246–1251.

43

Prescribing in infection: antifungals and antivirals

D Gbesemete and S Faust

Introduction

Although less widely prescribed than antibacterial drugs, antifungal and antiviral agents also form an important part of the antimicrobial armamentarium used for treating common infections in children.

The learning objectives of this chapter are:

➤ to know the key classes of antifungal and antiviral drugs
➤ to understand the spectrum of activity of different agents and how this affects their suitability for different types of infection
➤ to recognise important adverse effects associated with specific antifungal and antiviral drugs.

Antifungal drugs

Superficial fungal infections

- Fungal pathogens commonly cause superficial infections of the skin or mucous membranes.
- In immunocompetent non-hospitalised children, fungal infections are usually mild and can be treated effectively with topical antifungal agents.
- Oral agents are required if the hair or nails are affected or in more widespread, intractable or recurrent infection or in the immunocompromised host.[1]

Table 1 summarises the topical and oral antifungal agents frequently used in superficial fungal infections.

Table 1 Antifungal agents used in superficial infections[1–3]

Class	Drug	Route	Spectrum of activity	Uses	Important adverse effects
Polyenes	**Nystatin**	Topical Oral suspension (topical treatment for gastrointestinal (GI) mucosa)	*Candida* spp.	Oral/cutaneous candidiasis	–
Imidazoles	**Ketoconazole** **Miconazole** **Clotrimazole**	Topical	Dermatophytes *Candida* spp.	Tinea corporis, pedis, cruris Pityriasis versicolor Cutaneous candidiasis	–
Triazoles	**Itraconazole**	Oral	Dermatophytes *Candida* spp.	Tinea corporis, unguium, capitis	Risk of drug interactions Mild GI upset Transient hepatotoxicity Unpalatable but suspensions have better bioavailability than tablets in children.
	Fluconazole	Oral	*Candida* spp. Dermatophytes	Intractable or recurrent candidiasis	Mild GI upset Transient hepatotoxicity
Allylamine	**Terbinafine**	Topical	Dermatophytes *Candida* spp.	Tinea corporis	–
		Oral		Tinea capitis Tinea unguium	GI upset Taste disturbance Transiently raised liver enzymes
	Griseofulvin	Oral	Dermatophytes – *Microsporum* spp.	Tinea capitis	GI upset more common than newer agents Headache Risk of teratogenicity – males and females

Invasive fungal infections

- Invasive fungal infections cause significant mortality and morbidity in patients whose host defences have been compromised by disease, by immunosuppressive treatment or by invasive procedures.[4]
  - Most common cause is the yeast *Candida albicans*.
  - Other yeasts may be responsible (e.g. non-albicans *Candida* spp. and *Cryptococcus neoformans*), filamentous fungi (e.g. *Aspergillus fumigatus*) and occasionally dimorphic fungi (e.g. *Histoplasma capsulatum*).[4]
  - It is important to identify the causative organism in order to ensure that an effective treatment is used.

Amphotericin

- Amphotericin has a broad spectrum of activity and is often used in invasive fungal infections.
  - It is associated with serious adverse effects, particularly nephrotoxicity, which is often seen at therapeutic doses, and acute adverse reactions.
  - Lipid associated formulations such as liposomal amphotericin and amphotericin lipid complex alter the drug distribution and substantially reduce the risk of adverse effects.
  - Lipid formulations are now frequently used to minimise the risks of toxicity.
    - Significantly more expensive
    - Not (yet) found to be more efficacious
  - Factors associated with an increased risk of toxicity include pre-existing renal impairment, hyponatraemia, hypovolaemia and the concomitant use of other potentially nephrotoxic drugs.[1,4]

Triazole agents

- Triazole agents may be used in invasive infection – most commonly fluconazole, which has good activity against most *Candida* spp. but not against some rarer pathogens.
  - Good safety profile.
  - However, due to interaction with cytochrome P450 enzyme system, can interact with many other drugs including many drugs potentially used in the same patient groups, e.g. immunosuppressive treatments, fentanyl, midazolam.[1,4]
  - Especially true of itraconazole, with further disadvantage of very variable oral absorption making plasma concentration unpredictable.
    - In children, itraconazole suspension gives more reliable plasma concentrations than tablet formulations.
  - Second generation agents have improved spectrum of activity; useful in unusual or resistant pathogens.[1]

Echinocandins

- Echinocandins (including caspofungin, micafungin, anidulafungin) have a more limited spectrum of action but have a good safety profile with minimal drug interactions.
  - Rapidly fungicidal, so are useful in critically unwell patients with invasive candidiasis or aspergillosis[1,4]

Further details of all these agents are summarised in Table 2.

Resistance

- As with antibacterial agents, resistance can develop in fungal species.
- This is seen in *Candida* spp. developing fluconazole resistance with some cases of cross-resistance to other azoles.
- Sensitivity testing should be discussed with the microbiology team where required.[1]

Combination antifungal therapy

- Antifungal agents are usually used as monotherapy.
- The exception to this is flucytosine, in which resistance develops quickly if used as monotherapy, but due to having good cerebrospinal fluid (CSF) penetration and activity against yeasts it is a useful agent in cryptococcal meningitis in combination with amphotericin.
- Other combinations of antifungal therapy may be useful in selected complex situations, but therapy should be led by an expert in paediatric infectious diseases.[4,5]

Certain antifungal agents are very expensive, and there is growing interest in some larger hospitals in the development of antifungal stewardship programmes.

Antiviral drugs

Herpes simplex virus (HSV) and varicella zoster virus (VZV)

- HSV and VZV infections are usually self-limiting and do not require antiviral treatment.
- In certain situations, antiviral treatment is indicated.
  - Suspected or proven HSV encephalitis[7]
  - Neonatal HSV infection (disseminated, central nervous system (CNS) or cutaneous infection)[8]
  - VZV infection in immunocompromised individuals
  - Recurrent or persistent HSV infection in immunocompetent children and teenagers

Table 2 Antifungal agents used in invasive infections[1,4,6]

Class	Agents	Mechanism of action	Route	Activity	Uses	Absorption / distribution	Excretion	Main adverse effects
Polyenes	**Amphotericin**	Bind to ergosterol in fungal cell membranes causing leakage and cell death	IV	*Candida* spp. *Cryptococcus neoformans* *Aspergillus fumigatus* Dimorphic fungi	Invasive fungal infections	Poor oral absorption Highly protein and tissue bound Poor CSF penetration	Renal	Nephrotoxicity → ↓ in lipid associated formulations Hypokalaemia Anaemia
First generation Triazoles	**Fluconazole**	Block biosynthesis of ergosterol, resulting in damage to fungal cell membranes	IV Cral	Most *Candida* spp. *Cryptococcus neoformans* No activity against aspergillus or zygomycetes Dimorphic fungi	Prophylaxis in high risk patients Treatment of fungal urinary tract infections	Good oral absorption Low protein binding so well distributed and good CSF penetration	Renal – reaches high concentration in urine	Cytochrome P inhibition leading to multiple drug interactions (particularly itraconazole and voriconazole) Mild GI upset Transient hepatotoxicity, rarely idiosyncratic and fulminant Unpalatable
	Itraconazole		Cral	As fluconazole plus active against *Aspergillus fumigatus*	Prophylaxis in high risk patients with risk of aspergillus Superficial fungal infections	Variable and unpredictable oral absorption Poor CSF penetration Good distribution to other tissues	Hepatic degradation Biliary elimination	Voriconazole: Visual and CNS disturbances (reversible)

(continued)

Table 2 (Continued)

Class	Agents	Mechanism of action	Route	Activity	Uses	Absorption / distribution	Excretion	Main adverse effects
Second generation Triazoles	**Voriconazole**		Oral IV	As itraconazole plus active against other filamentous fungi	Fluconazole resistance Invasive aspergillosis	Good oral absorption Good CSF penetration		
	Posaconazole		Oral	As voriconazole plus active against zygomycetes	Fluconazole resistance Zygomycetes	Good oral absorption Good CSF penetration		
Echinocandins	**Caspofungin**	Inhibition of glucan synthesis resulting in damage to fungal cell wall	IV	*Candida* spp. *Aspergillus* spp.	Invasive candidiasis or aspergillosis	Poor CSF penetration No active drug excreted in urine so not useful in candiduria	Hepatic degradation	Infusion related reactions → slow IV Transient mild hepatotoxicity
Pyrimidine analogues	**Flucytosine**	Inhibition of fungal DNA synthesis and incorporation into fungal RNA leading to abnormal protein synthesis	IV Oral	Yeasts only – *Candida* spp. *Cryptococcus neoformans*	Used in combination with amphotericin in cryptococcal meningitis	Good oral absorption Low protein binding so well distributed and good CSF penetration	Renal	Bone marrow toxicity at high levels → monitor levels Transient hepatotoxicity

Aciclovir and valaciclovir

- Aciclovir is active against the above herpes viruses (HSV and VZV) but has reduced activity against others, e.g. Epstein–Barr virus and cytomegalovirus (CMV).
  - It has limited oral bioavailability, so is most effective when given intravenously.
  - Oral and topical aciclovir are also used for mucosal and cutaneous HSV infections.[9]
  - It is a prodrug which is activated by herpes virus enzymes. Therefore, it has minimal adverse effects on host cells, but can cause nephrotoxicity due to crystallisation in the renal tract of patients with underlying renal disease.
- Valaciclovir is the L-valene ester of aciclovir and has improved oral absorption and bioavailability, allowing oral completion of treatment.[7,9]
- Recent evidence suggests that in neonatal HSV, 6 months of oral aciclovir suppressive therapy following completion of intravenous (IV) treatment improves outcomes in terms of neurodevelopment and cutaneous recurrences.[8]
- One-year suppression regimens of aciclovir or, in older children and teenagers, valaciclovir are sometimes used in recurrent or persistent HSV infections.[10]

Cytomegalovirus

- Cytomegalovirus is a very common infection of childhood and is often subclinical.
- Antiviral treatment is currently indicated in symptomatic neonatal/congenital infection involving the CNS and where it has been shown to reduce the risk of hearing impairment and improve neurodevelopmental outcomes.
- It can also be considered in significant non-CNS disease in the neonatal period.[11]
- It is also used for prevention and treatment of CNS infection in high risk patients, such as following solid-organ transplantation.[12]

Ganciclovir and valganciclovir

- Ganciclovir has a similar structure and mode of action to aciclovir but with a broader range of activity, particularly against CMV.[13]
  - It is not as selective in its toxicity as aciclovir and so has a significant risk of bone marrow suppression.
  - The oral bioavailability of ganciclovir is poor, so it is most effectively used intravenously.

- Valganciclovir is the L-valene ester of ganciclovir.
  - It has approximately 10 times the oral bioavailability of ganciclovir and so is increasingly being used for both prophylaxis and treatment of CMV.[9,12]

Influenza

- In previously healthy patients with uncomplicated influenza, treatment with antivirals is not recommended unless the patient is felt to be at high risk of complications.
- Treatment is recommended in high risk patients, those requiring hospitalisation and those with complicated influenza (lower respiratory tract or CNS involvement, exacerbation of underlying conditions).
- Treatment should be commenced prior to laboratory confirmation.
- Enteral oseltamivir and inhaled zanamivir are the only antivirals for influenza currently licensed in the UK.

Oseltamivir

- Oseltamivir is the recommended first line treatment in most situations and is most effective when started within 48 hours of onset, although it can be used at any stage.
  - It is well absorbed enterally.
  - Suitable for use in critically ill patients with adequate GI function.
- Oseltamivir can also be used as post-exposure prophylaxis in high risk individuals.

Zanamivir

- Inhaled zanamivir is licensed from 5 years and is used in oseltamivir treatment failure or in suspected or proven oseltamivir resistance.
- Immunosuppressed individuals should be commenced on zanamivir as soon as possible if the circulating strain has a higher risk of oseltamivir resistance (e.g. H1N1).
- Nebulised or IV zanamivir could be considered in those unable to take the inhaled drug or in critically ill patients.
- Zanamivir can be used as prophylaxis for high risk individuals following exposure to suspected or proven oseltamivir resistant strains.[14]

Further details of antiviral drugs are summarised in Table 3.

Antiretroviral drugs

- Patients with HIV should be managed under the care of specialist paediatric HIV teams.

Table 3 Antivirals 6,8,9,15

Agents	Mechanism of action	Route	Activity	Absorption / distribution	Excretion	Main adverse effects
Aciclovir	Inhibition of viral DNA polymerase and DNA chain termination following activation by viral enzymes	IV Oral Topical	HSV 1 and 2 VZV	Poor oral absorption Widely distributed	Renal excretion	Acute kidney injury if underlying renal impairment Neutropenia – monitor FBC during prolonged courses GI upset Rash
Valaciclovir	Oral prodrug of aciclovir	Oral		Good oral absorption		
Ganciclovir	Inhibition of viral DNA polymerase and DNA chain termination following activation by viral enzymes	IV Oral	CMV HSV 1 and 2 (aciclovir used preferentially due to safety profile)	Poor oral absorption	Renal excretion	Neutropenia – monitor FBC during prolonged courses Thrombocytopenia Hepatotoxicity
Valganciclovir	Oral prodrug of ganciclovir	Oral		Good oral absorption		
Oseltamivir	NANA analogue – inhibits viral neuraminidase so blocking	Oral	Influenza A and B	Good oral absorption	Renal excretion	GI upset
Zanamivir	cleavage of virus from host cell surface	Inhalation IV			Renal excretion	Rhinorrhoea Bronchospasm

- Management should follow the latest guidelines of the Children's HIV Association (CHIVA; www.chiva.org.uk) and the Paediatric European Network for the Treatment of AIDS (PENTA; www.pentatrials.org).
- The websites are invaluable resources, as these guidelines are updated regularly and modified in the light of new evidence and improvement in available treatments.[15]
- Key management principles at the time of writing are summarised below.
  - Guidelines currently recommend treatment regardless of immune function in the youngest groups of children (use in all <1 year; consider use in all < 3 years), plus treatment in any child with significant disease or co-infections, CD4 count reduction or high viral load.
  - Different CD4 count thresholds are advised for different ages, but in general treatment should start when approaching these thresholds rather than waiting for levels to fall below the threshold.
    - Treatment should also be considered in asymptomatic sexually active adolescents to reduce the risk of onward transmission.[15]
  - Specific antiretroviral therapy (ART) regimens are beyond the scope of this book and should be led by an expert in paediatric HIV management.
  - The general aim is to start at least three effective ART drugs, usually two or three of which are nucleoside reverse transcriptase inhibitors (NRTIs), together with either a protease inhibitor (PI) or a non-nucleoside reverse transcriptase inhibitor (NNRTI).
  - Consider the following factors.
    - Potential resistance patterns
    - Previous exposure to ART therapy, e.g. during failed prevention of mother to child transmission treatment
    - Availability of suitable formulations
    - Likely adherence
  - It is important to ensure that the dose given does not become sub-therapeutic (thereby leading to an increased chance of resistance) by rounding doses up rather than down.
    - Remember to increase doses with increased weight or body surface area at every clinical review.[15]
  - Drug toxicity is a common problem with antiretroviral therapy, although less frequent with modern agents.
    - Acute reactions can occur with any of the agents used. Commonly, these may be mild and transient (e.g. GI disturbance, headache).
    - Severe reactions can also arise (e.g. hypersensitivity reactions, Stevens–Johnson syndrome, liver dysfunction), necessitating discontinuation of the responsible agent(s).
    - Other toxic effects, such as bone marrow dysfunction, can develop after a longer period of treatment.

Table 4 Antiretrovirals[6,9,15]

Drug class	Examples	Mechanism of action	Comments	Adverse effects	Resistance
NRTIs – nucleoside reverse transcriptase inhibitors	Abacavir	Analogues of nucleosides Converted to triphosphates by cellular kinases Act as substrates for reverse transcriptase Inhibit viral reverse transcriptase by prevention of phosphodiester linkages → chain termination	Active against HIV-1 and HIV-2	Bone marrow suppression Peripheral neuropathy Lipoatrophy Lactic acidosis Abacavir – rare hypersensitivity reactions associated with HLAB5701 – potentially fatal subsequent reactions Tenofovir – reduced bone marrow density, nephrotoxicity	Drug resistance → cross-resistance to other NRTIs
	Didanosine (ddI)				
	Emtricitabine				
	Lamivudine (3TC)				
	Stavudine (d4T)				
	Zidovudine (AZT)				
	Zalcitabine (ddC)				
	Tenofovir (nucleotide analogue)				
NNRTIs – non nucleoside reverse transcriptase inhibitors	Nevirapine	Inhibits HIV-1 reverse transcriptase by binding at a non-active site	Rapid fall in HIV-1 RNA load Not useful in HIV-2 Non-competitive inhibitors of HIV-1 RT Can interfere with cytochrome P450 enzyme system and cause drug interactions	Rash → SJS Hepatitis	Single mutation → resistance to whole class
	Efavirenz			Vivid dreams, sleep disturbance, other neuropsychiatric symptoms Dyslipidaemia Abnormal fat distribution Gynaecomastia	

(continued)

Table 4 (continued)

Drug class	Examples	Mechanism of action	Comments	Adverse effects	Resistance
PIs – protease inhibitors	Atazanavir	Inhibits protease responsible for post-translational cleavage of polyproteins into structural proteins and enzymes required for viral replication	Very potent → rapid fall in HIV RNA load	Lipodystrophy	Well recognised
	Darunavir		Metabolised and excreted rapidly → require frequent dosing	Dyslipidaemia	Number of protease mutations result in cross-resistance
	Fosamprenavir	Results in immature defective viral particles	Active against HIV-1 and HIV-2	Glucose intolerance	Combinations result in less drug resistance
	Indinavir	Peptidomimetic inhibitors of viral protease		Diarrhoea	
	Lopinavir				
	Nelfinavir				
	Ritonavir				
	Saquinavir				
	Tipranavir				
Fusion inhibitor	Enfuvirtide	Inhibits fusion of viral and cell membrane by blocking conformational changes in gp41 necessary for membrane fusion	May be useful in patients with resistance to first line ART	Injection site reactions	Specific mutations cause resistance but may also decrease efficiency of viral fusion
CCR5 antagonist	Maraviroc	Prevents attachment of viral envelope proteins to CCR5 coreceptor thus inhibiting viral entry into cell	Not currently licensed in paediatrics. May be useful in patients with resistance to first line ART	Hepatic dysfunction. Severe skin/hypersensitivity reactions	Only effective in strains using CCR5 for entry – variable sensitivity. Resistance can develop by use of other coreceptors for entry or by mutation of envelope protein
Integrase inhibitor	Raltegravir, Dolutegravir	Prevents insertion of HIV DNA into host genome thus inhibiting viral replication	Recently licensed in children. HIV-1 only	Neuropsychiatric / CNS symptoms. Pancreatitis. Hepatic dysfunction	Mutations proximal to active site of enzyme. Cross-resistance within class

- It is important to be aware of the potential toxic effects to allow appropriate support of the patient and alteration of regimen when necessary, in order to maximise compliance and optimise long term outcome.[15]

Further details of antiretroviral drugs are summarised in Table 4.

Conclusions

In this chapter we have summarised the key principles to consider when prescribing antifungal and antiviral agents for children. For the management of complex infections, liaise with your local paediatric infectious diseases service, specialist pharmacists and/or microbiologists to discuss how to optimise the choice of agent, dose and treatment duration for individual patients.

References

1   Chen SC, Sorrell TC. Antifungal agents. *Med J Aust* 2007; 187(7): 404–409.
2   Andrews MD, Burns M. Common tinea infections in children. *Am Fam Physician* 2008; 77(10): 1415–1420.
3   Managing scalp ringworm in children. *Drug Ther Bull* 2007; 45(12): 89–92.
4   Paramythiotou E *et al*. Invasive fungal infections in the ICU: how to approach, how to treat. *Molecules* 2014; 19(1): 1085–119.
5   Drew RH *et al*. Recent advances in the treatment of life–threatening, invasive fungal infections. *Expert Opin Pharmacother* 2013; 14(17): 2361–2374.
6   Finch RG *et al*. *Antibiotic and Chemotherapy, Anti-Infective Agents and Their Use in Therapy*, 8th edn. Churchill Livingstone, 2003.
7   Thompson C *et al*. Encephalitis in children. *Arch Dis Child* 2012; 97(2): 150–161.
8   Pinninti SG, Kimberlin DW. Management of neonatal herpes simplex virus infection and exposure. *Arch Dis Child Fetal Neonatal Ed* 2014; 99(3): F240– F244.
9   De Clercq E. Antiviral drugs in current clinical use. *J Clin Virol* 2004; 30(2): 115–33.
10 Cernik C *et al*. The treatment of herpes simplex infections: an evidence-based review. *Arch Intern Med* 2008; 168(11): 1137–1144.
11 Swanson EC, Schleiss MR. Congenital cytomegalovirus infection: new prospects for prevention and therapy. *Pediatr Clin North Am* 2013; 60(2): 335–349.
12 Kotton CN. CMV: Prevention, diagnosis and therapy. *Am J Transplant* 2013; 13 Suppl 3: 24–40, quiz 40.
13 Whitley RJ. The use of antiviral drugs during the neonatal period. *Clin Perinatol* 2012; 39(1): 69–81.
14 Public Health England. PHE guidance on use of antiviral agents for the treatment and prophylaxis of influenza (2014–15), version 5.1. London, UK: Public Health England, January 2015.
15 Bamford A *et al*. Paediatric European Network for Treatment of AIDS (PENTA) guidelines for treatment of paediatric HIV-1 infection 2015: optimizing health in preparation for adult life. *HIV Med* 2015; 19(1): e1–e42.

Further recommended reading

Agrawal S *et al*. The role of the multidisciplinary team in antifungal stewardship. *J Antimicrob Chemother* 2016; 71 (suppl 2): ii37–ii42.
Anker M, Corales RB. Raltegravir (MK-0518): a novel integrase inhibitor for the treatment of HIV infection. *Expert Opin Investig Drugs*. 2008; 17(1): 97–103.

Goering R *et al*. *Mims' Medical Microbiology*, 5th edn. Saunders, 2013.

Haqqani AA, Tilton JC. Entry inhibitors and their use in the treatment of HIV-1 infection. *Antiviral Res*. 2013; 98(2): 158–70.

Liverpool Drug Interactions. HIV Drug Interactions. www.hiv-druginteractions.org

Penazzato M *et al*. Optimisation of antiretroviral therapy in HIV-infected children under 3 years of age. *Cochrane Database Syst Rev*. 2014; (5): CD004772.

Razonable RR. Antiviral drugs for viruses other than human immunodeficiency virus. *Mayo Clin Proc* 2011; 86(10): 1009–1026.

44

Endocrinology

S Edate and A Albanese

Introduction

There are a wide range of medicines used in paediatric endocrinology. This chapter focuses on the commonest medicines used in thyroid, hypothalamic/pituitary and adrenal diseases.

The learning objectives of this chapter are:

➢ to understand the core medications used in thyroid, hypothalamic/pituitary and adrenal diseases
➢ to understand the key side-effects to be aware of
➢ to understand how to monitor treatment efficacy.

Thyroid hormones

Levothyroxine sodium

Background

- Levothyroxine is the pharmaceutically synthesised form of thyroxine (T4). It is used to treat primary or central hypothyroidism.
- Primary hypothyroidism is due to an under-functioning thyroid, while central hypothyroidism can be either secondary (pituitary, due to thyroid-stimulating hormone (TSH) deficiency) or tertiary (hypothalamic, due to thyrotrophin-releasing hormone (TRH) deficiency).
- Thyroxine is essential for normal growth and development, especially in the first 3 years of life when it plays a key role in ensuring normal brain growth and nervous system development.
- By measuring TSH levels in all babies shortly after birth, newborn screening programmes can identify congenital primary hypothyroidism.
- The aim of newborn screening programmes is to start treatment with levothyroxine at the earliest opportunity before clinical symptoms manifest and when irreversible neurodevelopmental damage can be minimised; this is currently by 14 days of postnatal age.

Indications

Congenital hypothyroidism

- The starting dose of oral levothyroxine should be 10–15 micrograms/kg/day, with a maximum dose of 50 micrograms/day. There is conflicting evidence as to the benefit of relatively high dose T4 in early infancy. The high dose regimen leads to more rapidly normalised thyroid function and improved IQ scores but there is evidence of later subtle problems with attention and behaviour.[1–5]
- The dose of levothyroxine may need to be reduced if TSH is suppressed, free T4 is too high or if the baby is showing signs of overtreatment. Babies with some endogenous thyroid hormone production may need smaller initial doses.
- Treatment with levothyroxine should lead to normalisation of free T4 and a 50% reduction in TSH within days. However, TSH normalisation can take weeks. The aim of treatment is therefore to achieve free T4 close to the upper reference range within the first 2 weeks of treatment and to normalise the TSH within the first month.[6] Free T4 concentrations may exceed the normal reference range at the time of TSH normalisation, but if the infant is not symptomatic, levothyroxine dose reductions are not necessary. Significant or prolonged elevation of free T4 levels should be avoided.
- Regular dose adjustments may be required not only because growth and change in body size is at its most rapid, but also because this is a critical period for ongoing dendritic formation and neurological development and therefore treatment should be optimised.
- Once levothyroxine treatment has been started, TSH and thyroid hormone concentration should be checked at approximately 2 weeks, 4 weeks, 8 weeks, 3 months, 6 months, 9 months and 12 months after treatment is started, and every 4 months from 1 to 3 years of age and every 6 months until the child's growth is complete, or more frequently if stable blood levels are difficult to achieve.[3–5]
- Adequate calcium intake (800–1200 mg/day), ideally from dietary sources, should be ensured, as thyroid hormones influence bone remodelling.[6]

Acquired hypothyroidism

- In children with severe acquired hypothyroidism with low or undetectable free T4, an initial low dose of levothyroxine should be used (e.g. 25 micrograms daily) and then increased slowly.
- It takes about 8–12 weeks for the TSH level to fully respond, hence thyroid function should be rechecked after 8 weeks and the dose increased or decreased by 12.5–25 micrograms per dose as required.

Hyperthyroidism

- Levothyroxine is also used in the treatment regimen for hyperthyroidism that is known as 'block and replace'.

Absorption and excretion

- Levothyroxine is incompletely and variably absorbed from the gastrointestinal tract. It is extensively metabolised in the thyroid, liver, kidney and anterior pituitary. Some enterohepatic recirculation occurs. Only a portion of the levothyroxine is metabolised to the active hormone triiodothyronine (T3). Levothyroxine is excreted in the urine and faeces, partly as free drug and partly as conjugates and deiodinated metabolites.[7,8]
- Ideally, levothyroxine should be taken on an empty stomach for better absorption. If, however, it is taken after food, it is important that the timing of the dose in relation to mealtimes is consistent; adjustments can be made to the dose to maintain the desired thyroxine level.
- Generic preparations of levothyroxine may differ in their bioavailability. Repeat thyroid function tests might be needed when changing between levothyroxine from different manufacturers.

Metabolism

- Levothyroxine has a half-life of 7 days in euthyroid patients, but this may be shortened to 3–4 days in hyperthyroidism or prolonged to 9–10 days in hypothyroidism.[8] (Note that the half-lives of the drugs discussed in this chapter are largely taken from adult studies, and half-lives might be different in children – but few paediatric data are available in most cases.)
- Levothyroxine is almost completely bound to plasma protein, mainly thyroxine binding globulin, with approximately 0.03% of levothyroxine unbound. The unbound levothyroxine is converted to T3.[8]
- In some cases, clinical effects can be seen after 2 weeks. In babies with severe hypothyroidism, clinical improvement will be seen within a few days to 1 week. Due to the half-life, it takes about 3.5 weeks for serum T4 levels to reach a steady state, therefore repeat laboratory testing is usually done about 6–8 weeks after initial treatment and/or dosage adjustment.[9]

Toxicity

- The following side-effects are usually due to accidental or excessive dosage and are equivalent to the symptoms of hyperthyroidism:[8]
  - Arrhythmias, anginal pain, tachycardia, disorders of menstruation, pseudotumor cerebri, cramps in skeletal muscles, headache, restlessness, excitability, flushing, sweating, diarrhoea, excessive weight loss and muscular weakness, insomnia, tremor, fever, vomiting, palpitations and heat intolerance

- Hypersensitivity reactions, including rash, pruritus and oedema, have also been reported.
- Thyroid crisis has occasionally been reported following massive or chronic intoxication, and cardiac arrhythmias, heart failure, coma and death have occurred.

Important/common drug interactions

- Sucralfate, sodium polystyrene sulfonate or colestyramine reduce the absorption of levothyroxine by binding within the gut.[8]
- Cimetidine, aluminium hydroxide, calcium carbonate, soya, multivitamin tablets and ferrous sulfate also reduce the absorption of levothyroxine from the gastrointestinal tract.
- In the above situations, levothyroxine should be administered at least 4 hours apart from the drugs. If thyroid function tests show that TSH is raised, the levothyroxine dose can be increased by 25–50 micrograms per dose.[8]
- The concurrent use of carbamazepine, phenytoin, phenobarbital, primadone or rifampicin with levothyroxine has been found to increase levothyroxine metabolism. If these medications are required, the dose of levothyroxine can be increased by 25–50 micrograms per dose.
- Hypothyroidism affects glycogenolysis and insulin, leading to reduced insulin requirements. Once euthyroidism is achieved by levothyroxine, it leads to higher blood glucose levels. Diabetic patients should be monitored for increased requirements of insulin or oral hypoglycaemic agents.[10]

General drug advice

In neonates, crushed tablets or liquid levothyroxine can be used, but the same formulation should be used for consistency. If crushed tablets are used, they should ideally be given with a spoonful of lukewarm water or breastmilk, and should be given on a spoon or with a medicine dispenser pipette so that the baby receives the whole dose. The crushed tablet should not be added to a feeding bottle, as it is important the baby gets the whole dose of levothyroxine and that none remains in any unfinished milk.[10,11]

Levothyroxine is best taken as a single dose on an empty stomach, usually half an hour before breakfast. As mentioned above, if administration with food is preferred, the same routine should be used every day, and a higher dose may be required. In children with Crohn's disease, coeliac disease, short gut syndrome or malabsorption, or post bariatric surgery, there may be poor absorption of levothyroxine also necessitating a higher dose.

Patients with central hypothyroidism may have adrenal insufficiency. It is extremely important to consider cortisol deficiency before starting levothyroxine in these patients, as the therapy will speed up cortisol metabolism, which could precipitate an adrenal crisis. Cortisol reserve can be assessed with an early morning cortisol measurement or appropriate dynamic tests.

If a child on oral levothyroxine is unable to tolerate enteral fluids, an intravenous preparation of liothyronine sodium (T3) can be used. Liothyronine has a rapid effect and is metabolised quickly. A quantity of 20–25 micrograms of liothyronine is equivalent to approximately 100 micrograms of levothyroxine. Liothyronine is given intravenously in two or three divided daily doses. Its effect develops after a few hours and disappears within 24–48 hours. Efficacy is determined by measuring free T3 levels and doses adjusted accordingly. Once the child is able to tolerate enteral fluids, then oral levothyroxine can be restarted.[6]

Formulations

The formulations of levothyroxine and other medicines discussed in this chapter are summarised in Table 1. These may vary in different countries.

Table 1 Formulations of drugs commonly used in paediatric endocrinology				
Drug name (generic)	Solid formulations (for oral administration)	Liquid formulations or melts (for oral administration)	Intravenous formulations	Other
Levothyroxine	Tablets: 25 µg, 50 µg and 100 µg	Liquid: 25 µg/50 µg/100 µg per 5 mL		
Carbimazole	Tablets: 5 mg and 20 mg			
Desmopressin	Tablets: 100 µg, 200 µg	Oral lyophilisates (melts) for sublingual use: 60 µg, 120 µg, 240 µg	Injection: 4 µg/mL	Intranasal solution: 100 µg/1 mL of the solution. Vials contains 2.5 ml Nasal spray: either 2.5 µg (on a named-patient basis) or 10 µg/metered spray
Somatropin			Injections	
Hydrocortisone	Hydrocortisone tablets 10 mg, 20 mg	Granules: 0.5 mg, 1 mg, 2 mg, 5 mg	Efcortesol IM injection 100 mg IV injection 100 mg/1 mL	

Antithyroid drugs

Carbimazole

Background

- Some antithyroid medications used to treat hyperthyroidism work by reducing the formation of thyroid hormones in the thyroid gland itself.
- Carbimazole is the drug mainly used in the UK, while methimazole tends to be preferred in Europe and the USA. Propylthiouracil (PTU) is considered second line drug therapy except in patients who are allergic to or intolerant of carbimazole/methimazole.
- In 2009 the US Food and Drug Administration (FDA) issued a safety alert regarding the use of PTU in adult and paediatric patients, notifying healthcare professionals of a risk of serious liver injury, including liver failure and death.[11] PTU also very infrequently causes antineutrophil cytoplasmic antibody (ANCA) positive small vessel vasculitis, with a risk that appears to increase with time – in contrast to adverse effects seen with the other antithyroid drugs that typically occur early during treatment.
- When substituting carbimazole, 1 mg is considered equivalent to PTU 10 mg, but the doses need adjusting according to response.

Indications

- Hyperthyroidism due to Graves' disease and associated with toxic multinodular goitre, thyrotoxicosis or a toxic adenoma ('hot nodule')
- Preparation for thyroidectomy in patients with hyperthyroidism
- Therapy prior to and post radioiodine treatment

Principles of treatment

- **Children:** The usual initial daily dose of carbimazole is 0.75 mg/kg/day, maximum 30 mg, in two or three divided doses adjusted according to response. The half-life of carbimazole is around 5 hours. Once stability is achieved with a particular dose, it can be changed to a single dose administered once a day.
- **Teenagers:** The initial dose of carbimazole is between 20 mg and 60 mg, taken as two to three divided doses. Again, the dose can be changed to a single daily dose once stability is achieved. The dose can be increased or decreased incrementally by 2.5–5 mg.
- Subsequent therapy can be administered in one of two ways.[12]
    - 'Block and replace' regimen: this approach aims to completely prevent endogenous thyroxine production. Carbimazole is usually started at the higher dose and a replacement dose of levothyroxine is added as the patient becomes hypothyroid.

The potential main advantages are:
- Improved stability with fewer episodes of hyper or hypothyroidism
- A reduced number of venepunctures and visits to hospital
- Dose titration regimen: this approach aims to maintain a euthyroid state by adjusting the carbimazole dose to suppress the thyroid over-activity to a normal level based on blood thyroid function tests. If the patient is over-suppressed, i.e. to hypothyroid blood thyroid function levels, then the daily carbimazole dose will be reduced by 2.5–5 mg, while if under-suppressed, i.e. to hyperthyroid blood thyroid function levels, the carbimazole will be increased by 2.5–5 mg.
  The potential main advantages are:
  - Fewer side-effects with a lower antithyroid drug dose
  - Improved compliance due to there being one rather than two medications
- It is important to note that the antithyroid drugs will not block the release of any thyroid hormone already synthesised in the gland, which will continue to be released after the medication has been started. It can take as long as six to eight weeks, therefore, for the elevated thyroid hormone levels to normalise and symptoms of hyperthyroidism to subside.

Pharmacology

- Carbimazole (a prodrug) is rapidly metabolised to its active metabolite, thiamazole. The mean peak plasma concentration of thiamazole is reported to occur 1 hour after a single dose of carbimazole. It is possible that the plasma half-life may also be prolonged by renal or hepatic disease. Over 90% of orally administered carbimazole is excreted in the urine as thiamazole or its metabolites. The remainder appears in faeces. There is 10% enterohepatic circulation.[7]

Administration

- Antithyroid drugs work best when there is a stable level in bloodstream. To achieve this, it is important that the antithyroid drugs are taken at the correct times, and if tablets are taken more than once a day, that they should be evenly spaced. Generally, carbimazole is taken in single or divided daily doses, while PTU is taken three to four times per day.

Toxicity

- **Agranulocytosis:** As fatal cases of agranulocytosis with carbimazole have been reported and early treatment of agranulocytosis is essential, it is important that patients should always be warned about the onset of sore throats, bruising or bleeding, mouth ulcers, fever or malaise, and should be instructed to stop the drug and seek medical advice immediately. In such patients, check the white blood cell count, especially if there is evidence of clinical infection. A baseline full blood count should be done at diagnosis of thyrotoxicosis before starting carbimazole, to identify any associated or pre-existing leucopenia, thrombocytopenia or aplastic anaemia.[7,12]

- **Hepatic failure:** Carbimazole should be used with caution in patients with mild to moderate hepatic insufficiency. Baseline liver function tests should be done before starting the medication. If any signs or symptoms of liver dysfunction develop (pain in the upper abdomen, anorexia, general pruritus), the drug should be stopped and liver function tests performed immediately. Early withdrawal of the drug will increase the chances of complete recovery. The medication should also be discontinued if transaminase levels reach two to three times the upper limit of normal. After the drug is discontinued, liver function tests should be monitored weekly until there is resolution. If resolution is not evident, prompt referral to a gastroenterologist or hepatologist is warranted.[7,12]

- Carbimazole should be stopped temporarily at the time of administration of radioiodine (to avoid thyroid crisis).

- Hypersensitivity and allergic reactions: angioedema and multisystem hypersensitivity reactions such as cutaneous vasculitis, liver, lung and renal effects can occur.

- Other side-effects:[7] headache, nausea, mild gastrointestinal disturbance, fever, malaise, skin rashes, pruritus, urticaria. Isolated cases of myopathy have been reported. Patients experiencing myalgia after the intake of carbimazole should have their creatine phosphokinase levels monitored.

Important drug interactions

- *Anticoagulants (oral):* the efficacy of oral anticoagulant medications may be potentiated by carbimazole.

- *Beta-blockers:* for some patients, their dose of beta-blockers may need to be reduced when thyroid function returns to normal after antithyroid drug treatment.

- *Digitalis glycosides:* there can be an interaction between thyrotoxicosis or carbimazole and concomitant administration of digitalis glycosides. Monitoring of blood digoxin levels, which can either increase or decrease, is therefore recommended, with appropriate dose adjustments of the digitalis glycoside treatment.

- *Theophylline:* antithyroid drug treatment may reduce the dose of theophylline required for asthma management.[7]

Synthetic vasopressin analogues

Desmopressin

Background

Desmopressin is a synthetic analogue of antidiuretic hormone (ADH) vasopressin, used to treat central diabetes insipidus, which is characterised by decreased ADH secretion, typically causing polyuria, with the passage of large volumes of dilute urine (< 300 mOsm/kg). Desmopressin has potent antidiuretic activity and a weak vasopressor effect.

Indications

- **Diabetes insipidus.** Specialist management is required for the treatment of central diabetes insipidus and also during a water deprivation test.
- **Primary nocturnal enuresis**

Absorption

- Absorption from the nasal mucosa may be erratic in the presence of an upper respiratory tract infection or allergic rhinitis.

Distribution

- Given intranasally or orally, desmopressin maximum plasma concentrations are reached in 40–55 minutes. The half-life of the drug is 3.5 hours. Generally, urine output will decrease 1–2 hours after administration, and the duration of action will range from 8 to 24 hours.[7]

Toxicity

- Overdose can lead to free water retention, causing a decrease in plasma osmolality and hyponatremia. Symptoms of hyponatremia include headache, nausea, vomiting and seizures. Untreated, these symptoms can lead to coma and death. However, asymptomatic mild hyponatremia can also occur.[7]
- Rare side-effects with intranasal delivery of desmopressin include eye irritation, headache, dizziness, rhinitis or epistaxis, coughing, flushing, nausea, vomiting, abdominal pain, chest pain, palpitations and tachycardia.
- Desmopressin is contraindicated in patients with cardiac problems or taking diuretics.
- In patients with hypoadrenalism and diabetes insipidus, desmopressin should be temporarily stopped during episodes of acute illness requiring hydrocortisone emergency cover and the patient advised to drink water only if thirsty and to seek urgent medical attention.

Formulations

- Desmopressin has variable antidiuretic activity, lasting from 8 to 24 hours depending on the preparation used and the disease severity. The efficacy and duration of a given dose must be established separately for each patient, because of significant individual variation.
- The duration of action can be established clinically by the reappearance of polyuria and polydipsia, e.g. the night-time dose is that required to prevent nocturia and polyuria. The morning and evening doses should be adjusted separately.
- If for any reason the route of administration needs to be changed, it should be noted that the dosages of the different formulations of desmopressin are not directly interchangeable.

Recombinant human growth hormone

Somatropin

Background

- Growth hormone (GH, also known as somatotrophin) is an anterior pituitary hormone that promotes growth of body tissues as one of its main effects. It also regulates body composition, muscle and bone metabolism. It is released into the circulation in a pulsatile fashion. The largest and most predictable of these GH peaks occurs about an hour after the onset of sleep.
- IGF-I (insulin-like growth factor 1) is the main effector of GH action on linear growth. Recombinant human growth hormone (somatropin) is the biosynthetic GH analogue used to promote growth in children and young adults with growth failure.[13]
- Somatropin is administered by daily subcutaneous injection, preferably in the evening, just before bedtime.

Indications

- Somatropin is indicated and licensed in the UK for children with growth failure in association with the following conditions.[13]
  - Growth hormone deficiency
  - Turner syndrome
  - Prader–Willi syndrome
  - Chronic renal insufficiency
  - Growth disturbance in short children born small for gestational age who fail to show catch-up growth by 4 years of age or later (see NICE guidelines from 2010)
  - Short stature homeobox-containing gene (SHOX) deficiency

Possible side-effects

- *Orthopaedic complications:* slipped capital femoral epiphysis and worsening of scoliosis
- *Otitis media:* increased incidence, especially in patients with Turner syndrome
- *Glucose intolerance or diabetes:* somatropin induces transient insulin resistance, leading to increased levels of insulin but not necessarily glucose. Several cases of pancreatitis associated with somatropin have been reported. Patients with limited insulin reserve may develop glucose intolerance. Type 2 diabetes has been reported in a few adolescents treated with somatropin.
- *Pseudo-tumour cerebri:* headaches are more frequently seen in children on GH treatment, with the incidence of 1/1000 children treated. This side-effect is not dose-dependent. Symptoms of raised intracranial pressure and papilloedema usually resolve after therapy is discontinued. Only some patients who resume therapy experience recurrent headaches and papilloedema.
- *Sudden death in Prader–Willi Syndrome:* the majority of reported deaths have occurred within 6 months of starting somatropin. Risk factors associated with sudden death are morbid obesity, obstructive sleep apnoea and respiratory tract infections.
- *Impaired thyroid function:* somatropin enhances T4 to T3 conversion, leading to a decrease in serum T4 and increase in T3 levels. Therefore there is a risk of overt hypothyroidism in central subclinical hypothyroidism and mild hyperthyroidism in patients on levothyroxine.
- *Small for gestational age:* this condition implicates an intrinsic increased risk of cardiovascular disease and insulin resistance in adulthood. However, at the moment, there are no published data reporting increased risk of any specific side-effect of somatropin in this population. Since the dose of somatropin used in this condition is higher than in GH deficiency, long term safety data are needed.
- *Oncogenesis:* there were case reports of leukaemia in the 1980s in Japan in patients on GH therapy. Subsequent rigorous studies in Western countries and Japan have not confirmed this finding. Somatropin should be used carefully in conditions with increased risk of cancer, such as Fanconi anaemia, Bloom syndrome and neurofibromatosis type 1.

Contraindications

- *Prader–Willi Syndrome:* in cases with severe obesity, uncontrolled diabetes, untreated severe obstructive sleep apnoea, active cancer and active psychosis
- *Oncological patients:* active cancer

Formulations

- GH is available only as an injection for subcutaneous use. An up-to-date list of the different brands available in the UK can be found in the current *British National Formulary for Children* (BNFC).
- Each brand of somatropin is administered using brand specific pen devices. The pen devices are delivered free of charge to the family after registration with the brand related homecare service.

GH therapy monitoring

- The routine follow-up of paediatric patients on GH should be performed by a paediatric endocrinologist in partnership with the paediatrician or primary care physician. Children should be evaluated every 4–6 months. Specialist nurses from the hospital or from allocated homecare services will support the family during initiation and can be contacted by the family in case of any problems.
- For checking concordance with the prescribed therapeutic regimen and for safety monitoring, yearly serum IGF-1 levels are useful. IGF-1 based GH dosing regimens may lead to improved growth responses, but supraphysiological levels (> +2 SD (standard deviation)) of IGF-1 for healthy age-matched controls should be avoided. If, on repeated measurement, IGF-I levels exceed +2 SD of reference values for age and pubertal status, the GH dose should be reduced.
- Thyroid function, namely free T4 and TSH, should be tested at initiation and then monitored yearly if normal to detect GH therapy induced hypothyroidism, which needs to be treated.
- The effect of GH on glycaemia should be monitored periodically by measurement of random blood glucose and haemoglobin A1C. When impaired glucose tolerance is suspected, or in an at-risk individual, a formal oral glucose tolerance test should be performed. In children small for gestational age on GH treatment, fasting insulin and blood glucose should be measured before start of GH and annually thereafter.
- Scoliosis may progress during phases of rapid growth. GH treatment itself does not increase the incidence or severity of scoliosis. If scoliosis is noted, then the child should be referred to an orthopaedic surgeon without altering the dose of GH if the latter is appropriate for the child.
- In at-risk groups (Turner and Prader–Willi syndrome) patients and carers should be advised of the changes to look out for, and a diagnosis-orientated clinical surveillance programme should be followed.
- Sudden onset of a limp or of hip/knee pain that is not explained by a preceding trauma should be investigated with radiological imaging of the hip to rule out a slipped capital epiphysis.
- In children with Prader–Willi syndrome, before starting somatropin the following recommendations are applicable.

- Ear, nose and throat clinic referral if history of sleep-disordered breathing or snoring, or if enlarged tonsils and adenoids are present. Tonsillectomy and adenoidectomy where indicated
- Referral to respiratory specialist/sleep clinic. Sleep oximetry in all patients, preferably completed by polysomnographic evaluation
- Scoliosis evaluation and referral to orthopaedic surgeon if indicated
- Effective weight control before and during GH
- Discontinuation of GH is indicated in:
  - acute critical illness
  - Prader–Willi syndrome associated with severe obesity/upper airways obstruction
  - overt diabetes in small for gestational age children
  - active cancer
  - hypersensitivity to the active substance or to any of the excipients
  - chronic renal disease at renal transplantation.

Hydrocortisone replacement

Background

- Cortisol is a natural steroid hormone which is produced by the zona fasciculata in the adrenal cortex of the adrenal gland.
- Cortisol maintains blood glucose, controls blood pressure and supports the body in dealing with stress and infection.
- Cortisol secretion has a circadian rhythm, with peak levels in the morning on waking, and falling throughout the day with nadir values at midnight.
- Hydrocortisone is used for replacement in cortisol deficiency.
- The aims of treatment are to reduce signs and symptoms of hypocortisolism, to prevent acute adrenal crisis and to mimic the normal circadian rhythm of cortisol secretion. The lowest possible daily dose of hydrocortisone that ensures an adequate quality of life should be used.
- The hydrocortisone replacement dose is 8–12 mg/m^2/day orally in three divided doses. The largest dose is given on waking before breakfast; the second dose should not be later than 6 hours after the first dose, to prevent cortisol levels falling below the normal range; and the third and last dose should be 5–6 hours before bedtime to avoid an overexposure to cortisol during the night.

Indications

- Hypocortisolism can be due to primary (adrenal), secondary (pituitary, due to ACTH (adrenocorticotropic hormone) deficiency) or tertiary (hypothalamic, due to CRF (corticotrophin-releasing hormone) deficiency) failure. In secondary and tertiary cortisol deficiency, the pituitary is not producing ACTH, hence the adrenal glands are not stimulated to produce cortisol.

- Congenital adrenal hyperplasia (CAH). In this case, cortisol is not produced, due to an enzymatic defect in the synthetic pathway in the adrenal gland. Lifelong treatment is required not only for replacement, but also to prevent the overproduction of androgens resulting from the position of the enzyme deficiency in the metabolic pathway.

Absorption

- It takes about an hour for oral hydrocortisone to be absorbed. Absorption can be affected by milk, vomiting and diarrhoea. The dose should be given 1 hour before a milk feed.

Toxicity

- The adrenal glands produce between 5 and 10 mg/m^2 of cortisol per day, with a circadian rhythm. The dose of administered hydrocortisone is calculated to replicate the normal adrenal production and so is unlikely to cause side-effects.
- Side-effects will only tend to occur if hydrocortisone is taken above the level produced by the body, and if this is over a prolonged period. If clinically indicated, the hydrocortisone regimen can be monitored with a 24 hour blood cortisol profile with regular venous blood samples to document the pharmacological profile of the hydrocortisone therapy (including absorption, peak concentration, duration of action, etc.).

Education

- Both clinicians and patients need to understand how to manage acute illness in a setting of hypocortisolism, and when it is necessary to increase the dose of hydrocortisone, as summarised in Table 2 and Table 3.

Table 2 Management of acute illness in hypocortisolism[14,15]
➢ Treatment of the underlying illness
➢ Doubling or trebling of regular hydrocortisone dose for duration of the illness, and an extra dose of hydrocortisone at 5 am should be considered.
➢ Parental hydrocortisone, if oral administration not possible or if illness is severe, should be given intravenously/intramuscularly 6- to 8-hourly
➢ Carbohydrate, sodium and fluid replacement
➢ Treatment of hypoglycaemia
➢ *Children with hypocortisolism should have open access to local hospital, wear a MedicAlert or similar identification tag, and carry a steroid card with treatment details*

Table 3 Situations when the hydrocortisone regimen should be increased (hydrocortisone emergency cover)[14,15]

Vomiting	If there is one vomit within 1 hour of taking an oral dose of hydrocortisone, then that dose should be repeated, but if the vomit happens more than an hour after taking the dose then that dose does not need repeating. If the child vomits more than once, the oral hydrocortisone dose should be doubled or trebled and an extra dose of hydrocortisone at 5 am can be added. If vomiting persists, the patient/parents/carers should be instructed to see the GP, local paediatric department or specialist treatment centre.
Diarrhoea	If diarrhoea develops, there is a risk that the oral hydrocortisone will not be absorbed. The oral dose of hydrocortisone should be doubled or trebled until the diarrhoea resolves. If the patient has both diarrhoea and vomiting, or if they become clinically unwell with either symptom alone, then an intramuscular injection of hydrocortisone should be administered and an ambulance called to take the child to hospital immediately.
Hypoglycaemia	If the child develops symptoms of hypoglycaemia, e.g. is pallid, clammy, drowsy, confused, dazed and is not responding normally, then Glucogel® (or equivalent) and an intramuscular injection of hydrocortisone should be administered immediately and an ambulance called to go straight to hospital.
Temperature	If fever suggestive of an infection occurs, hydrocortisone doses should be doubled or trebled for the first few days until the temperature resolves and the patient is back to normal. An increased dose of hydrocortisone can be considered for a temperature associated with immunisations.
General anaesthetics	If a general anaesthetic is required for any reason, extra hydrocortisone given either intramuscularly or intravenously will be required.
Accidents and injuries	If there is a serious injury with fracture or loss of consciousness with head injury, an intramuscular injection of hydrocortisone should be administered and an ambulance called for immediate transportation to hospital.
Dentists	If the child needs minor dental work (such as a check-up or cleaning), then no extra hydrocortisone is required. If fillings or any other treatment are required, then the hydrocortisone dose should be doubled or trebled for 24 hours around the appointment. If there is the unexpected need for an injection of local anaesthetic for fillings or other treatment, the dose of oral hydrocortisone should be doubled or trebled as soon as possible and for the next 24 hours. Major dental work such as having teeth removed should be carried out in hospital and a stress dose of intravenous hydrocortisone will be needed.
Acute illness	Parents/carers of patients, and patients themselves with adrenal insufficiency and diabetes insipidus on replacement hydrocortisone and desmopressin should be instructed to give extra oral hydrocortisone during an acute illness and withhold desmopressin. Drinking should only be in response to thirst followed by assessment in hospital and check of the patient's electrolytes.

Conclusion

In summary, paediatric endocrine drugs need close monitoring and should be prescribed and monitored with advice from tertiary paediatric endocrine specialists and paediatric clinical pharmacy services.

References

1   Jacob H, Peters C. Screening, diagnosis and management of congenital hypothyroidism: European Society for Paediatric Endocrinology Consensus Guideline. *Arch Dis Child Educ Pract Ed* 2015; 100(5): 260–263.
2   Hindmarsh PC. Optimisation of thyroxine dose in congenital hypothyroidism. *Arch Dis Child* 2002; 86: 73–75.
3   Public Health England. Newborn blood spot screening programme: supporting publications. http://newbornbloodspot.screening.nhs.uk/cht
4   UK standards and guidelines: https://assets.publishing.service.gov.uk/government/uploads/system/uploads/attachment_data/file/698364/NBS06_CHT_confirmed_final_100418.pdf
5   The Child Growth Foundation. *Thyroid Disorders: A Guide for Parents and Patients.* London: The Child Growth Foundation, 2000. www.childgrowthfoundation.org/CMS/FILES/15_Hypothyroidism.pdf
6   Jacob H, Peters C. Screening, diagnosis and management of congenital hypothyroidism: European Society for Paediatric Endocrinology Consensus Guideline. *Arch Dis Child Educ Pract Ed* 2015; 100(5): 260–263.
7   Electronic Medicines Compendium (eMC). www.medicines.org.uk/emc
8   Drugs.com. Levothyroxine sodium. www.drugs.com/pro/synthroid.html
9   Sinha SK, Sasigarn A. Pediatric Hypothyroidism Treatment & Management. Medscape website (2016). Available at: http://reference.medscape.com/article/922777-treatment [last accessed 28 June 2018].
10 Johnson JL. Diabetes control in thyroid disease. *Diabetes Spectr* 2006; 19(3): 148–153.
11 US Food & Drug Administration. FDA Drug Safety Communication: New boxed warning on severe liver injury with propylthiouracil. www.fda.gov/Drugs/DrugSafety/PostmarketDrugSafetyInformationforPatientsandProviders/ucm209023.htm
12 Cheetham TD *et al*. Treatment of hyperthyroidism in young people. *Arch Dis Child* 1998; 78: 207–209.
13 NICE. Human growth hormone (somatropin) for the treatment of growth failure in children. Technology appraisal guidance TA188, 2010. www.nice.org.uk/guidance/ta188
14 Great Ormond Street Hospital for Children. Cortisol deficiency. www.gosh.nhs.uk/medical-information/search-for-medical-conditions/cortisol-deficiency/cortisol-deficiency-information
15 Child Growth Foundation. *Congenital Adrenal Hyperplasia: A Guide for Parents and Patients*. London: The Child Growth Foundation, 1996. www.childgrowthfoundation.org/CMS/FILES/06_CongenitalAdrenalHyperplasia.Pdf

Further recommended reading

Deal CL *et al*. Growth Hormone Research Society workshop summary: consensus guidelines for recombinant human growth hormone therapy in Prader–Willi Syndrome. *J Clin Endocrinol Metab* 2013, 98(6): E1072–E1087.
Ooi HL *et al*. Desmopressin administration in children with central diabetes insipidus: a retrospective review. *J Pediatr Endocrinol Metab* 2013; 26(11–12): 1047–1052.
Souza FM, Collett-Solberg PF. Adverse effects of growth hormone replacement therapy in children. *Arq Bras Endocrinol Metab* 2011; 55(8): 559–565.

45

Diabetes mellitus

C de Beaufort

Introduction

The rising prevalence of diabetes mellitus in children during recent decades makes the understanding of this complex condition increasingly important for paediatricians.[1] The management of paediatric diabetes mellitus presents numerous challenges because of the multifaceted interaction between normal growth and development, pathophysiology and behavioural issues.

The learning objectives of this chapter are:

➢ to know the current pharmacological management strategies available for paediatric diabetes mellitus
➢ to understand the different regimens of subcutaneous insulin administration
➢ to introduce dose determination for insulin regimens
➢ to recognise the role of blood glucose measurements
➢ to be familiar with the management of diabetic emergencies.

Diabetes mellitus: overview

Diabetes mellitus is a chronic disease, characterised by hyperglycaemia. Hyperglycaemia can be caused by insulin deficiency, insulin resistance or both. Different forms require different therapeutic approaches.

The most common forms (Table 1) are type 1 diabetes mellitus (T1DM) and type 2 diabetes mellitus (T2DM), although it remains important to identify monogenic diabetes (maturity onset diabetes of the young; MODY). As treatment will differ, it is important to make the right diagnosis.

For full definitions and further details, see the 2018 clinical practice consensus guidelines (CPCG) of the International Society for Pediatric and Adolescent Diabetes (ISPAD).[2]

Table 1 Characteristics of different forms of diabetes

	T1DM	T2DM	Monogenic
Age at onset	Most > 6 months	> 10 years	< 6 months and after puberty
DKA[*]	11–40%	<25 %	Rare
Obesity	Population dependent	Most	Population dependent
Autoimmunity	> 80%	No	No
Acanthosis nigricans	Population dependent	Frequent	Population dependent
Positive family history	10–25%	> 80%	> 90%

*DKA, diabetic ketoacidosis

For all forms of diabetes, the same overall targets are applicable:

- Near normal metabolic control, without acute complications
- Near normal psychosocial development
- Optimal quality of life

Type 1 diabetes mellitus: overview

The only life-saving drug for the treatment for type 1 diabetes (T1DM) is insulin, given via non-enteral administration. Different insulin formulations exist and allow the administration of insulin that results in a profile as close to normal physiology as possible. Treatment of children with any form of diabetes should be supervised by an experienced multidisciplinary team (physician, nurse educator, dietitian, psychologist). The target for all age groups is glycated haemoglobin (HbA1c) $\leq$ 7.0% (53 mmol/mol), while avoiding large glycaemic variation and taking quality of life into account. Reaching these goals requires a flexible approach tailored to the patient and his or her age, and culturally appropriate education (see Figure 1) is the cornerstone of management.

Many different insulins are available. Good knowledge of the profiles of action is needed to ensure optimal use in relationship to the lifestyle and food intake of patients.

- Short and very short acting insulins (both can be used in continuous sub-cutaneous (SC) insulin infusion pumps):
  - Very short acting insulin analogues are used as a meal bolus
    - Onset within 10–15 minutes
    - Peak after 30–90 minutes
    - Maximum duration of 3–4 hours
  - Recombinant human insulin can also be used as meal bolus
    - Onset after 30–60 minutes

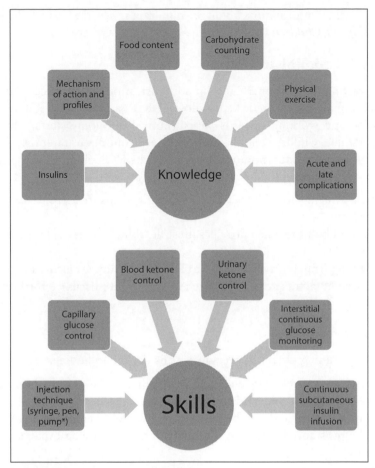

Figure 1 Diabetes education: knowledge and skills
*This may not yet be available in all clinics.

- Peak around 2–4 hours
- Duration 6–8 hours
- Intermediate acting isophane insulins
  - With protamine (neutral protamine Hagedorn; NPH) and/or zinc to prolong effect
    - Later peak: 3–8 hours
    - Long duration: 12–15 hours
- Long acting insulin analogues
  - Almost no peak
  - Duration between 12–24 hours
- For most insulins, the quantity administered will influence its duration of action
  - Smaller dose, shorter duration
- All insulins can be administered with syringes and pens

For further information about insulin types, see the *British National Formulary for Children* (BNFC) or the ISPAD CPCG.[2,3]

SC insulin administration

When starting patients on SC insulin administration, either directly at diagnosis (minimal or no diabetic ketoacidosis; DKA) or after initial stabilisation, education and working towards patient/family autonomy starts. This process takes time. Children and their families need continuous multidisciplinary input until a stable, autonomous phase is reached, which may take years.

For general principles:

- The treatment should be made to measure and ensure a proactive approach.
- The basal bolus regimen provides most flexibility and is the treatment of choice.
- Switching from intravenous (IV) to SC is not a simple calculation, and several factors need to be taken into account (discussed further below).

Insulin regimens

When determining the insulin regimen, consider the following:

- Newly diagnosed (where endogenous insulin may be secreted over first days or weeks) or 'old' and completely insulin deficient patient
- Insulin resistance induced by duration of hyperglycaemia and DKA
- Insulin resistance induced by obesity (can be seen in type 1 diabetes obesity)
- Sensitivity for insulin (age dependent)
- IV insulin requirements over the previous 24 hours, to normalise blood glucose levels
- Meal content
- Physical activity

Basal bolus insulin treatment (at least four injections per day by syringe or by pen; both can be used in all age groups) is started, which includes three short/very short acting insulin doses before each meal and one long acting insulin dose before bedtime. In some situations, the long acting insulin may be needed twice daily and/or injected in the morning. In general, a total dose of 0.8 units/kg/day is used, but this may vary from close to 0 (in the so-called remission phase) to 1.5 units/kg/day after ketoacidosis or during adolescence, characterised by insulin resistance.

Different insulin regimens can be applied, with many different names. A recent classification has sought to simplify this (see Table 2).[4] Fixed doses, although limiting injection frequency to twice daily, impose a regular lifestyle, which is rarely pragmatic for children/adolescents; metabolic outcome is also worse, therefore fixed doses should only be used in exceptional situations.

Table 2 Classification of insulin regimens: summary overview	
Category I:	**Fixed insulin dose regimens**
Definition:	Set insulin dosage not adjusted or minimally adjusted to daily varying meals. Insulin dosage defines the subsequent mealtimes and their amount of carbohydrates.
Insulin administration:	1–2 injections per day
Includes:	Basal insulin only/premixed insulin only/free-mixed insulin combinations
Category II:	**Glucose- and meal-adjusted injection regimens**
Definition:	Administration of insulin according to results of self-monitoring of glucose and intended time of meal intake (no set dose). Insulin dosage allows a varying amount of carbohydrates following the injections.
Insulin administration:	3 or more injections
Includes:	Intensified conventional therapy/basal bolus concept/multiple daily injections/flexible insulin treatment[*]
Category III:	**Pump therapy**
Definition:	Continuous SC insulin infusion and administration of insulin according to results of self-monitoring of glucose and intended time of meal intake. Insulin dosage allows a varying amount of carbohydrates following the injections.
Insulin administration:	Continuous insulin administration for basal insulin

*These terms are all used in literature, but without clear definitions.

Capillary blood glucose measurements are needed to evaluate the treatment, and currently at least four controls per day are requested. All glucose values need to be useful, and therefore testing before and 2 hours after the meals will allow appropriate insulin adjustment for the meals.

For children with diabetes, healthy eating should be targeted. Regular review of healthy food intake is necessary to meet the constantly changing needs and requirements of the developing child.

Insulin dose determination

In glucose- and meal-adjusted insulin regimens (Table 3), pre-meal insulin doses depend on:

- B – basal needs (base, without food intake, including potential activities, stress or physical activity, when not covered by a second long acting insulin injection)
- F – food intake (carbohydrate counting)
- C – correction dose, when applicable

Table 3 Glucose- and meal-adjusted injection regimens: an overview

Time	Insulin administration	Insulin type	Dose calculation
Morning	Bolus	Short or very short acting insulin	BFC
Midday	Bolus		BFC
Evening	Bolus		BFC
Snacks between meals (any time)	Yes /no	With insulin coverage from the preceding dose or give extra insulin dose[*]	
Bedtime	Basal	Long acting insulin analogue	

*Is a snack eaten? If so, what size and has it been planned for and calculated in the prior meal dose or should extra insulin be given? For example, insulin should be administered with snacks that require more than 1 unit according to carbohydrate content.

The final dose will be the addition of B + F + C.

- Note the pre-bedtime long acting insulin will be administered before bedtime or at the same time as the evening premeal dose, but *only* NPH can be mixed in the same syringe with short/very short acting insulins without changing the profile of action.
- The pre-bedtime long acting dose's effectiveness will depend on the body weight (and endogenous insulin secretion).
- Usually the night dose will be maximally 30% of the total daily dose.
  - Typical maximum 0.3 × patient weight (in kg)
- Bolus doses will be about 70% of the total daily dose (divided over meals).
- Dose selection should be discussed with a specialist, as dose will vary according to the age of the child (particularly in infancy/adolescence).
- Regular adjustments will remain necessary, based on blood glucose measurements and changes in growth and lifestyle (e.g. during puberty).
- New long acting analogues have less peak effect → less risk of nocturnal hypoglycaemia.
- Note: expect a reduction in all doses in all patients due to:
  - changes in insulin resistance (e.g. during puberty)
  - increased mobility
  - increased endogenous insulin secretion in newly diagnosed patients with normoglycaemia (the so-called remission phase, or honeymoon period).

Most patients will eat huge quantities during the first weeks after diagnosis (restoration of weight lost). The duration of this period varies, but the insulin dose needs to be appropriate to cover the food intake. This phase (although sometimes worrying for parents) is in general self-limiting, except when the medical team insists on maintaining the same insulin doses over time.

Flexibility and understanding how to adjust the doses are key to successful treatment. When a much lower/higher basal insulin dose is needed, look for potential explanations such as remission (the remaining beta cells may start to transiently secrete insulin), or hyperglycaemia (toxic for beta cells), puberty (insulin resistance), omission of bolus doses (e.g. during school time) or nocturnal hypoglycaemia (03:00 is usually the glucose nadir). Without checking, this nocturnal hypoglycaemia may be missed due to lack of symptoms. It is advised to carry out a monthly nocturnal blood glucose check, which should be continued over time.

This meal-adjusted insulin regimen will allow a proactive approach. It will ensure flexibility around food intake (three opportunities/day, at least, at which the dose can be changed), flexibility around physical activity and quick correction when a previous dose was inappropriate. Acute complications such as hypoglycaemia and hyperglycaemia are better prevented or quickly corrected.

Previously, twice-daily premixed insulin was injected, with lifestyle and food intake adjusted to insulin administration, and there was no flexibility following each insulin injection. This proved difficult – especially as children should, ideally, be able to participate in as many activities as possible with their peer group – and, once again, supports the use of glucose- and meal-adjusted injection regimens or pumps.

Continuous SC insulin infusion

In very young children (<6 years of age), many centres use continuous SC insulin infusion as the treatment of choice, based on age specific characteristics.

It is important to remember in such young children:

- Increased insulin sensitivity
- Small doses are used, which have a shorter effect
- Limited space for injections
- Unpredictable food intake
- Increased intercurrent infections
- Short remission

Acceptance is good when insulin is started at diagnosis after initial stabilisation. Some centres wait several weeks before introducing this regimen, to ensure that parents can first use pens/syringes.

In pumps, only human or very short acting analogues are used. A basal rate (units/h) will be set and can be changed over 24 hours to get the best fit for the patient. In general, the basal rate is about 30% of the total insulin dose in children.

For every meal, an insulin bolus can be administered, and the parents/patient can be guided by the device (bolus wizard) regarding the best dose to administer. Different parameters are recorded in the device to help the diabetes team and family optimise the insulin dose advice provided each day by the bolus wizard:

- Insulin sensitivity factor (ISF)
  - ISF: 1 unit of insulin decreases glucose values with x mg/dL or mmol/L
- Insulin/glucose ratio (also known as insulin carbohydrate ratio; ICR)
  - 1 unit of insulin is needed for x g carbohydrate intake
- Glycaemic targets (individualised)

At home, the patient/parents enter the measured blood glucose value and the planned carbohydrate intake, which leads to the bolus dose recommendation, with the device only requesting validation (one extra manual confirmation) before the dose is administered. Regular discussion on these pre-set factors is needed to adjust them.

In these devices, which are suitable for all age groups, only short acting insulin can be used, which means there is no insulin depot of any significance. Although rare, technological defects or user problems and the subsequent absence of insulin administration can lead rapidly to complete insulin deficiency and DKA; this happens more quickly than with basal bolus treatment.

All pumps and glucose meters include a memory of a limited time period. The use of these in clinics or by mail exchange has become a key source of information during any clinic visit and helps to improve understanding of the treatment and its impact.

Nutrition composition and carbohydrate counting

- Daily dietary requirements comprise:
  - Carbohydrate 50–55%
    - Moderate sucrose intake (up to 10% total energy)
  - Fat 25–35%
    - <10% saturated fat + trans fatty acids
    - <10% polyunsaturated fat
    - >10% monounsaturated fat (up to 20% total energy)
  - Protein 15–20%
- Carbohydrate counting is an adjunct to improve clinical and metabolic outcomes.
- For each meal/snack, carbohydrate content is calculated.

- Individualised carbohydrate (in grams) to insulin (in units) ratios are determined:
  - usually during inpatient/outpatient visits.
- Ratio is used to calculate insulin dose needed for the food.
  - Ratio is usually between 5–25 grams/1 unit.
- The ratio is subject to regular adjustment – based on age and endogenous insulin secretion.
- Adapt nutrition education and lifestyle counselling to individual needs.

Blood glucose measurements

To ensure good metabolic control and thereby reduce diabetic complications:

- Measure glucose before each meal and before bedtime (as a minimum).
  - Using results, adjust insulin boluses.
  - Correct high values appropriately.
- If glucose is measured within 2 hours following a meal:
  - Interpret with caution.
  - The value cannot automatically be used to adjust the pre-meal insulin.
- Check blood glucose around 03:00 at least monthly.
  - Detects nocturnal hypoglycaemia
  - Ensures appropriate adjustment of evening long acting insulin dose

Continuous glucose monitoring systems

The advent of continuous interstitial glucose monitoring has dramatically improved our understanding of insulin treatment. Glucose trends and warning signals for impending hypoglycaemia have become valuable tools, providing more information with fewer finger pricks. The next-generation sensor-augmented pumps include mechanisms for stopping basal insulin administration when hypoglycaemia is detected.

Emergency presentations

Hypoglycaemia

- Treatment related complications include hypoglycaemia.
  - May lead to loss of consciousness and seizures
- Triggers can include:
  - Decreased food intake (or increased insulin : food ratio)
  - Increased physical activity
  - Time spent in sauna (or equivalent warm environment), which improves circulation

- Emergency management:
  - Administer 1 mg glucagon intramuscularly.
      Or:
  - Give or 10% glucose intravenously (2 mL/kg).

Previously, the risk of hypoglycaemia was thought to increase with improved metabolic outcome, but recent studies clearly show the opposite. Children with better controlled diabetes have no increased risk of hypoglycaemia. With new technology and more frequent glucose checks, this phenomenon is becoming less frequent.

When strenuous exercise has taken place in the afternoon or evening, reduction of the evening (long/intermediate acting) insulin can prevent nocturnal hypoglycaemia, as 6–12 hours after intensive activity blood glucose values may drop. Confirmation of the right dose adjustment should be done by nocturnal (03:00) and morning glucose checks.

Diabetic ketoacidosis

- T1DM can be complicated by DKA at onset (as can T2DM).
- Most DKA patients have considerable fluid depletion.
- Current guidelines advise to commence fluid replacement with normal saline (0.9% NaCl), starting with 10 mL/kg over 1 hour.
  - If needed, repeat this maximally twice over 1–2 hours.
- After some restoration of the peripheral circulation, start IV short acting insulin: 0.05–0.1 units/kg/h (max 0.1 units/kg/h).

As young children may be very sensitive to insulin, recent guidelines have recommended a lower starting dose. For adults, a solution using a syringe with 50 mL normal saline and 50 units of short acting insulin can be used (1 mL = 1 unit). However, for children, this may lead to the inadvertent administration of unsuitably high doses, e.g. while flushing a line (total dose per hour for a 10 kg child: 0.5–1 unit/h), and therefore the recommendation below (Box 1) provides an alternative option that reduces this risk. It is very important to document clearly which solution is used.

Box 1 Preparing intravenous insulin

In 50 mL syringe:
  50 mL of 0.9% sodium chloride
  with 0.5 × patient weight (in kg) of short acting insulin (units):
→ 5 mL/h = 0.05 units/kg/h

For preparing insulin, as with any intravenous medication, your local hospital guidelines (if available) should always be consulted.[5]

Rehydration can be limited to 50% of calculated losses over 48 hours, in combination with maintenance. Potassium replacement will be needed in most cases, except in renal failure. Consider adding potassium to the infusion fluid after the initial vascular repletion. Hyperkalaemia and hypokalaemia may both be life-threatening (risk of cardiac arrhythmias), so potassium levels require close monitoring. (Correction of the acidosis will be associated with a potassium shift from extracellular to intracellular.)

During DKA management:

- Closely monitor:
  - blood pH
  - serum electrolytes
  - glucose levels
  - clinical (particularly neurological) symptoms
  - beta-hydroxybutyrate levels (if available/recommended locally).
- Do not stop children drinking (if they want to).
  - Limit oral fluids to small quantities of water.
- Avoid excessively rapid rehydration.
- Avoid fast drops in blood glucose levels.
  - Decrease should not exceed 50–100 mg/dL/h (= 2.8–5.6 mmol/L/h).
- Bicarbonate administration is no longer advised, except for life-threatening hyperkalemia.[6]
- In uncomplicated DKA, start SC insulin treatment 24–48 hours after initial diagnosis.

Cerebral oedema

A major risk for morbidity and mortality with DKA is cerebral oedema (7% of DKA), the pathophysiology of which is an ongoing research topic (investigating vasogenic versus cellular causes).

- Clinical signs include neurological changes (altered consciousness, bradycardia, rapid drop in heart rate (> 20 beats/min in 1 hour, not explicable by fluid administration) incontinence, lethargy, vomiting and headache).
- Pre-existing risk factors (young age) as well as treatment related factors may be involved, such as excessively rapid rehydration, excessive insulin administration and bicarbonate administration. As mentioned above, bicarbonate administration is no longer recommended.
- If there is clinical evidence of cerebral oedema, mannitol (1 g/kg = 5 mL/kg 20% mannitol over 15–20 minutes) or hypertonic saline (3%) (5 mL/kg over 5–10 minutes) should be given, and ongoing care should be in a paediatric intensive care unit.

T2DM

Lifestyle and diet remain the cornerstones of T2DM management in all age groups. In children, depending on the initial metabolic disturbances, insulin may, however, be the first treatment. Once the diagnosis is confirmed and the patient is stabilised, the transition towards oral medication starts, taking 2–6 weeks. The same metabolic target, namely HbA1c $\leq$ 7.0% (53 mmol/mol), should be met in this population, combining metformin (see below) at increasing dosage (maximum 2000 mg) with lifestyle changes. If the goal is not met, or metformin is poorly tolerated, subsequent insulin treatment – either only long acting before bedtime or basal bolus – might be needed. Diabetic complications (cardiovascular, renal and retinal) can be observed early, necessitating an intensive approach from diagnosis onwards.

Metformin

- Oldest oral drug: biguanide oral hypoglycaemic
- Mechanisms of action:
  - Inhibits gluconeogenesis and glycogenolysis ($\rightarrow$ decreasing hepatic glucose production)
  - Improves muscle insulin sensitivity ($\rightarrow$ enhances peripheral glucose uptake)
  - Delays intestinal glucose absorption
- Currently metformin is the only oral drug approved in children with T2DM
- Beneficial effect on both metabolic control and chronic complications
- Does not stimulate insulin secretion: no risk of hypoglycaemia
- Gastrointestinal adverse events occur
- Main serious adverse event is lactic acidosis (0.06/1000 patient years)
  - Risk increased in patients with renal impairment, chronic liver disease, hypoxia and alcoholism

At the time of writing, many new glucose lowering drugs are under development or partially approved for adult patients. Many paediatric trials are in progress. The most advanced are the glucagon-like peptide 1 (GLP1) analogues and dipeptidyl peptidase-4 (DPP4) inhibitors. Newer drugs such as sodium/glucose cotransporter 2 (and 1) (SGLT 2-1) inhibitors, sympatholytic D2 dopamine analogues (bromocriptine) and G protein coupled receptor (GPR40) activators may also improve treatment outcomes.

Monogenic diabetes

Neonatal diabetes

- This is a separate form of diabetes.
- An underlying genetic mutation is frequently detected.

- Insulin is the treatment of choice (insulin pump where possible).
- Treatment may only be needed for a few months (e.g. in transient neonatal diabetes) – although diabetes may reappear later in life.

MODY

- This is uncommon.
- 1–4% of patients with diabetes.
- Genetic defects or mutations lead to abnormal pancreatic development, abnormal β cell function or β cell destruction.
- Enquire about family history.
- Genetic testing provides final diagnosis.
- Management options: no treatment (diet only: MODY 2), oral (sulfonylurea MODY 1 and 3) or insulin administration (MODY 5) may be necessary, depending on the mutation.

Cystic fibrosis and diabetes

- Diabetes is a frequent complication of cystic fibrosis (CF).
- Diabetes is caused by loss of pancreatic α and β cells, combined with variable periods of insulin resistance due to infections, corticosteroid use and liver disease.
- Changed gut motility and delayed gastric emptying also contribute.
- Cystic fibrosis is rarely associated with DKA.
- Progresses insidiously, leading towards insulin deficiency.
- Start annual glucose tolerance testing from age 10 in all CF patients.
  - Do not limit to 2 hours post glucose administration, as mid-test values may be more useful.
- The main treatment is insulin.
- High calorific, high salt and high fat dietary intake recommended.
- Carbohydrate counting is needed.

Conclusions

Diabetes mellitus is a chronic disease necessitating lifelong treatment. Different causes may need a different therapeutic approach, although T1DM is more common in childhood. The treatment target should be to achieve near normoglycaemia to ensure normal physical and psychological development and to prevent acute and chronic complications. Patient and family education is crucial to the success of diabetes management.

References

1   Patterson C *et al*. Incidence trends for childhood type 1 diabetes in Europe during 1989–2003 and predicted new cases 2005–20: a multicentre prospective registration study. *Lancet* 2009; 373: 2027–2033.

2   ISPAD Clinical Practice Consensus Guidelines 2018. *Pediatric Diabetes* 2018; 19 (Suppl. 27): 1–338. https://www.ispad.org/page/ISPADGuidelines2018

3   Danne *et al*. Insulin treatment in children and adolescents with diabetes. *Pediatric Diabetes* 2018; 19 (Suppl. 27): 115–135.

4   Neu A *et al*. Classifying insulin regimens – difficulties and proposal for comprehensive new definitions. *Pediatric Diabetes* 2015; 16: 402–406.

5   Appendix 2, How to make up special intravenous fluids. In: BSPED Recommended Guideline for the Management of Children and Young People under the age of 18 years with Diabetic Ketoacidosis 2015. www.bsped.org.uk/media/1557/dkaguidelinenov18.pdf

6   Wolfsdorf JL *et al*. Diabetic ketoacidosis and hyperglycemic hyperosmolar state. *Pediatric Diabetes* 2018; 19 (Suppl. 27): 155–177.

46

Adolescent medicine

H Fonseca and H Braga Tavares

Introduction

The UN uses the term 'adolescents' for people aged 10–19 years.[1] The developmental transformations during adolescence, associated with changes in body size and composition, have a great impact on both drug distribution and biotransformation during this period. Adolescents are a particularly vulnerable group in this domain, as they are more exposed to and influenced by many marketing campaigns and are at risk of misuse of both illicit and over-the-counter drugs. A better understanding of the physiological and psychosocial factors that define this unique period of life will enhance the safe and effective use of medications, as well as the development of new drugs. Adolescents have specific needs and should neither be viewed as small adults nor big children.

The learning objectives of this chapter are:

➤ to recognise the impact of adolescence specificities on adherence to pharmacological treatments
➤ to understand the transition to adult services and healthcare
➤ to gain insight into factors affecting adolescent participation in clinical trials
➤ to recognise key issues relating to contraception in adolescence.

Compliance/adherence to pharmacological treatment

Adherence is an essential component of any therapeutic intervention. The term 'adherence' is preferred over 'compliance', as it relates better to what adolescence is, involving a dynamic negotiation through promotion of autonomy and self-responsibility, leading to active and maintained choices and encouragement to choose self-management options. The need to exercise autonomy and the desire to fit in with peers may lead to insufficient adherence to medical treatment and can constitute a health-threatening problem in chronic illness.

During the second decade of life, adolescents may suffer not only from common chronic diseases acquired during childhood, but also from conditions that are acquired during adolescence, which may limit the full potential quality and quantity of their lives. Although puberty is complete within the 10- to 19-year time frame, attainment of brain maturation can take as long as three decades. This discordance between physical and mental development can make adolescents vulnerable to behaviours and choices that may have negative effects on their health. Among the barriers to medication adherence identified by chronically ill adolescents are: confusion about how to take the medicine or changes in regimen, number of pills per dose, the perception of taking medicine too many times a day, not understanding the purpose of the prescribed medicine, and not knowing who to ask about medication problems.[2]

Adherence to therapeutic regimens is crucial and has been considered as a significantly modifiable risk factor for optimising therapy.[3] As knowledge alone may not always drive behaviour, some strategies have been defined for improving adherence:

- Development of age appropriate communication
- Assurance of confidentiality
- Simplification of the regimen whenever feasible, using the optimal dosage form and schedule
- Use of compliance aids (alarms, app-based approaches, etc.)
- Provision of medication counselling, including behavioural techniques (goal setting, self-monitoring, skills training and positive reinforcements)
- Reinforcement of support from family and other caregivers

Transition to adult services/care

Strengthening adolescents' independence and self-management competencies, combined with early preparation and repeated discussions on transition, seem to be useful strategies to increase adolescents' readiness for transfer to adult care.[4] The survival of young people with chronic conditions has increased significantly during the last decades, with chronic conditions currently representing a global public health concern (around 10% of adolescents live with a chronic condition). Living with a chronic condition encompasses a set of behaviours that need to be added to daily routines; taking medication is one of them. A progressive transition from parental to self-management should happen throughout adolescence.

The promotion of self-efficacy and autonomy in healthcare seem crucial for an effective transition into adult services. At this time, there is a risk of dropping out from healthcare. It should be ensured that young people continue to engage with health services. Most adult providers have not been sufficiently trained to assess the developmental and psychosocial challenges faced by young adults with chronic conditions. Paediatricians play a crucial role here by intensifying transition efforts and initiating a transitional plan from a very early stage. A well-timed, well-planned and well-executed transition to adult orientated healthcare should be a standard part of providing care for all youth. Every adolescent, regardless of whether they have a special healthcare need, should have an individualised transition plan.[5]

Participation of adolescents in clinical trials

Participation of adolescents in clinical trials (CTs) is deemed necessary, because most medications currently used have never been studied in paediatric patients. Adolescents may have pharmacokinetic/pharmacodynamic specificities and a distinct adverse reaction profile. There are several international ethical recommendations regarding adolescent involvement in CTs (see chapter 27). Nevertheless, country specific legislation applies and ethics committees have a very important role in deciding on youth participation in CTs.

- Important CT definitions include:
  - Legal representative: parent(s) or legal representative(s), defined as those who are able to consent on behalf of the minor until he or she becomes legally competent.
  - Informed consent: written, dated and signed authorisation given by legal representative (or adolescent if legally competent) for participation in a CT. It should be taken freely after information on the goal, implications and risks has been provided in an age appropriate way.
  - Assent: the expression of a legally incompetent patient of his or her will to participate in a CT. It depends on the assessment of his or her maturity, developmental stage and intellectual capacities. It should be supplemented by informed consent of the legal representative. Age of assent is defined locally, but its assessment should be considered for all adolescents, even more when sensitive information is collected in the context of a CT.
- Mature minors (as defined by local legislation) may be capable of giving autonomous consent. In some countries, by the age of 16 years old adolescents are considered competent to decide on matters regarding their health and also on participation in CTs (unless proven otherwise).
- An adolescent, by emancipation or reaching adulthood, may become legally competent to make decisions and to give informed consent during his or her participation in a CT. This should, especially, be considered in long term trials, with a need for monitoring of the maturation progression and ability for assent.

- Independently of the adolescent competency status, all information obtained in the context of the young person's participation in a CT is confidential, and this should be explained (along with its limits) to the adolescent and legal representatives.
- In case of conflict of opinions (adolescent versus legal representative):
  - The investigator should listen and try to understand the different perspectives.
  - An adolescent's strong and definitive objection to be involved in a CT should be respected.
  - If, by not participating or by early drop-out from a CT, the life of the adolescent is threatened (therapeutic studies for life-threatening conditions), the best interest of the patient should be considered and the opinion of the investigator and parent(s)/legal guardian is considered sufficient to allow/maintain participation in the CT, even if it conflicts with that of the adolescent. Nevertheless, every effort should be made to reach a consensus.
- Similar to the treatment of other paediatric patients:
  - All efforts should be made to minimise pain, distress, hospital admissions, blood draws.
  - Use of a placebo should be cautious, never compromising the offer of an effective treatment, especially for serious or life-threatening conditions.

Contraception in adolescence

According to World Health Organization (WHO) recommendations on contraception:[6]

- Adolescence is a period of sexual maturation and exploratory behaviour, when most youths engage in sexual experiences.
- Contraception comprises the adoption of behaviours and/or medicines/devices used to prevent a pregnancy.
- Adolescent pregnancy and sexually transmitted infections (STIs) are significant public health issues.
- Every contact with adolescents should be seen as an opportunity for screening and counselling on sexual behaviour.
- Adolescents should take an active part in the choice of the best-suited contraceptive option.
- Irrespective of the contraceptive option, prevention of STIs should be discussed and ensured through correct and consistent condom use.

- As most adolescents are healthy, past medical and family history plus blood pressure and body mass index (BMI) assessment are the only requisites before deciding on the best contraceptive method (except for intrauterine devices (IUD), which require a gynaecological examination on insertion).
- Return to fertility is immediate for most of the contraceptive options once stopped. An exception is depot medroxyprogesterone acetate (DMPA), which has a median delay in return to fertility of 10 months from the date of the last injection. Male and female sterilisation are permanent methods and not an option for adolescents.

Contraceptive options

Natural methods

These are not generally recommended, because they are inherently unreliable in preventing pregnancy as well as offering no protection against STIs. They require a highly trained and motivated adolescent, with regular menstrual cycles and who agrees to have periods of abstinence.

Barrier methods

- Condom (male and female)
- Diaphragm
- Cervical cap

Hormonal methods

- Combined (progestogen + oestrogen)
  - Oral combined contraceptive pill
  - Transdermal patch (21 days on, 7 days off)
  - Vaginal ring (21 days on, 7 days off)
- Progestogen only (amenorrhoea or irregular/unpredictable menses more frequent)
  - Oral progestogen-only pill
  - Injectable (intramuscular) – DMPA (every 3 months)
  - Intramuscular – levonorgestrel implants (every 3 years)
  - Levonorgestrel-releasing intrauterine devices (every 5 years)

Other methods

- Copper-bearing IUD (every 10 years)
- Spermicides (foams, creams, gels, vaginal suppositories, vaginal film)
- Sponge
- Surgical – vasectomy and tubal ligation (definitive methods are not an option for adolescents)

Emergency contraception

- As soon as possible after unprotected intercourse
- Options:
  - Levonorgestrel pill
    - 1.5 mg single dose *or* two 0.75 mg pills 12 hours apart (if not available, two doses of ethinyloestradiol (100 µg) + levonorgestrel (0.50 mg) pills, 12 hours apart)
    - Ideally within 72 hours. Efficacy depends on administration timing: 24 h, 95%; 48 h, 85%; 72 h, 58%
  - Ulipristal acetate pill
    - 30 mg single dose
    - Less emesis
    - Efficacious until 120 hours after unprotected intercourse
  - Copper-bearing IUD – up to 5 days after unprotected intercourse, and if this method is foreseen thereafter
- In case of emesis within 3 hours of taking the pill, treatment should be repeated together with an anti-emetic.
- If no menstrual bleeding within 3 weeks of emergency contraception, refer for medical evaluation/pregnancy test.

Adolescent specificities in contraception

Ability to comply with the chosen contraceptive method and understanding of the consequences of non-compliance should be assessed and discussed with the adolescent. This may influence the final method choice.

Some contraceptive methods may represent a secondary benefit for adolescents.

- Condoms – prevention of STI (condom use should be advocated throughout the whole adolescence)
- Hormonal methods:
  - Control of blood loss, dysmenorrhoea
  - Oral combined contraceptive pill – menstrual cycle regularisation
  - Antiandrogenic progestins (included in many oral combined contraceptive pills) – control of acne and hirsutism

When used for long periods, DMPA may have a negative impact on bone mineral density. As such, its use in adolescence is recommended only for short periods (with exceptions made for patients with epilepsy, for whom the benefits of long term use may overcome the risks).

Specific conditions affecting contraception

- Disabilities (psychomotor delay and/or cognitively impaired adolescents) – a long term method not dependent on the adolescent's compliance is preferred
- Progestogen-only methods or an IUD should be chosen when methods containing oestrogen are either contraindicated or not recommended:
  - Thromboembolic events or thrombophilia
  - Migraine with aura
  - Hypertension
  - Type 1 or 2 diabetes mellitus if associated with kidney or eye disease
  - Cardiovascular disease (stroke, ischaemic heart disease)
- Use of hormonal contraception is not recommended, and an IUD should be considered in:
  - systemic lupus erythematosus with positive antiphospholipid antibodies
  - hepatic tumour, acute viral hepatitis or cirrhosis
  - adolescents taking medications known to be hepatic enzyme inducers.
- Some medications (mainly some antiepileptics, antiretrovirals and antibiotics) may impair or increase hormonal contraceptive hepatic metabolism. Their use should be checked, and the best contraceptive option should be discussed on a case by case basis.

Conclusions

A well-timed, well-planned and well-executed transition to adult orientated healthcare should be a standard part of care provision for all young people. Improved understanding of the physiological and psychosocial factors that characterise adolescence promotes the effective use of medications in this age group. Adherence to therapeutic regimens is crucial and is a significantly modifiable risk factor for optimising therapy.

Most available contraceptive options may be readily used by adolescents, but when selecting the method, consider: adolescent's choice, availability, specific medical conditions and possible secondary benefits. The need for concomitant use of condoms for STI prevention should always be emphasised.

The age cut-off for legal competence in taking health-related decisions varies across countries, however adolescents should always be asked for their assent for participating in a CT irrespective of their competence. Those legally competent or assessed as mature should be asked for informed consent.

References

1   UN. *Report of the Expert Group Meeting on Adolescents, Youth and Development.* New York: UN-DESA, 2011. www.un.org/esa/population/meetings/egm-adolescents/ EGM%20on%20Adolescents_Youth%20and%20Development_Report.pdf
2   Hanhoj S, Boisen KA. Self-reported barriers to medication adherence among chronically ill adolescents: A systematic review. *J Adolesc Health* 2014; 54(2): 121–138.
3   Jones BL, Kelly KJ. The adolescent with asthma: fostering adherence to optimize therapy. *Clin Pharmacol Ther* 2008; 84(6): 749–753.
4   Staa AL *et al.* Readiness to transfer to adult care of adolescents with chronic conditions: exploration of associated factors. *J Adolesc Health* 2011; 48(3): 295–302.
5   American Academy of Pediatrics *et al.* Supporting the health care transition from adolescence to adulthood in the medical home. *Pediatrics* 2011; 128(1); 182–200.
6   WHO. *Sexual and Reproductive Health - Medical eligibility for contraceptive use.* Geneva: WHO, 2015. Available at: https://apps.who.int/iris/bitstream/handle/10665/ 181468/9789241549158_eng.pdf?sequence=1 [last accessed February 2019].

47

Nephrology

N Webb, A Lunn and A Wignell

Introduction

Kidney disease may affect drug handling through multiple mechanisms, including impaired kidney function, hypoalbuminaemia, alteration in total body water and altered acid–base status.[1] In children, prescribing in renal disease can be particularly challenging because of the difficulties in accurately monitoring renal dysfunction, especially in neonates, and the limited pharmacokinetic and pharmacodynamic data available in these special populations to guide optimal dosing.

The learning objectives of this chapter are:

- ➤ to understand the physiological and pharmacological principles underlying changes in drug pharmacokinetics and pharmacodynamics in renal dysfunction
- ➤ to recognise the consequent need to review drug dosing in acute kidney injury (AKI) and chronic kidney disease (CKD), particularly with respect to nephrotoxic agents
- ➤ to recognise common nephrotoxic medications used in paediatrics
- ➤ to understand the importance of prompt recognition and management of AKI secondary to nephrotoxic medications.

Background

Kidney function may be reduced because of either AKI or CKD.

AKI describes an acute reduction in kidney function resulting in a failure to maintain fluid, electrolyte and acid–base homoeostasis. The rate of deterioration in kidney function may be rapid. Despite being in routine use, plasma creatinine is a poor measure of kidney function, particularly in early AKI; plasma creatinine levels only rise above baseline once 25–50% of kidney function has been lost. AKI is usually associated with a degree of recovery of renal function. Prompt recognition and treatment will reduce the severity of AKI and increase the likelihood of full renal recovery. Long term follow-up is recommended, however, as increasing evidence indicates that an episode of AKI is a risk for future CKD.[2]

CKD describes irreversible reduction in kidney function and occurs as a result of multiple causes. The commonest causes of CKD in children and neonates are congenital abnormalities of the kidney and urinary tract.[3] CKD is a continuum, and a formal staging system is used (see Table 1).[4]

It is important to remember that glomerular filtration rate (GFR) matures over the first 2 years of life (mean GFR: at birth, $20.3\,\text{mL/min/1.73 m}^2$; 6 months, $77\,\text{mL/min/1.73 m}^2$; 12 months, $115\,\text{mL/min/1.73 m}^2$; 2 years, $127\,\text{mL/min/1.73 m}^2$). Neonates, particularly those born prematurely, therefore have immature renal function. An estimate of GFR (eGFR) can be made using the modified Schwartz formula:

$$\text{eGFR}\ (\text{mL/min/1.73 m}^2) = \text{height (cm)} \times k/\text{plasma creatinine}\,(\mu\text{mol/L})$$

The most recently validated value for k is 36.2;[5] however, the figure used depends upon local factors, including the technique used for measuring plasma creatinine. Many centres use 40. For neonates, a commonly used k value is 30.

Table 1 Definitions of CKD stages 1–5		
Stage 1 CKD	GFR > 90 mL/min/1.73 m²	Normal kidney function, but urine findings or structural abnormality or genetic trait point to kidney disease
Stage 2 CKD	GFR 60–89 mL/min/1.73 m²	Mildly reduced kidney function and other factors (above) point to kidney disease
Stage 3 CKD **Often divided into** **Stage 3a and 3b**	GFR 30–59 mL/min/1.73 m² 3a: GFR 45–59 mL/min/1.73 m² 3b: GFR 30–44 mL/min/1.73 m²	Moderately reduced kidney function
Stage 4 CKD	GFR 15–29 mL/min/1.73 m²	Severely reduced kidney function
Stage 5 CKD	GFR <15 mL/min/1.73 m²	End stage renal failure; generally requires dialysis and kidney transplantation

Prescribing considerations in impaired kidney function

General principles: reducing drug dosing in impaired kidney function

- Problems can arise when medicines are prescribed to children with impaired kidney function. Reduced excretion of a renally cleared drug may result in accumulation and toxicity with more side-effects. Sensitivity to some drugs is increased, even if elimination is unimpaired.[1]
- Drugs that are renally excreted may require dose alteration in the presence of reduced kidney function. In general, dose reduction is not necessary for drugs metabolised by the liver, providing there are no concomitant alterations in hepatic function or active metabolites that are renally excreted (e.g. the morphine glucuronides, which accumulate to prolong analgesia and may cause respiratory depression).
- Changes in the clearance of renally excreted drugs become more significant in the more advanced stages of CKD and in severe AKI. Problems are most likely to occur with drugs that are both renally excreted and nephrotoxic, e.g. the aminoglycosides.
- Renal function may be rapidly changing, particularly in AKI. Wherever possible (and particularly with the aminoglycosides), therapeutic drug monitoring should be performed.
- Great care needs to be taken when prescribing in renal failure. The *British National Formulary for Children* (BNFC)[6] provides detailed information about dose modification in various degrees of CKD; however, a number of drugs in regular use are not listed. If in doubt, always seek expert advice from a paediatric nephrologist or paediatric pharmacist with renal expertise. Locally, drug monographs have been developed to provide additional information regarding particularly high risk drugs such as gentamicin and vancomycin.[7]

General principles: other changes occur with drug handling in renal impairment and other renal disease

- In advanced renal impairment, there is reduced motility in the gastrointestinal tract, with nausea and vomiting. This may affect **drug bioavailability** (the fraction of the administered dose that reaches the systemic circulation).
- Both AKI and CKD may result in volume overload with peripheral oedema and ascites, with a resultant effect on the **volume of distribution**. This particularly affects agents such as the aminoglycosides that preferentially distribute into body water.

- Renal disease may be associated with hypoalbuminaemia, either as a result of albuminuria in glomerular disease or of malnutrition in CKD. Drugs that are heavily **protein bound**, e.g. phenytoin, may have high levels of free drug as a result of this, despite apparently normal blood levels. Protein binding may also be affected by acid–base balance and inflammation. Uraemia induces changes in albumin structure, so acidic drugs bind less avidly.[1]
- Patients with impaired renal function, particularly those with CKD, are likely to be taking multiple medications. This increases the risk of **drug interactions** occurring. **Drug absorption** may be limited by binding in the gut lumen to other non-absorbable drugs (e.g. phosphate binders such as calcium carbonate or sevelamer).
- **Non-adherence** with prescribed therapy is common in the CKD population, as is the case in many childhood chronic disorders. It is always important to consider this diagnosis in the child or young adult with suboptimal drug levels or where there appears to be poor treatment efficacy.
- Where patients are receiving renal replacement therapy (dialysis or haemofiltration) this may affect **drug clearance**. This is dependent upon the molecular weight of the drug and its degree of protein binding. Drugs that have a large volume of distribution (these tend to be lipid soluble) are not confined to the circulation; these are generally less well cleared by haemodialysis. Peritoneal dialysis is much less efficient at drug clearance than haemodialysis, unless the drug has a low volume of distribution and low protein binding.

AKI and nephrotoxic medication

General principles: presentation of medication induced nephrotoxicity

- There are many prescribed medications that are associated with nephrotoxicity, including antibiotics (particularly aminoglycosides), antifungal, antiviral and non-steroidal anti-inflammatory medications, and cancer treatments (see Table 2).
- Some medications that are used in the management of CKD can cause AKI, particularly in the setting of intravascular depletion, e.g. angiotensin converting enzyme (ACE) inhibitors and calcineurin inhibitors.
- Many children who are admitted to hospital are prescribed nephrotoxic medication.
- There are multiple mechanisms by which medication can cause renal damage, and hence multiple ways in which it can present. These include Fanconi's syndrome, nephrotic syndrome, thrombotic microangiopathy and glomerulonephritis. The most common presentations in childhood, however, are AKI through reduction in renal blood flow (e.g. non-steroidal anti-inflammatory drugs; NSAIDs), acute tubular necrosis (e.g. aminoglycosides) or acute interstitial nephritis (e.g. penicillins).

Table 2 Some common nephrotoxic medications	
Class of medication	**Examples**
NSAIDS	Ibuprofen
	Diclofenac
Calcineurin inhibitors	Tacrolimus
	Ciclosporin
Antibiotics	Gentamicin
	Vancomycin
Antifungals	Amphotericin B
Antivirals	Valaciclovir
	Valganciclovir
	Aciclovir
	Ganciclovir
ACE inhibitors	Captopril
	Lisinopril
	Enalapril
Chemotherapy	Cisplatin
	Ifosfamide
Intravenous contrast agents	Iodixanol
	Iohexol
	Iopamidol
	Ioversol

- Nephrotoxicity can be prevented by avoiding concurrent use of multiple nephrotoxic agents and, where possible, monitoring drug levels. Ensuring adequate hydration is also important, particularly in the case of medication that causes AKI through reduction in renal blood flow.
- If identified early enough, AKI will improve through simple supportive care and removal of the nephrotoxic medication.

General principles: early identification of AKI secondary to nephrotoxic medication

- The incidence of AKI secondary to nephrotoxic medication is rising, although this may in part reflect increased awareness.
- In many children, multiple nephrotoxic medications are prescribed.
- The risk of developing AKI increases with the number of nephrotoxic agents that a child is receiving.
- Urine output and plasma creatinine should be monitored in patients who are on multiple nephrotoxic drugs or who receive aminoglycosides for more than 3 days. However, as plasma creatinine is an insensitive method of detecting AKI in children, an estimated GFR using the Schwartz formula should also be calculated.
- A paediatric modification of the RIFLE (risk, injury, failure, loss, end stage) criteria for AKI – pRIFLE (see Table 3) – can be used to identify children with AKI.
- The severity of AKI increases down the scale, i.e. failure is worse than injury, etc.
- The mortality risk increases with a more severe pRIFLE score.
- If AKI is identified in patients receiving nephrotoxic medication, then the following steps should be undertaken.[9]
    1. Doses of all medications should be adjusted according to the level of renal function (eGFR).
    2. Where possible, nephrotoxic medication should be stopped and alternative medication used.
    3. If the medication is known to cause injury through reduced renal blood flow, then adequate hydration should be ensured.
    4. Strict monitoring of fluid intake, urine output, blood pressure and plasma creatinine should take place.

Table 3 pRIFLE criteria[8]		
Risk	eGFR decrease by 25%	< 0.5 mL/kg/h for 8 hours
Injury	eGFR decrease by 50%	< 0.5 mL/kg/h for 16 hours
Failure	eGFR decrease by 75% or eGFR less than 35 mL/min/1.73m^2	< 0.3 mL/kg/h for 24 hours or anuric for 12 hours
Loss	Persistent failure > 4 weeks	
End stage	Persistent failure > 3 months	

From Akcan-Arikan et al.[8]

5 Early discussion should be had with a paediatrician experienced in the management of children with renal disease if there is no improvement once the medication has been discontinued or if the RIFLE criterion 'injury' or more severe is met.

General principles: reducing drug dosing in AKI

• The principles of dose reduction apply equally to AKI and CKD. Regardless of the aetiology of AKI, reduced excretion of a renally cleared drug may result in accumulation and toxicity.

• If the drug itself is nephrotoxic, this can exacerbate the AKI and delay recovery. When possible, the drug levels of any nephrotoxic drugs should be monitored, particularly aminoglycosides.

• In AKI, consideration should be given to monitoring aminoglycoside levels earlier than usual practice and delaying further dosing until normal trough levels have been achieved.

• AKI can also resolve quickly, and this can then result in normal clearance of medication that has been dose reduced because of the AKI.

• A regular review of medication and renal function is important in this situation to prevent toxicity, but also to prevent inadequate treatment of the underlying medical condition.

If in doubt, always seek expert advice from a paediatric nephrologist or paediatric pharmacist with renal expertise.

Conclusions

In summary, there are a number of key practical points that should always be considered when prescribing for children with renal impairment. It is important to avoid known nephrotoxins wherever possible, especially in combination. Given that potassium excretion is usually reduced in renal impairment, exercise extreme caution in using drugs that raise serum potassium. The calculated eGFR should be used to adjust doses according to BNFC recommendations. As many antibiotics are renally excreted, renal dose adjustments are frequently necessary. The BNFC usually reflects manufacturers' recommendations and consequently can be relatively conservative; in severe sepsis, higher doses may be justified, so seek specialist advice in order to avoid undertreatment. For medications that routinely have therapeutic drug monitoring, use this to guide dosing. This is especially important for the aminoglycoside and glycopeptide antibiotics, where the most appropriate course of action is often to give a single dose but no further doses until the trough level is back in range. Make use of other resources, such as *The Renal Drug Handbook*,[10] which are available to supplement BNFC guidance. As a general rule, when initiating long term medication, start with low doses and titrate slowly.

References

1   Geary D, Schaefer F (eds). *Comprehensive Paediatric Nephrology*, 1st edn. Philadelphia: Elsevier Inc., 2008

2   Greenberg *et al*. Long-term risk of chronic kidney disease and mortality in children after acute kidney injury: a systematic review. *BMC Nephrol* 2014; 15: 184.

3   Hamilton *et al*. UK Renal Registry 18th Annual Report: Chapter 4 Demography of Patients Receiving Renal Replacement Therapy in Paediatric Centres in the UK in 2014. *Nephron* 2016; 132 Suppl 1: 99–110.

4   The Renal Association. *CKD stages*. www.renal.org/information-resources/the-uk-eckd-guide/ckd-stages#sthash.F4TTZFMM.dpbs

5   Schwartz GJ *et al*. New equations to estimate GFR in children with CKD. *J Am Soc Nephrol* 2009; 20: 629–637.

6   Paediatric Formulary Committee. BNF for Children (online). London: BMJ Group, Pharmaceutical Press and RCPCH Publications.

7   EMEESY Children's Renal Network. Medicines news. www.emeesykidney.nhs.uk/professional-area/pharmacy-information

8   Akcan-Arikan A *et al*. Modified RIFLE criteria in critically ill children with acute kidney injury. *Kidney Int* 2007; 71(10): 1028–1035.

9   UK Renal Registry. Think Kidneys – Guidance for clinicians managing children at risk of, or with, acute kidney injury. www.thinkkidneys.nhs.uk/aki/guidance-clinicians-managing-children-risk-acute-kidney-injury

10 Ashley C, Currie A (eds). *The Renal Drug Handbook*, 3rd edn. Oxford: Radcliffe Publishing, 2009.

48

Prescribing blood and blood components

L Gibb and N Ghara

Introduction

Blood components, by custom and practice, are referred to as being prescribed. The term 'prescription' in this context is the written authorisation for a blood component transfusion. The responsibility for prescribing blood and blood components rests, in most organisations, with the medical staff, and is an important role for all paediatricians. There are some senior nurses who are able to make the clinical decision and give the written authorisation for a blood transfusion in their specialist clinical area. Blood and blood components should be prescribed in accordance with an individual hospital's local clinical guidelines, which should also reflect national guidelines.[1]

The learning objectives of this chapter are:

➤ to understand the key components of a safe prescription for blood transfusion
➤ to understand how to identify suitable volumes and infusion rates
➤ to understand the importance of accurate documentation
➤ to know how to discuss consent for or refusal of blood components
➤ to be able to determine when there are special requirements for blood components.

Background

For the purposes of this chapter, blood components are formally defined as 'any therapeutic substance derived from human blood, including whole blood, labile blood components and plasma-derived medicinal products'.[2] This definition encompasses (but is not limited to) the following:

- Blood components prepared in blood transfusion centres:
  - Packed red blood cells
  - Platelets

- Fresh frozen plasma (FFP)
- Cryoprecipitate
- Granulocytes
- Derivatives of human plasma that are manufactured in plasma fractionation centres (and prepared from pooled plasma donations):
  - Human normal immunoglobulin
  - Anti-D immunoglobulin
  - Anti-tetanus immunoglobulin
  - Blood coagulation factors (factor VIII, prothrombin complex concentrate)
  - Human albumin solution
- Commercially produced pooled plasma
  - Solvent/detergent treated plasma

The following abbreviations are used throughout this chapter:

Rh/RhD: an antigen found on the surface of red blood cells. Red blood cells with the antigen are said to be Rh positive (Rh+). Those without the surface antigen are said to be Rh negative (Rh−).

ABO: a system for classifying human blood on the basis of antigenic components of red blood cells and their corresponding antibodies. The ABO blood group is identified by the presence or absence of two different antigens, A and B, on the surface of the red blood cell. The four blood types in this grouping, A, B, AB, and O, are determined by and named for these antigens.

CMV: cytomegalovirus, a common virus that belongs to the herpes family of viruses. It is spread through bodily fluids, such as saliva and urine, and can be passed on through a blood transfusion. CMV can cause a potentially life-threatening infection in patients who cannot form an effective immune response. CMV disease is the commonest infection problem in the post transplant period.

Documentation

Prescribing blood components for administration

Blood components, including albumin and immunoglobulins, for administration on the ward must not be administered unless prescribed on the child's blood transfusion prescription chart or using an agreed alternative, e.g. electronic prescribing. Blood components administered in a theatre setting must be annotated on the anaesthetic record or agreed alternative, e.g. an electronic anaesthetic record.

The blood transfusion prescription chart must contain:[3]

- Child's full details – Family name, first name, hospital number, date of birth, body weight, allergies (there should be a policy in place to identify patients in an emergency)

- Consultant and ward
- Details of special requirements and consent
- Type of blood component to be administered
- Date and time infusion required
- Volume to be infused (see Table 1):
  - It is essential that all blood components are ordered and prescribed in millilitres (mL) if the volume prescribed comes to less than 200 mL.
  - Volumes greater than 200 mL can be rounded to the nearest unit.
  - Volume ordered and prescribed should not exceed that normally ordered for an adult in a similar situation.
- A suitable infusion rate in mL/hour (see Table 1)
- An infusion time of 4 hours or fewer to reduce risk of infection
- Any special instructions to enable the clinical area to plan adequately
- Concomitant drug, e.g. hydrocortisone/chlorphenamine/furosemide, to prevent adverse reactions in children who have reacted previously
- Printed name and signature of prescriber

Accurate documentation of the transfusion episode should be entered into the patient's medical record, and the child and family should be informed. The indication for the transfusion, type of component used, the quantity and the date and time should also be clearly recorded.

Platelets for children from 1 year of age must be ABO and RhD identical or compatible with the recipient and obtained by apheresis from a single donor where possible (recipients born on or after 01/01/96 should be provided with apheresis platelets when possible, as a variant Creutzfeldt–Jakob disease

Table 1 Volume and rate to be infused		
Component	**Volume to be infused**	**Rate**
Red cells	3–4 mL/kg will raise haemoglobin by 10 g/L	5 mL/kg/h (max 150 mL/h)
Platelets	< 15 kg: 10–20 mL/kg (max 1 apheresis unit) >15 kg: 1 apheresis unit	10–20 mL/kg/h
Non UK MB fresh frozen plasma (FFP)/solvent detergent FFP	Usually 12–15 mL /kg; up to a maximum of 20 mL/kg	10–20 mL/kg/h
Non UK MB cryoprecipitate	5–10 mL/kg (max 2 'adult' pools can be used for larger children)	10–20 mL/kg/h
Granulocytes	10–20 mL/kg (max 2 pools)	10–20 mL/kg/h
Neonatal red cell exchange	Approximately 160 mL/kg (double volume exchange)	Dependent on the stability of the child

(vCJD) risk reduction measure). Human leucocyte antigen (HLA) matched platelets and platelets in additive solution are specialist components and may require notice to the local blood service to provide them.

FFP is available either from the blood service (single donor, methylene blue treated) or is commercially available (pooled, solvent detergent treated). Plasma for children born on or after 01/01/96 is supplied from outside the UK due to the risk of vCJD.

Adjusted paediatric transfusion volume calculation

As highlighted by the 2013 Serious Hazards of Transfusion (SHOT) report, the change in reporting of Hb units from g/dL to g/L needs to be taken into account when calculating and prescribing paediatric red cell transfusion volumes, in order to avoid significant over- or under-transfusion.[4] A common formula for calculating the volume is:

$$\text{volume to transfuse (mL)} = (\text{desired Hb (g/L)} - \text{actual Hb (g/L)}) \times \text{weight (kg)} \times \text{factor}^*/10$$

*It is reasonable to use a factor of 4 (practice varies between 3 and 5), but this should be assessed on an individual patient basis.

Infusion rate and volume

It is important to prescribe the exact rate in mL/hour (see Table 1) as well as the volume to be given and the time over which the transfusion should be administered. All blood components must be transfused within 4 hours of removal from storage. Cryoprecipitate must be transfused within 4 hours of thawing.

Transfusion rates are for guidance only. They are based on current practice and will depend on the exact volume given and the clinical status of the child, and local recommendations.[5]

Patient consent

The Advisory Committee on the Safety of Blood, Tissues and Organs (SaBTO) has issued guidance for clinical staff on consent for blood transfusion.[6] It states that valid consent should be obtained prior to any planned transfusion and documented in the patient's medical record. Consent should be obtained by those 'with parental responsibility' or the patient if he or she has 'sufficient understanding and intelligence to enable him or her to understand fully what is proposed'.

Refusal of consent must be documented and legal advice and guidance obtained to ensure correct management of children for whom blood and blood components are refused.

Special requirements

Patients with certain clinical conditions will require special components. It is imperative that the reason for transfusion and the diagnosis of the patient's condition is stated on all request forms. The blood transfusion laboratory must be informed of new special requirements or any changes to them. Special requirements must also be flagged in the patient's medical record.

The blood transfusion laboratory relies on the information provided by the medical team, and lack of information, or incorrect information, regarding special requirements has the potential for errors, especially for new and shared care patients.

If components are not available to meet the special requirements of the patient, then in the event of an emergency, patients must be supported with standard components.

Irradiated blood components

Engraftment of viable lymphocytes transfused with blood components can cause fatal transfusion associated graft versus host disease (TA-GvHD) in patients who are immunocompromised. Irradiation at 25 gray (Gy) inactivates any residual donor lymphocytes, which may be present in very small numbers even after leucocyte depletion.

All patients with one of the conditions listed below are at risk of TA-GvHD and therefore must have irradiated blood components.[7]

Indications for irradiated blood components

- Allogeneic bone marrow or peripheral stem cell recipients: from the start of conditioning. This should be continued while the patient continues to receive graft versus host disease (GvHD) prophylaxis, i.e. usually for 6 months post transplant or until lymphocytes are $> 1 \times 10^9$/L
- Allogeneic blood transfused to bone marrow donors and peripheral blood stem cell donors: 7 days prior to or during the harvest
- Patients undergoing bone marrow or peripheral blood stem cell harvesting for future autologous reinfusion: during and for 7 days before the bone marrow/stem cell harvest
- All patients undergoing autologous bone marrow transplant or peripheral blood stem cell transplant from initiation of conditioning chemotherapy/radiotherapy until 3 months post transplant (6 months if total body irradiation was used in conditioning)

- Hodgkin's lymphoma
- Patients treated with purine analogue drugs (e.g. fludarabine) or purine antagonists (e.g. clofarabine), alemtuzumab (anti-CD52) therapy
- Aplastic anaemia patients receiving immunosuppressive therapy with anti-thymocyte globulin and/or alemtuzumab
- All donations from first or second degree relatives
- All HLA-selected components
- All granulocyte components
- All blood for intrauterine transfusion (IUT) and for neonatal exchange transfusion (ET) if there has been a previous IUT, until 6 months after the expected delivery date (40 weeks gestation), or if the donation has come from a first or second degree relative
- For other neonatal ET cases, irradiation is recommended provided this does not unduly delay transfusion
- All severe T lymphocyte immunodeficiency syndromes (once the suspicion of this diagnosis is raised, irradiated components should be given while further tests are being undertaken to rule out the possibility)

There is *no* indication for routine irradiation of cellular blood components in the following infants or children:

- Those who are suffering from a common viral infection
- Those who are HIV antibody positive or who have AIDS
- Patients with acute leukaemia, except for HLA-selected platelets or donations from first or second degree relatives
- Those with solid tumours, autoimmune diseases or after solid organ transplantation (unless alemtuzumab (anti-CD52) has been used in the conditioning regimen)
- Premature or term infants, unless either there has been a previous IUT or the donation has come from a first or second degree relative
- Infants undergoing cardiac surgery, unless clinical or laboratory features suggest a coexisting T lymphocyte immunodeficiency syndrome
- Patients with asplenia without T lymphocyte immunodeficiency syndrome

Cryopreserved red cells after deglycerolisation, fresh frozen plasma, cryoprecipitate and fractionated plasma components are never irradiated.

CMV negative blood components

Cytomegalovirus (CMV) is an important cause of mortality and morbidity in certain groups of patients, including premature infants. However, the risk of transmission has been greatly reduced by the provision of leucodepleted and/or CMV seronegative blood components (i.e. components that have been screened and found negative for CMV antibody). Only very specific groups of patients need to receive CMV seronegative blood components. All fetal, neonatal and infant red cells and platelets are routinely provided as CMV negative, as are those provided for elective transfusions during pregnancy, regardless of the maternal CMV serostatus due to potentially serious outcomes in the very select population cohorts, because of the extremely small but distinct possibility of CMV transmission via plasma in leucodepleted components. CMV seronegative red cell and platelet components should be provided for intrauterine transfusions and for neonates (i.e. up to 28 days post expected date of delivery),[8] but it is important to check local guidelines, as some hospitals may not have fully adopted the SaBTO recommendations. This includes some transplant centres.

Granulocyte components should continue to be provided as CMV seronegative for CMV seronegative patients. Granulocyte components cannot be leucodepleted.

In the SaBTO review, no relevant literature was found that supported the use of CMV seronegative blood for immunodeficient patients, including HIV antibody positive and organ transplant patients. These patients should receive leucodepleted blood.

Hepatitis E negative blood components

The hepatitis E virus (HEV) is found throughout the world in both humans and animals, especially pigs. The most common route of infection in the UK is from eating raw or undercooked meat (particularly pork products) and shellfish; however, HEV can be transmitted via blood transfusion and solid organ transplantation.

While the risk of HEV to the general population is negligible, SaBTO has also now recommended that certain patient groups who are immunocompromised/immunosuppressed should receive HEV negative blood components.[9] Unlike screening for cytomegalovirus (CMV), this recommendation is being applied to both cellular components (i.e. red cells, platelets and granulocytes) and plasma components (fresh frozen plasma and cryoprecipitate).

Indications for HEV negative components.

- Solid organ transplant (SOT) recipients: HEV screened blood components should be given to all SOT recipients taking immunosuppressive medication.
- Potential SOT recipients: from 3 months prior to date of elective SOT, potential recipients should only receive HEV screened blood components.
- Any patient who is receiving immunosuppressive therapy before SOT should receive HEV screened blood components.

- Extracorporeal procedures: HEV screened blood components should be used for extracorporeal circulatory support for patients undergoing SOT and for SOT patients receiving immunosuppressive medication.
- Allogeneic haematopoietic stem cell transplantation (HSCT): HEV screened blood components should be given to potential allogeneic HSCT recipients from 3 months prior to the date of planned HSCT until 6 months following allogeneic HSCT, or for as long as the patient is immunosuppressed. For patients with high transfusion burden due to diseases with a significant likelihood of proceeding to allogeneic HSCT over a period of a few months (such as acute leukaemia or aplastic anaemia), this should be from the time of diagnosis.

At present, there is no convincing evidence to support using HEV screened blood components for all recipients of autologous HSCT.

Neonatal red cells, neonatal platelets and methylene blue treated FFP and cryoprecipitate are routinely provided as HEV negative. Red cells and platelets for IUT and neonatal exchange units and large volume red cells are also provided as HEV negative. Granulocytes will be HEV screened and confirmed as negative prior to distribution.

Haemoglobinopathies

Children with haemoglobinopathies, such as sickle cell disease and thalassaemia, may require regular lifelong transfusions. Some of these children may, on occasion, also need exchange transfusion. Blood should be HbS negative and match the Rh phenotype of the patient (ideally extended phenotyping should take place prior to the first transfusion). Blood should also be fresh, i.e. < 14 days old for a top up transfusion and < 7 days old for exchange transfusion.

Necrotising enterocolitis (NEC)

Blood components for children with NEC may include:

- red cells in SAGM solution (saline, adenine, glucose, mannitol)
- platelets in additive solution.

Blood components for exchange transfusion

Red cell exchange

The complications of sickle cell disease constitute the commonest group of disorders for which red cell exchange transfusion is indicated. Other indications include severe malaria, haemolytic disease of the fetus and newborn (HDFN) and prevention of RhD immunisation after incompatible red cell transfusion.

Plasma exchange

Plasma exchange may be indicated for ABO mismatched heart and renal transplant, acute vasculitis, Guillain–Barré syndrome, multi-organ failure, systemic lupus erythematosus, haemolytic uraemic syndrome and thrombotic thrombocytopenic purpura.

Management of exchange transfusion

Exchange transfusion requires planning to ensure that appropriate and sufficient numbers of components are available.

It is also important that the clinical area has sufficient numbers of appropriately trained staff available, as there are a number of potential complications associated with exchange transfusion. These include hypothermia, oxygen desaturation, hyperkalaemia, hypocalcaemia, metabolic acidosis, arrhythmia, thrombocytopenia, infections and line complications.

Conclusions

Blood components are a precious resource and their use should be rational. This chapter provides an introduction to recent guidelines on blood component prescribing for children. The information is not intended to be comprehensive, and the most up-to-date guidelines should always be consulted. Administration of blood and its components is both a life-saving and potentially life-threatening procedure. It is imperative that all medical staff should be confident and competent in prescribing blood components.

References

1 Harris AM *et al. Administration of Blood Components*. British Committee for Standards in Haematology (BCSH), UK, 2009.
2 The World Health Assembly Resolution on availability, safety and quality of blood products (WHA 63.12), Adopted May 2010. http://apps.who.int/medicinedocs/documents/s19998en/s19998en.pdf
3 New HV *et al. Transfusion for Fetuses, Neonates and Older Children'?* British Committee for Standards in Haematology (BCSH), UK. 2016.
4 Bolton-Maggs PHB (ed.) *et al.* on behalf of the Serious Hazards of Transfusion (SHOT) Steering Group. The 2013 Annual SHOT Report, 2014. www.shotuk.org/shot-reports/report-summary-supplement-2013
5 Joint UKBTS Joint Professional Advisory Committee (JPAC). Effective transfusion in paediatric practice. www.transfusionguidelines.org.uk/transfusion-handbook/10-effective-transfusion-in-paediatric-practice
6 Advisory Committee on the Safety of Blood, Tissues and Organs (SaBTO). *Patient Consent for Blood Transfusion*, 2011. www.gov.uk/government/publications/patient-consent-for-blood-transfusion
7 Treleaven J *et al. Guidelines on the use of Irradiated Blood Components*. British Committee for Standards in Haematology (BCSH), UK, 2010.

8   Advisory Committee on the Safety of Blood, Tissues and Organs (SaBTO). Provision of cytomegalovirus tested blood components position statement, 2012 www.gov.uk/government/news/provision-of-cytomegalovirus-tested-blood-components-position-statement-published
9   SaBTO/BSBMT Recommendations on the use of HEV-screened blood components. 2016. http://hospital.blood.co.uk/media/28241/hev-sabto-recommendations-march-2016.pdf

Further recommended reading

Bolton-Maggs PHB (ed.) *et al.* on behalf of the Serious Hazards of Transfusion (SHOT) Steering Group. The 2016 Annual SHOT Report, 2017. www.shotuk.org/wp-content/uploads/SHOT-Report-2016_web_11th-July.pdf

JPAC. Transfusion Handbook, Blood products. www.transfusionguidelines.org/transfusion-handbook/3-providing-safe-blood/3-3-blood-products

McCelland DBL (ed.). *Handbook of Transfusion Medicine*, 5th edn. London: HMSO, 2014.

NHS Blood and Transplant. Cytomegalovirus (CMV) Negative Blood Components – Information for Healthcare Professionals. http://hospital.blood.co.uk/media/27175/blc707_cmv_factsheet.pdf

Woolley S. *Children of Jehovah's Witnesses and adolescent Jehovah's Witnesses: what are their rights? Arch Dis Child* 2005; 90: 715–719.

49

Oncology: cytotoxic drugs

K Cooper, E Evans and B Pizer

Introduction

This chapter will provide background information useful for the prescribing and monitoring of commonly used cytotoxic drugs in children.

The learning objectives of this chapter are:

➤ to know the main classes of cytotoxic drugs
➤ to understand common side-effects of cytotoxic drugs
➤ to gain insight into the indications, risks and monitoring of key cytotoxic agents
➤ to recognise the need for specialist training in prescription and administration of chemotherapy.

While the prescription of cytotoxic agents is reserved for those working in the relevant paediatric subspecialties, a sound understanding of cytotoxic therapy and its potential side-effects is essential for those practising in general paediatrics or (paediatric) emergency medicine, or for doctors working in the community who may be responsible for the care of a child receiving any of these drugs.

Introductory overview of cytotoxic drugs

Cytotoxic drugs have anti-tumour effects but can also damage normal healthy tissue and therefore need to be prescribed with a high degree of precision and expertise. Chemotherapy in children is generally prescribed as part of a treatment protocol or clinical trial – a series of treatment courses at defined intervals.

There are multiple modes of action of cytotoxic drugs, many acting by targeting steps in DNA synthesis. Cells must be actively cycling in order for these drugs to be effective. Treatment protocols therefore involve multiple courses of chemotherapy in order to target cell populations in different phases of the cell cycle. Chemotherapy drugs are often used in combination, exploiting different modes of action and toxicity profiles.

There are several different classes of cytotoxic drugs, which are summarised briefly in Table 1. Each drug class is discussed in more detail later in this chapter. For further drug specific information, please see the summary of product characteristics (which are often available online, e.g. via the Electronic Medicines Compendium www.medicines.org.uk).

Dose calculation methods

- Doses for cytotoxic drugs are usually calculated using body surface area.[1]
- Dose reductions may apply for patients less than 1 year old or less than 10 kg (12 kg in some protocols).
- Further dose reductions may apply for patients less than 5 kg.
- Dose modifications are often necessary following toxicity.
- Individual protocols should be consulted for further information.

Table 1 Different classes of cytotoxic drugs			
Drug class	**Examples**	**Example mechanisms of action**	**Toxicities**
Alkylating agents	Ifosfamide Cyclophosphamide	Formation of inter- and intra-strand crosslinks with DNA	Nephrotoxicity Neurotoxicity Haemorrhagic cystitis
Anthracyclines	Doxorubicin Daunorubicin	Cause DNA strand breaks by intercalating into DNA and binding to topoisomerase II	Cardiotoxicity
Antimetabolites	Cytarabine	Inhibit enzymes essential for DNA synthesis	Conjunctivitis Fever
	Methotrexate		Nephrotoxicity Hepatotoxicity Mucositis
Antineoplastic antibiotics	Dactinomycin	Form a complex with DNA, preventing DNA and RNA synthesis	Veno-occlusive disease
Platinum compounds	Cisplatin Carboplatin	Formation of inter- and intra-strand crosslinks with DNA	Nephrotoxicity Ototoxicity
Podophyllotoxin derivatives	Etoposide	Complex formation between topoisomerase II and DNA	Anaphylaxis
Vinca alkaloids	Vinblastine Vincristine	Bind to tubulin, thus preventing the formation of spindle fibres essential for mitosis	Neurotoxicity Ileus

Side-effects common to cytotoxic drugs

- Nausea and vomiting
  - Acute: during chemotherapy
  - Delayed: more than 24 hours after chemotherapy
  - Anticipatory: prior to treatment, usually when patients have suffered severe nausea and vomiting previously
- Alopecia
  - Usually begins 1–3 weeks after first dose of chemotherapy
- Myelosuppression
  - Onset, duration and severity vary with individual cytotoxic drugs and combinations
- Infection
  - Patients are at higher risk of infection during treatment
- Electrolyte abnormalities
  - Acute: usually resolve within weeks of treatment
  - Chronic: related to nephrotoxicity
- Oral mucositis
  - May occur 7–10 days after chemotherapy
- Skin and nail changes
  - Usually occur weeks after starting chemotherapy and resolve after treatment is complete

Alkylating agents

Alkylating agents kill cells by forming inter- and intra-strand crosslinks with DNA.

Cyclophosphamide and ifosfamide

Cyclophosphamide and ifosfamide are both prodrugs that must be metabolised in the liver to produce the active cytotoxic compound. This metabolism also produces acrolein, which is thought to be responsible for haemorrhagic cystitis; Mesna (sodium 2-mercapto-ethanesulfonate) protects against this complication by binding to acrolein.

Use of Mesna

Doses of cyclophosphamide above $1 \, g/m^2$ and all doses of ifosfamide require prophylactic Mesna. Mesna is given to prevent urothelial toxicity (e.g. microhaematuria, macrohaematuria or haemorrhagic cystitis). It is usually administered in intravenous hydration containing Mesna at 120% of the daily cyclophosphamide or ifosfamide dose. Hydration should be infused at a rate of $3 \, L/m^2$/day, commencing 3 hours prior to cyclophosphamide or ifosfamide and continuing for 24 hours after the last dose. Mesna may be given as intravenous boluses or orally according to specific protocols. The oral bioavailability of Mesna is 50%.

Cyclophosphamide and ifosfamide should be used with caution in patients with concurrent urinary tract infection or urothelial damage caused by radiotherapy or previous chemotherapy.

Strict fluid balance is required. Urinalysis should be done routinely to check for blood. It should be noted that Mesna can cause false positive results for ketone bodies in dipstick tests.

Nephrotoxicity

Ifosfamide is nephrotoxic. Glomerular filtration rate (GFR) should be measured by radioisotopic clearance, e.g. by chromium 51 EDTA (51Cr-EDTA), prior to the first cycle of ifosfamide and then periodically during and after treatment according to individual protocols. Dose adjustment or substitution of ifosfamide may apply if GFR is below 60 mL/min/1.73 m^2.

Neurotoxicity

Ifosfamide is associated with encephalopathy. The mechanism is unclear but is possibly linked to the chloroacetaldehyde metabolite. Risk factors for encephalopathy include low serum albumin, high creatinine and pelvic tumours. Signs of encephalopathy can range from mild (somnolence, agitation) to severe (seizures, coma, psychosis).

Methylthioninium chloride (formerly called methylene blue) has been used in the treatment and prophylaxis of ifosfamide induced encephalopathy.[2,3]

Temozolomide

Temozolomide is given orally. Doses should be taken on an empty stomach. Treatment with temozolomide has been associated with hepatic failure. Liver function tests should be checked before every cycle.

Anthracyclines

Anthracyclines (e.g. doxorubicin and daunorubicin) intercalate into DNA and bind to topoisomerase II. This causes DNA strand breaks. Anthracyclines form complexes with copper and iron. These complexes generate free radicals that may contribute to cardiotoxicity.

Cardiotoxicity

Cardiotoxicity of anthracyclines is related to cumulative dose. Anthracycline doses in paediatric protocols rarely exceed 450 mg/m^2. Left ventricular function (e.g. shortening fraction) should be measured by echocardiogram prior to treatment, before alternate cycles of chemotherapy until a cumulative dose of 300 mg/m^2 is reached, and then before every cycle thereafter.[4]

Antimetabolites

Antimetabolites inhibit enzymes essential for DNA synthesis.

Cytarabine

Cytarabine can be given by intrathecal, subcutaneous or intravenous injection. High doses are given by intravenous infusion. Steroid eye drops should be given with doses of cytarabine above 1 g/m^2 to prevent conjunctivitis. Fever is commonly observed during and within 12 hours of infusion. Cytarabine is primarily metabolised by the liver, and dose reductions apply in liver impairment.

Mercaptopurine

Mercaptopurine is given by the oral route only. It is metabolised by thiopurine methyltransferase (TPMT). Some individuals will be deficient in TPMT and will be unable to tolerate conventional doses of mercaptopurine. TPMT status should be assessed prior to treatment. Individuals who are deficient in TPMT will require massive dose reduction and close monitoring of full blood count.

Methotrexate

Low dose methotrexate can be given orally once a week. Intermediate and high dose methotrexate is given by intravenous infusion and requires specific supportive care. Methotrexate can also be given intrathecally.

Supportive care for high dose methotrexate

Hyperhydration with sodium bicarbonate is necessary to alkalinise urine and promote excretion of methotrexate. Urine pH should be above 7 prior to commencing methotrexate infusion. Calcium folinate rescues normal tissue from methotrexate toxicity. Scheduling of calcium folinate depends on the duration of methotrexate infusion and is dictated by individual protocols. Creatinine and methotrexate concentrations are measured at least daily. High methotrexate levels require increased doses of calcium folinate.

In the event of renal failure or severely delayed methotrexate clearance, the enzyme glucarpidase is given, which inactivates methotrexate. Methotrexate should not be given to patients with renal impairment. Concurrent drugs that impair methotrexate clearance should be avoided.

Antineoplastic antibiotics

Dactinomycin

Dactinomycin forms a complex with DNA preventing DNA and RNA synthesis. By preventing DNA synthesis, dactinomycin increases side-effects of radiotherapy. Dactinomycin should be omitted from chemotherapy cycles given during radiotherapy.

Dactinomycin can cause hepatic veno-occlusive disease (VOD). This can be life threatening. Patients should have liver function tests checked prior to every dose of dactinomycin and be monitored for clinical signs of VOD, i.e. jaundice, hepatomegaly and ascites.

Platinum compounds

Platinum compounds interact with DNA in a similar manner to alkylating agents. The formation of inter- and intra-strand crosslinks prevents DNA replication.

Carboplatin

Clearance of carboplatin has been related to glomerular filtration rate. Desired exposure to the drug or area under the curve (AUC) can be calculated on renal function. The Newell formula using 51Cr-EDTA half-life is the preferred method of calculation. The Newell formula is a complex calculation. Treatment protocols provide tables for the intended AUC. Carboplatin doses are read from the table according to weight (kg) and 51Cr-EDTA half-life (minutes). Therapeutic drug monitoring is recommended for patients with renal impairment. Carboplatin causes more myelosuppression than cisplatin. High doses of carboplatin require stem cell rescue.

Cisplatin

Cisplatin is usually given by intravenous infusion over 6–24 hours. Hyperhydration is required from 3 hours before until 24 hours after completion of infusion. Strict fluid balance is necessary. Mannitol should be used to force diuresis if necessary. Furosemide should be avoided due to additive ototoxicity and nephrotoxicity.

Monitoring

Platinum compounds are both ototoxic and nephrotoxic. Baseline audiology and GFR measurement should take place and be repeated periodically throughout treatment as dictated by individual protocols.

Podophyllotoxin derivatives

Etoposide

Etoposide blocks replication of DNA by forming a complex between the enzyme topoisomerase II and DNA.

Administration

Etoposide is usually given by intravenous infusion over 1–4 hours. Rapid infusion can result in hypotension. Patients should be observed for signs of anaphylaxis.

Etoposide can also be given orally (doses dictated by individual protocols). The injection solution can be given orally (unlicensed use) if capsules are not tolerated. It should be noted that the bioavailability of capsules and injection solution is not equivalent. Use 70% of the capsule dose if administering the injection solution orally.

Vinca alkaloids

Vinca alkaloids (vinblastine, vincristine and vinorelbine)

Vinca alkaloids bind to tubulin, thus preventing the formation of spindle fibres essential for mitosis.

Administration

Vinca alkaloids are severe vesicants (they have the potential to cause serious tissue damage or necrosis if extravasation occurs). They should be administered via established secure venous access.

Administration of vinca alkaloids is via the intravenous route only. Inadvertent intrathecal administration is nearly always fatal. Intrathecal therapy with other agents should be scheduled on a different day from vinca alkaloid administration.

Neurotoxicity

Dose limiting symptoms often include peripheral paraesthesia, loss of deep tendon reflexes and paralytic ileus. Symptoms may improve with dose reduction. Peripheral paraesthesia may respond to gabapentin. Constipation should be treated with laxatives as appropriate.

Metabolism

Vinca alkaloids are metabolised by the CYP450 enzyme system. Caution should be used when prescribing concurrent medication. CYP450 enzyme inhibitors, e.g. azole antifungals, reduce the metabolism of vinca alkaloids and increase toxicity.

Dose reductions apply in hepatic impairment.

Condition specific management

This section gives a brief overview of selected conditions seen in oncology where chemotherapy plays an important role.

Acute lymphoblastic leukaemia

Acute lymphoblastic leukaemia (ALL) is the most common malignancy of childhood. Treatment has rapidly improved due to multiple progressive randomised controlled trials. The treatment involves an initial period of intense chemotherapy involving three phases of chemotherapy: remission induction, consolidation and delayed intensification. This is followed by a lower-intensity maintenance therapy, with a total treatment lasting 2–3 years. Intrathecal methotrexate is used throughout treatment to prevent central nervous system (CNS) relapse.

Chemotherapy agents used include steroids, methotrexate (intravenous, oral and intrathecal), vincristine, asparaginase, cytarabine, cyclophosphamide, daunorubicin, doxorubicin and 6-mercaptopurine.

Infant ALL is a distinct subgroup that accounts for approximately 4% of all childhood ALL and is treated with a more intense protocol.[5]

Tumour lysis syndrome (TLS)

Patients with ALL, particularly those with a high white cell count ($> 50 \times 10^9$/L) and/or bulky disease are at risk of TLS. This is a life-threatening condition that can occur in all malignancies but is more common in ALL, Burkitt lymphoma, other non-Hodgkin lymphomas and acute myeloid leukaemia (AML). Biochemical derangements occur due to tumour cell necrosis. Features include:

- Hyperuricaemia – consider dialysis if levels continue to rise > 0.5 mmol/L.
- Hyperphosphataemia
- Hyperkalaemia – give calcium resonium; if electrocardiogram (ECG) changes, use calcium gluconate, glucose and insulin. Dialysis may be required if no response to medication.
- Hypocalcaemia – give calcium gluconate if patient is symptomatic.

Frequent monitoring of electrolytes is essential. Prevention of TLS involves hydration fluids (without potassium) and allopurinol, both of which should be started at least 12 hours prior to chemotherapy. Allopurinol blocks the conversion of hypoxanthine to xanthine and of xanthine to uric acid. For high risk patients, rasburicase is used, which converts uric acid to allantoin, a soluble compound more easily excreted via the kidneys.

Acute myeloid leukaemia

AML represents approximately 15% of childhood leukaemias and arises from a heterogenous group of non-lymphocytic bone marrow progenitor cells. Prognosis depends on the cell of origin and molecular factors. As opposed to ALL, AML is treated with four or more pulses of intensive multi-agent chemotherapy, including the drugs daunorubicin, etoposide, cytarabine, etoposide and mitoxantrone. Limited intrathecal chemotherapy is given. Survival overall is around 65%.

Lymphoma

Hodgkin's lymphoma

Hodgkin's lymphoma accounts for 40% of paediatric lymphomas. It has a favourable prognosis due to a good response to both radiotherapy and chemotherapy. Two to six chemotherapy cycles are required, dependent on the stage of disease, which is classified by lymph node involvement.

- Stage I – single lymph node group
- Stage II – two or more lymph node groups on the same side of the diaphragm
- Stage III – lymph node involvement on both sides of diaphragm
- Stage IV – remote extranodal disease

Radiotherapy is often used, particularly for patients who have an inadequate response to initial chemotherapy.

Chemotherapy agents used include vincristine, etoposide, prednisolone, dacarbazine, cyclophosphamide and doxorubicin.[5]

Non-Hodgkin's lymphoma

Non-Hodgkin's lymphoma can be divided into lymphoblastic lymphoma, Burkitt lymphoma, anaplastic large cell lymphoma and diffuse large cell lymphoma.

B-cell disease, e.g. Burkitt lymphoma, is treated with four to eight cycles of intensive chemotherapy. Cytotoxic drugs include vincristine, prednisolone, doxorubicin, methotrexate (intravenous and intrathecal), cyclophosphamide, cytarabine and etoposide. For endemic Burkitt lymphoma, a common malignancy of sub-Saharan Africa, a cure can be achieved with relatively low intensity chemotherapy (cyclophosphamide, vincristine, methotrexate, prednisolone), especially in low stage disease.

T-cell lymphoma is generally treated according to protocols used for T-cell ALL and has a good prognosis.

Wilms' tumour

Wilms' tumour (also known as a nephroblastoma) is an embryonal renal tumour, usually arising in young children. It is generally very sensitive to both chemotherapy and radiotherapy. After a diagnosis made on biopsy or radiological grounds, short course neoadjuvant chemotherapy is given with vincristine and dactinomycin (together with doxorubicin for metastatic cases). The tumour together with affected kidney is then removed and risk adapted chemotherapy is given with additional radiotherapy in stage 3 cases (residual disease or lymph node involvement). Prognosis is generally very good, although adverse prognostic factors include anaplastic histology or a preponderance of blastemal cells on the tumour nephrectomy specimen.[6]

Rhabdomyosarcoma

Rhabdomyosarcoma (RMS) is the most common paediatric soft tissue sarcoma, of which there are two major histological types: embryonal (accounts for approximately 75%) and alveolar. RMS incidence is highest in children between the ages of 1 and 4 years. Li-Fraumeni, retinoblastoma gene mutation and neurofibromatosis type 1 can predispose to RMS. Treatment stratification is dependent on several risk factors, with the following being poorer prognostic features.

- Primary tumour site
  - Higher risk sites: parameningeal and limbs
  - Favourable sites: orbit, paratesticular, vagina
- Stage: residual or metastatic disease
- Histology: alveolar type
- Tumour size > 5 cm
- Age > 10 years

Chemotherapy agents used in first line therapy include vincristine, dactinomycin, cyclophosphamide, ifosfamide and doxorubicin. Neoadjuvant chemotherapy is the most common strategy, with subsequent local therapy with surgery, radiotherapy or both.[7]

Bone tumours

Osteosarcoma and Ewing's sarcoma are the most common bone tumours in childhood, accounting for approximately 8% of childhood tumours. They occur mainly in adolescence and early adulthood. Both types of tumours need local and systemic treatment. Treatment for osteosarcoma consists of a combination of surgery and neoadjuvant and adjuvant chemotherapy. Ewing's sarcoma is treated with chemotherapy, surgery and radiotherapy depending on the extent of disease. Both treatment regimens are associated with substantial toxicity, including cardiomyopathy, nephrotoxicity and infertility.

Chemotherapy agents used for osteosarcoma include cisplatin, doxorubicin, methotrexate, ifosfamide and etoposide. For Ewing's sarcoma, drugs employed include vincristine, ifosfamide, cyclophosphamide, etoposide, doxorubicin and dactinomycin.[8,9]

Brain tumours

Brain tumours are the most common group of solid tumours in children. They can be classified according to the site of the lesion and histological diagnosis. General principles of treatment involve surgery, radiotherapy (including proton beam therapy) and chemotherapy. Symptomatic treatment may initially be required for the treatment of hydrocephalus, e.g. insertion of external ventricular drain, endoscopic third ventriculostomy or ventriculo-peritoneal shunt. Dexamethasone is frequently given at the time of diagnosis where there is evidence of raised intracranial pressure.

Posterior fossa tumours

Medulloblastoma
Medulloblastoma is an embryonal tumour arising in the posterior fossa. It can be divided into standard and high risk groups dependent on the presence or absence of metastases and postoperative residual tumours, and on age, histological and biological factors. Surgery is important followed by risk adapted craniospinal radiotherapy and chemotherapy. In those under 3 years old, radiotherapy is generally avoided. In standard risk cases, chemotherapy generally includes vincristine, cisplatin, lomustine and cyclophosphamide.

Ependymoma
Ependymoma accounts for 10% of brain tumours. It is derived from ependymal cells that line ventricles – 70% infratentorial and 30% supratentorial. Surgical treatment is crucial, with total resection being the most significant prognostic factor. Radiotherapy (including proton beam therapy) is usually given postoperatively. Chemotherapy is sometimes used, particularly in very young children, and may include cisplatin, cyclophosphamide, etoposide, vincristine, carboplatin and methotrexate.

Supratentorial tumours

Low grade glioma
This group accounts for 30–40% of childhood brain tumours. The gliomas most frequently arise from the cerebellar or cerebral cortex or from the visual pathways. Neurofibromatosis type 1 is associated with 30% of visual pathway tumours and confers a better outcome. Surgery, if possible, is curative, but chemotherapy is frequently used, particularly for young children with unresectable tumours. First line chemotherapy is with a combination of carboplatin and vincristine.

High grade glioma
High grade gliomas account for around 10% of childhood brain tumours. Prognosis is poor and depends on the degree of resection and grade (World Health Organization grade III or IV). Radiotherapy is given postoperatively.

Chemotherapy with temozolomide is given as standard treatment but has questionable benefit.

Other CNS embryonal tumours (previously CNS primitive neuroectodermal tumours)

This group comprises 3–5% of paediatric brain tumours. The tumours arise from the cerebral cortex (poor prognosis) or less frequently pineal region (better prognosis). Treatment includes surgery, craniospinal radiotherapy and multi-agent chemotherapy in a similar fashion to that used for high risk medulloblastoma.

Germ cell tumours

Germ cell tumours include teratomas, germinomas, embryonal carcinomas and yolk sac tumours. Malignant tumours are classified into germinomas and tumours secreting markers such as alpha-fetoprotein (AFP) and human chorionic gonadotrophin. These are treated with risk adapted focal or craniospinal radiotherapy. Chemotherapy is generally used, including carboplatin, etoposide, cisplatin and ifosfamide.

Clerking in oncology

When taking a history in the emergency department from a child presenting with acute illness during or after chemotherapy, always remember to ask about the key information summarised in Box 1.

Box 1 Top tips for practice when clerking oncology patients

1 Primary diagnosis and date of diagnosis
2 Primary treatment centre and lead consultant
3 Date(s) of most recent chemotherapy/radiotherapy/other treatments or surgery
4 Details of which regimen (including which chemotherapeutic agents) being used if known
5 Details of any concurrent medication, e.g. antifungals, anti-emetics
6 Ask to see the patient's personal chemotherapy record, if available, which may include recent blood test results

---

Chemotherapy and cytotoxics: prescription and administration

All professionals involved in cytotoxic chemotherapy require specialist training.

- Only prescribers who have undertaken appropriate training and demonstrated competency may prescribe cytotoxic chemotherapy.

- Chemotherapy should be prescribed electronically (if facilitated by local resources).
- All prescriptions for cytotoxic chemotherapy must be verified by an appropriately trained pharmacist.
- Nursing staff must be assessed and demonstrate competency prior to administering cytotoxic chemotherapy.
- All staff involved in the preparation and administration of chemotherapy must be aware of health and safety procedures.

Conclusions

Cytotoxic chemotherapy has revolutionised the treatment of childhood cancer. For example, 80% of children diagnosed with ALL are now cured, and advances in survival have been made in many paediatric solid tumours. Cytotoxic chemotherapy has a significant toxicity profile, with many drugs having a narrow therapeutic index. Children undergoing treatment with chemotherapy should be managed in specialist centres by a multidisciplinary team of professionals who have expert knowledge in this complex field. National treatment protocols should be followed. Specialist training is essential for the safe prescribing and verification of chemotherapy prescriptions.

References

1 BNFC 2016. https://bnfc.nice.org.uk/guidance/body-surface-area-in-children-image.html
2 Patel PN. Methylene blue for management of ifosfamide-induced encephalopathy. *Ann Pharmacother* 2006; 40: 299–303.
3 Pelgrims J *et al.* Methylene blue in the treatment and prevention of ifosfamide-induced encephalopathy: report of 12 cases and a review of the literature. *Brit J Cancer* 2000; 82(2): 291–294.
4 Hale JP, Lewis IJ. Anthracyclines: cardiotoxicity and its prevention. *Arch Dis Child* 1994; 71: 457–462.
5 Bailey S, Skinner R (eds). *Paediatric Haematology and Oncology*. Oxford: Oxford University Press, 2010.
6 Malkan AD *et al.* An approach to renal masses in pediatrics. *Pediatrics* 2015; 135(1): 142–158.
7 Hawkins DS *et al.* What is new in the biology and treatment of pediatric rhabdomyosarcoma? *Curr Opin Pediatr* 2014; 26(1): 50–56.
8 Lawless ER, Sorensen PH. Twenty years on: what do we really know about Ewing sarcoma and what is the path forward? *Crit Rev Oncog* 2015; 20(3–4): 155–171.
9 Isakoff MS *et al.* Osteosarcoma: current treatment and a collaborative pathway to success. *J Clin Oncol* 2015; 33(27): 3029–3035.

50

Immunosuppressive agents in paediatric solid organ transplantation

H de Jong, T van Gelder and K Cransberg

Introduction

Transplantation is the treatment of choice for end-stage organ failure, including the kidney, pancreas, liver, heart, lung and intestine. Successful solid organ transplantation requires the suppression of immune reactivity against the alloantigens of the transplanted organ. Currently this is achieved by downregulating the recipient's immune system with immunosuppressive agents. Combinations of immunosuppressive agents are used for induction (intense immunosuppression in the initial days after transplantation), maintenance and reversal of established rejection. In this chapter, we give an overview of current knowledge of important immunosuppressive agents.

The learning objectives of this chapter are:

➢ to understand the classification and mode of action of immunosuppressant therapies
➢ to know important side-effects and drug–drug interactions relevant to immunosuppressive therapy
➢ to recognise the role of therapeutic drug monitoring.

Background

Over the last two decades the number of immunosuppressive drugs available in solid organ transplantation has increased substantially. Before 1995, only ciclosporin, prednisolone and azathioprine were on the market. In contrast, today we can choose from at least 12 different drugs (see Table 1). The range of available agents, the complexity of side-effects and drug–drug interactions, and the specific pharmacokinetic challenges in children make the treatment of this specific patient group a multidisciplinary effort of paediatricians together with pharmacists and/or pharmacologists.

Table 1 Classification of immunosuppressant therapy

Type of immunosuppressant	Class of immunosuppressant	Drugs
Non-specific cytokine inhibition	Corticosteroids	Prednisolone, methylprednisolone
Small molecule drugs	Calcineurin inhibitors	Ciclosporin, tacrolimus
	Motor inhibitors	Sirolimus, everolimus
	Nucleotide synthesis inhibitors	Mycophenolate mofetil, enteric coated mycophenolic acid, leflunomide (FK778)
	Antimetabolites	Azathioprine
	Proteosome inhibitor	Bortezomib
Protein drugs	Depleting polyclonal antibodies	Depletes all T-lymphocytes: anti-thymocyte globulin – ATG (horse or rabbit)
	Depleting monoclonal antibodies	Depletes all T-lymphocytes: anti-CD3 (muromonab-CD3)(OKT3) Depletes all mature lymphocytes: anti-CD52 (alemtuzumab) Depletes all B-lymphocytes: anti-CD20 (rituximab)
	Non-depleting antibodies	IL2 receptor blocker: anti-CD25 (basiliximab) Anti-complement C5 (eculizumab)
	Fusion protein	Contains CTLA4 – CD152 (belatacept)
Intravenous immunoglobulin (see chapter 56)		IV-Ig

Normal immune cell activation and the mode of action of the immunosuppressive agents

An alloimmune response is the result of a cascade of at least three signal pathways that can be blocked by different immunosuppressive drugs (see Table 1 and Figure 1).[1] The first signal consists of an antigen in the context of a human leukocyte antigen molecule on the surface of an antigen-presenting cell activating a CD4+ T-cell via the T-cell receptor (TCR)–CD3 complex. Signal 2, the co-stimulatory signal, is formed by CD80 and CD86 on the antigen-presenting cells engaging with CD28 on the T-cell. Signal 1 and 2 together activate three signalling transduction pathways intracellularly – the calcineurin pathway, the mitogen activated protein (MAP) kinase pathway,

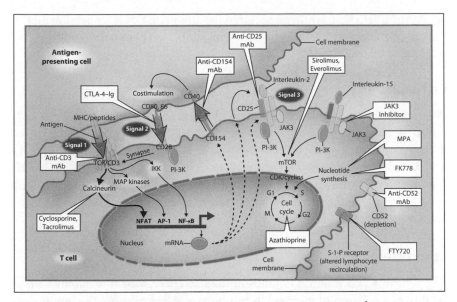

Figure 1 Mode of action of immunosuppressive drugs in the cellular 'synapse'.[1] Reproduced from Halloran PF. Immunosuppressive drugs for kidney transplantation. *N Engl J Med* 2004; 351(26): 2715–2729.

and the nuclear factor-kB pathway – which in turn trigger the expression of many new molecules, including interleukin-2, CD40 ligand (CD154) and IL2-receptor (CD25). The third signal is formed by IL-2 and other cytokines together with CD25 on the T-cell membrane, via the mTOR pathway, leading to T-cell proliferation.

Blockade of signal 1:

Although not commonly used in clinical practice, the activation of the TCR–CD3 complex can be blocked by anti-CD3 monoclonal antibody (mAb). Downstream of signal 1, the calcineurin pathway can be downregulated by calcineurin inhibitors, which results in partial blockade of the signal.

Blockade of signal 2:

The co-stimulatory signal can be suppressed by treatment with CTLA-4-Ig or belatacept. CTLA-4, also known as CD152, is a mainly inhibitory part of the co-stimulatory signal to the T-cell.

Blockade of signal 3:

Signal 3 is also called the proliferation pathway. It can be blocked at various sites.

- At the cell surface by IL-2 receptor antibodies (basiliximab)
- At the signal transduced by the IL-2 receptor ligation by mTOR inhibitors such as sirolimus, everolimus
- At the JAK3 level with JAK3 inhibitors (tofacitinib); currently this drug is only used in cancer and inflammatory diseases

- At the nucleotide synthesis required for adequate DNA replication and cell proliferation by mycophenolate mofetil (MMF) or leflunomide
- At the cell cycle itself, by azathioprine

Cell depletion strategies

Apart from the effects of drugs upon the cellular 'synapse', there are cell-based strategies aiming to deplete certain cell populations. Depletion of T-cells can be achieved with anti-thymocyte globulin (ATG), depletion of T- and B-cells with alemtuzumab (anti-CD52 mAb), and depletion of B-cells with rituximab (anti-CD20). These cell depletion strategies are currently only used as induction therapy and/or as a treatment option for a steroid-resistant acute rejection episode.

Corticosteroids

These have a generalised immunosuppressive effect, which is mainly caused by down-regulation of interleukin promotors. After entering the immunoresponsive cell and binding to the intracellular glucocorticoid receptors, phosphorylated steroids are transported to the nucleus, where they activate or repress various genes. This results in either release or decrease of a vast number of interleukins and growth factors, ultimately leading to a dramatic immunosuppressive effect.

Guidelines versus individualised maintenance immunosuppression

Most guidelines for maintenance immunosuppression recommend a combination of a calcineurin inhibitor (signal 1) and an anti-proliferative agent (signal 3), with or without corticosteroids. The total immunosuppressive dose differs according to the type of organ transplanted; e.g. in liver transplantation the amount of immunosuppression required is less than in heart, kidney and intestine transplantation. Although guidelines help the clinician to decide which combinations of immunosuppressive drugs work best in the majority of patients, they do not take into account the specific needs of the individual patient. Individualised treatment is of great importance when side-effects force the clinician to switch immunosuppressants.

Although the incidence of acute rejection episodes has dropped dramatically since the introduction of the newer immunosuppressive agents, the long term graft survival has only slightly improved. The primary cause of graft loss has moved from acute rejections towards chronic allograft nephropathy, a phenomenon secondary to long term toxic side-effects of the immunosuppressants on the graft, in combination with low grade immunological processes. New therapeutic strategies are in development (e.g. regulatory cell infusions, transplantation combined with stem cell transplantation) to create transplant tolerance without the use of such toxic long term maintenance immunosuppression.[2,3]

Therapeutic drug monitoring and adequate drug dosing

Fixed dosing (mg/kg body weight or mg/m^2 body surface area) of immunosuppressive drugs in children has been proven to result in varying exposure due to inter-individual and intra-individual variability of drug handling in paediatric solid organ transplantation.[4,5] This dictates the use of therapeutic drug monitoring and adequate dosing algorithms to achieve accurate drug dosing.[6] Drug monitoring can be performed by the assessment of the area under the concentration–time curve (AUC 0–12) or by trough levels as an indicator of the AUC (C0 concentration). In some cases the AUC can be estimated from a limited number of samples (e.g. for MMF samples at 0, 30 and 120 minutes after ingestion).[6] An additional indication for intensive therapeutic drug monitoring is the possibility of drug non-adherence, especially in adolescent patients.

Dosing recommendations for immunosuppressive agents in children generally are derived from studies in adult patients. However, children, depending on their age, have different pharmacokinetic profiles from adults – especially infants, who have different rates of absorption and metabolism. For ciclosporin and MMF, for instance, it is known that younger children require a higher relative dose and dosing frequency than older children and adults to achieve a comparable exposure. For these drugs in children less than 3 years of age, a three times daily instead of twice-daily dosing schedule is recommended.[7,8] Tacrolimus should be dosed higher in the youngest children, but can be given twice daily. Furthermore, MMF has been proven to be more accurately dosed when the dose is calculated in relation to body surface area rather than according to body weight.[5] Finally, appropriate dosing also depends on co-medication, as is shown below.

The domain of pharmacogenetics adds to the understanding of inter-patient variability in the pharmacokinetic profile. The genes encoding the enzymes that metabolise calcineurin inhibitors have polymorphisms affecting the rate of metabolism. The presence of the CYP3A5*3 allele, for example, results in the absence of enzyme activity, whereas CYP3A5*1 gives rise to higher enzyme activity demanding higher tacrolimus dosage. In addition, the ATP binding cassette protein B1 (ABCB1) gene encoding the permeability glycoprotein (P-gp) has been reported to influence the variability of calcineurin inhibitor concentration in blood. However, at the time of writing, pharmacogenetic tests to further individualise drug therapy are rarely used, despite reported associations between drug dose requirement and genotype. This may be explained by the lack of evidence that use of a pharmacogenetic test will improve transplantation outcome.[9] The cost-effectiveness of such tests also needs consideration.

Side-effects of immunosuppressants

Apart from the general immunosuppressive effect and consequently a higher risk of infections and malignancies, most immunosuppressive agents have a number of specific side-effects, as shown in Table 2. The burden of

Table 2 Side-effects of immunosuppressive drugs	
Immunosuppressive agent	**Side-effects**
Prednisolone	Cushingoid face, obesity Excessive appetite Higher risk of glucose intolerance Neuropsychiatric effects, e.g. aggressive behaviour, rarely psychosis Growth retardation Osteoporosis Peptic ulcer Cataract
Ciclosporin	Gingival hyperplasia Hirsutism High blood pressure Nephrotoxicity Diabetes mellitus
Tacrolimus	Hyperglycaemia, diabetes mellitus High blood pressure Nephrotoxicity Neurotoxicity QT interval prolongation
Sirolimus/everolimus	Anaemia High serum cholesterol Proteinuria
MMF	Gastrointestinal complaints, diarrhoea Anaemia Neutropenia
Azathioprine	Liver enzyme disturbance Bone marrow depression
Basiliximab	Allergic effects
Alemtuzumab	Leucopenia, lymphocytopenia Opportunistic infections
Belatacept	Post-transplant lymphoproliferative disorder

side-effects may be a reason to switch immunosuppressants in the individual patient.

Drug – drug interactions

Calcineurin inhibitors (ciclosporin/tacrolimus)

Both calcineurin inhibitors are metabolised by the enzymes CYP3A4 and CYP3A5. Other drugs that induce or inhibit these enzymes have a direct effect on the concentrations of ciclosporin and tacrolimus, as is shown in Table 3. Furthermore, the concomitant use of corticosteroids will result in a slight decrease in the ciclosporin and tacrolimus levels, and during corticosteroid withdrawal the opposite will occur, indicating the importance of regular monitoring of the trough level.[10]

MMF

MMF is dosed differently in combination with either of the two calcineurin inhibitors. Ciclosporin interferes with the enterohepatic circulation of MMF, while tacrolimus does not. Therefore, in combination with ciclosporin, MMF has to be dosed higher, in general $1200 \, mg/m^2/day$, while with tacrolimus it can be dosed lower, at $600-900 \, mg/m^2/day$.

mTOR inhibitors (sirolimus, everolimus)

The mTOR inhibitors are, like the calcineurin inhibitors, metabolised by CYP3A4. The interactions described in Table 3 also interfere with the mTOR blood level. In case of the combination of ciclosporin and an mTOR

Table 3 Medication that induces or inhibits CYP3A4 and CYP3A5 enzymes in calcineurin inhibitors

Interaction	Medication
Elevation of calcineurin inhibitor serum level (CYP3A4 inhibitors)	Grapefruit juice, ketoconazole, fluconazole, itraconazole, voriconazole, erythromycin, clarithromycin, calcium antagonists, metoclopramide
Decrease in calcineurin inhibitor serum level (CYP3A4 inducers)	Rifampicin, phenytoin, carbamazepine, oxcarbazepine, phenobarbital, clindamycin, cotrimoxazole, hypericum (St John's Wort)
Decrease of calcineurin inhibitor serum level (due to decreased absorption)	Cholesterol synthesis lowering medication (colesevelam, colestyramine), anti-retroviral therapy (especially protease inhibitors)

inhibitor, the level of both medications is higher, because both drugs compete for the same metabolising enzymes. This effect is not seen during concomitant use of tacrolimus and an mTOR inhibitor.

Basiliximab

Apart from sporadic allergic reactions or a cytokine release syndrome, no specific side-effects have been described. Basiliximab may cause a rise in the tacrolimus level when used simultaneously with tacrolimus.[11] The decreasing presence of basiliximab in the months after transplantation may lead to lowering of the tacrolimus level.

Conclusions

In conclusion, immunosuppressive therapy is effective in reducing immuno-logical reactions towards transplanted solid organs. Safe management of this medication, however, is a complex matter and depends on multiple factors including age, interactions with co-medication and genetics.

References

1 Halloran PF. Immunosuppressive drugs for kidney transplantation. *N Engl J Med* 2004; 351(26): 2715–2729.
2 Golshayan D, Pascual M. Drug-minimization or tolerance-promoting strategies in human kidney transplantation: is Campath-1H the way to follow? *Transpl Int* 2006; 19(11): 881–884.
3 Montgomery RA. One kidney for life. *Am J Transplant* 2014; 14(7): 1473–1474.
4 Tonshoff B *et al*. Pediatric aspects of therapeutic drug monitoring of mycophenolic acid in renal transplantation. *Transplant Rev (Orlando)* 2011; 25(2): 78–89.
5 Weber LT *et al*. Long-term pharmacokinetics of mycophenolic acid in pediatric renal transplant recipients over 3 years posttransplant. *Ther Drug Monit* 2008; 30(5): 570–575.
6 Andrews LM et al. Dosing algorithms for initiation of immunosuppressive drugs in solid organ transplant recipients. *Expert Opin Drug Metab Toxicol* 2015: 1–16.
7 Filler G. Value of therapeutic drug monitoring of MMF therapy in pediatric transplantation. *Pediatr Transplant* 2006; 10(6): 707–711.
8 Filler G *et al*. Cyclosporin twice or three times daily dosing in pediatric transplant patients - it is not the same! *Pediatr Transplant* 2006; 10(8): 953–956.
9 van Gelder T *et al*. Pharmacogenetics and immunosuppressive drugs in solid organ transplantation. *Nat Rev Nephrol* 2014; 10(12): 725–731.
10 Hesselink DA *et al*. Tacrolimus dose requirement in renal transplant recipients is significantly higher when used in combination with corticosteroids. *Br J Clin Pharmacol* 2003; 56(3): 327–330.
11 Sifontis NM *et al*. Clinically significant drug interaction between basiliximab and tacrolimus in renal transplant recipients. *Transplant Proc* 2002; 34(5): 1730–1732.

51

Nutrition and metabolism

BC Schwahn, S Bowhay and B Cochrane

Introduction

Prescribing micronutrients, food supplements and medical formula feeds is a common task both in primary care and hospital-based medicine. Apart from a few common scenarios such as mild iron or vitamin D deficiency, prescriptions need to be tailored to the individual patient and his or her actual needs. Effective prescribing requires good communication about the purpose and the practical details of treatment with the patient and family to achieve concordance with treatment goals and satisfactory outcomes.

The learning objectives of this chapter are:

> to understand how to prescribe micronutrient supplements for nutritional deficiencies
> to develop awareness of some common drugs used to treat metabolic disorders
> to recognise the central role of specialist teams when dealing with rare disorders.

Background

Complete special feeds, food supplements or molecularly defined nutritional supplements are frequently prescribed to children with malnutrition, nutrient malassimilation or chronic disease. Single or combined micronutrients are given either in physiological amounts to match daily requirements and prevent nutritional deficiencies or they may be prescribed in pharmacological doses to treat manifest deficiencies, to act as chaperones for cofactor-dependent enzymes or to overcome disorders of cofactor transport and processing. Common prescribing, e.g. of hypoallergenic infant formula, iron or vitamin D supplements, is usually directed by local guidelines.

A number of rare metabolic disorders are successfully treated by diets restricted in certain nutrients and require the use of specially formulated medical supplements and consumption of prescribable medical food items to replace staple foods.[1] In the UK, many necessary medical formulas, supplements and food items are endorsed for prescribing by the Advisory Committee on Borderline Substances (ACBS) and will be reimbursed. Due to the rarity of the conditions treatable by diet, the dietary prescriptions may initially cause confusion in primary care. However, as these foods and supplements are not able to be bought over the counter, it is imperative that sufficient product is supplied by prescription.

Metabolic diets must be initiated and monitored by specialised dietitians to avoid malnutrition with potentially devastating consequences. Close communication and cooperation between primary care, local paediatric teams and specialists is required to ensure the correct amount and type of each product is prescribed.

A small number of drugs and chemicals are used that were specifically designed to replace, enhance or inhibit metabolic reactions in individual metabolic disorders. Examples are: intravenous (IV) enzyme replacement therapies for lysosomal storage disorders; sodium benzoate or sodium phenylbutyrate as substrates for alternative nitrogen removal; betaine for hyperhomocysteinaemia; and nitisinone to prevent the accumulation of toxic metabolites in hepatorenal tyrosinaemia. Many of these drugs are exceptionally expensive, and some are still not licensed. They are generally prescribed by specialists, and treatment is overseen by specialists.

Anaemias

Microcytic anaemia

Microcytic hypochromic anaemia may be due to iron deficiency, altered iron utilisation or haemoglobinopathy. It is important to establish iron deficiency before supplementation and to restore iron depleted children prior to investigating for haemoglobinopathies.

Macrocytic or megaloblastic anaemia

In infants this will be commonly caused by maternal or nutritional deficiency of vitamin B12 or, rarely, of folates. Deficiency caused by malnutrition or malabsorption will be easily corrected with parenteral vitamin supplementation, usually given as intramuscular (IM) injection for a prolonged effect. If parenteral hydroxocobalamin is required urgently and IM injections are contraindicated, e.g. in children with coagulopathy or thrombocytopenia, it can also be safely administered by slow IV injection. Folic or folinic acid supplementation should only be started after exclusion or treatment of vitamin B12 deficiency.

If there is no history compatible with vitamin deficiency or if serum vitamin B12 and folate concentrations are not decreased, it is mandatory to search for genetic disorders of metabolism by measuring plasma total homocysteine and plasma methylmalonic acid or urinary organic acids, and to seek specialist advice. Such disorders may require long term high-dose parenteral hydroxocobalamin supplementation. Vitamin B supplementation is revisited in the section 'Vitamin B group'.

Oral nutrition

Foods for special diets

An increasing number of children are managed on special diets. Infant formulas with reduced lactose content can be helpful for children with lactose intolerance. Feeds based on partially or fully hydrolysed milk protein are used for infants with cow's milk protein allergy or chronic inflammatory bowel disease. There are a range of protein hydrolysate milk substitutes used in the management of cow's milk protein allergy. Liquid soya or nut milks may be used if they contain sufficient calories and calcium. Rice milk is not suitable for children under 5 years old due to natural contaminants. Complete amino acid and glucose based 'elemental' formulas are necessary to treat severe food allergies or malassimilation.

Local formularies have been developed that provide guidance for use of, and information on, products for the dietary management of more common conditions in children.

Highly specialised and individualised modular feeds are used for children with intestinal, liver or kidney failure and are often necessary to treat children diagnosed with genetic metabolic disorders (Table 1). Increasing evidence discouraging the use of soya formula for those with cow's milk protein allergy suggests that soya formula should also not be used for galactosaemia. Galactose free protein hydrolysates are the milks of choice for the management of galactosaemia, and medium-chain triglyceride (MCT)-based formulas are preferable for the initial treatment of children with impaired liver function.

It is very important to be clear about specialised dietary plans and to not mix up prescriptions. The use of special diets should be overseen by a qualified paediatric dietitian and may be aided by home delivery of dietary items as part of a care programme. In the UK, the Association of UK Dietitians (BDA) Paediatric Group and the British Inherited Metabolic Disease Group (BIMDG) can provide directions to specialist centres. A number of patient support organisations are available to provide advice and support for rare metabolic disorders.

Table 1 Examples of dietary treatment principles for rare genetic metabolic diseases

Metabolic disorder	Restricted nutrient	Diet principle
Galactosaemia	Galactose	Minimal lactose intake (plus galactose restriction)
Isovaleric acidaemia	Protein	Protein intake adjusted to safe minimum intake, carbohydrate emergency drinks for illness
Phenylketonuria	Phenylalanine	Low protein diet, amino-acid-based protein substitute and medical low protein foods
Medium-chain fatty acid oxidation defect (MCAD)	Medium-chain fats in excess	Regular meals, avoid prolonged fasting, carbohydrate emergency drinks for illness
Long-chain fatty acid oxidation defect (VLCAD[1], LCHAD[2], TFP[3])	Long-chain fats	Low fat diet, supplementation with MCT fats, carbohydrate emergency drinks for illness
Maple syrup urine disease	Branched-chain amino acids	Low protein diet, amino-acid-based protein substitute and medical low protein foods, carbohydrate emergency drinks for illness
Homocystinuria (CBS deficiency)	Methionine	Low protein diet, amino-acid-based protein substitute and medical low protein foods
Glutaric aciduria type 1	Lysine and tryptophan	Low-protein diet, amino-acid-based protein substitute and medical low protein foods, carbohydrate emergency drinks for illness
Fructosaemia	Fructose	Avoid sucrose and excess fructose
Glucose transporter type 1 deficiency	Carbohydrates	Ketogenic diet with very restricted carbohydrate and high fat content

[1] very long-chain acyl-CoA dehydrogenase
[2] long-chain 3-hydroxyacyl-CoA dehydrogenase
[3] trifunctional protein

Enteral nutrition

Food aversion or inability to feed is commonly observed in children affected with genetic metabolic diseases, which often requires enteral nutrition. Continuous overnight enteral feeding is an important part of the dietary management of some metabolic disorders such as glycogen storage disease type 1.

If a child refuses to eat or drink during times of illness, temporary enteral feeding can be useful to avoid hospital admission and IV infusions, especially in children with fasting intolerance due to metabolic disorders, e.g. in medium-chain fatty acid oxidation defect (MCAD) deficiency. Urgent hospital admission for IV therapy, however, becomes essential for almost every child with recurrent vomiting and a metabolic disease.

Emergency fluids based on glucose polymers (e.g. Maxijul®, Polycal®, SOS®) are used to prevent hypoglycaemia or increased catabolism with resultant accumulation of toxic metabolites such as ammonia or organic acids. Carers are advised on a suitable regimen, which is age dependent.

Fluids and electrolytes

A ready-made solution of 0.45% sodium chloride and 5% glucose is typically used as maintenance fluid for children. Children affected with metabolic disorders often require a solution containing 0.45% sodium chloride and 10% glucose to provide adequate energy and avoid excessive protein or fat catabolism. Such a solution can be prepared by removing 50 mL from a 500 mL bag of 0.45% NaCl/5% glucose and replacing it with 50 mL of 50% glucose. Alternatively, 7.5 mL of 30% NaCl can be added to a 500 mL bag of 10% glucose (see also advice on the website of the BIMDG). Children on a ketogenic diet are either maintained on 0.9% NaCl or, if they become hypoglycaemic, may require a solution of 0.45% NaCl and 2.5% glucose. This can be prepared by removing 25 mL from a 500 mL bag of 0.45% NaCl and replacing it with 25 mL of 50% glucose. The prescription and administration of such non-standard infusion solutions is normally governed by local guidelines, which should always be consulted.

Intravenous nutrition

Children suspected of a metabolic disorder on diets restricted in fat or protein and requiring parenteral nutrition should not be given standard total parenteral nutrition (TPN) without a metabolic specialist team being consulted. Such children may be provided with either altered proportions of regular parenteral nutrition (PN) constituents or may require a custom-made PN solution available from specialist providers. Children with disorders of fatty acid metabolism must not be infused with parenteral long chain triglyceride (LCT) lipids. Long term TPN can be associated with secondary micronutrient deficiency. A recognised problem is acquired thiamine deficiency, leading to lactic acidosis.

Minerals

Calcium and magnesium

Insufficient dietary intake of calcium is common in children whose diet is low in dairy products and meat. Table 2 shows the calcium content of some

Table 2 Selected sources of dietary calcium as alternatives to medication	
Food	**Serving in g or mL to provide 200 mg calcium**
Tahini (sesame) paste	30
Tofu (steamed)	40
Calcium fortified cereals, e.g. Coco-Pops®, Rice Krispies®, Cheerios®	60
Almonds	85
White bread (sliced)	120
Spinach (boiled)	140
Fruit yoghurt	150
Milk (all types)	165
Wholemeal bread	200
Soya milk + calcium	225
Baked beans	375
Concentrated orange juice (unsweetened)	575

food choices that may be suitable alternatives. Children on low protein diets or dairy free diets often require a pharmaceutical calcium supplement.

A list of suitable galactose-free calcium supplements for children with galactosaemia is available from a specialist dietitian. In addition, advice should be given on increasing the calcium content of the diet by use of calcium rich foods such as orange juice and soya alternatives such as yoghurt and cheese. Some hard cheeses may be suitable, and advice is available from the galactosaemia support group.

Phosphorus

When oral phosphate supplements are prescribed, diarrhoea may occur following high-dose supplementation, which can be ameliorated by dosing more frequently, e.g. every 4 hours instead of every 6–8 hours.

In hyperphosphataemia (e.g. during renal failure), phosphate binders are available in solid dose forms and as liquids. Dissolving solid formulations and administering them through feeding tubes is feasible but requires special precautions. It is advisable to consult pharmacists or specialist nurses

Table 3 Typical doses used in the UK for vitamins and cofactors used in the acute management of metabolic disorders in neonates and infants. Higher doses have been used for specific disorders or for older patients.[2,3]

Drug	Dose (mg)	Dosing interval (h)	Application
Biotin	5	12–24	PO/NG/IV
Carglumic acid	400–800	12	PO/NG
Folinic acid	15	24	PO/NG/IV
Hydroxocobalamin	1	24	IM/IV slow injection
Pyridoxine HCl	50–100	12	PO/NG/IV
Pyridoxal phosphate	30	8	PO/NG
Riboflavin	50	12	PO/NG/IV
Thiamine HCl	50	12	PO/NG/IV infusion
Ubidecarenone	100	12–24	PO/NG

PO, oral
NG, via nasogastric tube
IV, intravenous

over safe practice whenever medication is being administered in a non-licensed way.

Vitamins

Vitamin B group

- Thiamine, riboflavin, pyridoxine, pyridoxal phosphate, biotin or hydroxocobalamin may be required to treat acutely ill neonates with severe lactic acidosis, hyperammonaemia or seizures (see Table 3).
  - Under these circumstances, there might be limited intestinal absorption, and parenteral preparations are preferable.
- A number of oral and IV preparations are unlicensed in the UK and only available via specialist importation companies.
  - Advice on sourcing such products should be obtained from local hospital pharmacies.

Vitamin D

Plasma 25-hydroxycholecalciferol concentrations are often found to be low in children, in particular in strongly pigmented individuals living in sun-deprived regions or in children with chronic liver or kidney disease, and sometimes in exclusively breastfed infants. Symptomatic vitamin D deficiency is much rarer and requires different treatment.

- Asymptomatic vitamin D deficiency in otherwise healthy children responds well to oral supplementation with the precursors ergocalciferol (vitamin D2) or colecalciferol (vitamin D3).
  - These are metabolically activated according to need.
- Oral supplements to match daily demands are available over the counter or can be prescribed as calciferol, typically in a dose of 200–400 units (5–10 μg) per day.
- Symptomatic or severe vitamin D deficiency requires a short term high dose supplement of ergocalciferol or colecalciferol, typically as a daily dose of 10- to 20-fold the recommended dietary intake for a period of 4–8 weeks.
  - This should be followed by continued supplementation of 1- to 2-fold the daily requirement.
- If adherence to oral medication is an issue, the initial high dose course can be replaced by a single IM injection of 300,000 units ergocalciferol.
- High dose vitamin D therapy often requires an additional calcium supplement to avoid hypocalcaemia.
- Local guidelines or pharmacies can assist with safe prescribing.
- Children with chronic disease may require long term supplementation with activated forms of vitamin D3, such as 1-alpha-hydroxycholecalciferol in kidney failure or 1,25-dihydroxycholecalciferol in liver disease.
  - Those drugs are required in very small amounts only, and prescription requires careful monitoring of calcium metabolism to avoid adverse effects.

Vitamin E

- Bioavailability of oral vitamin E (and A) is greatly decreased in disorders associated with cholestasis or fat malabsorption.
- Success of oral or enteral high dose alpha tocopherol acetate supplementation depends critically on strict adherence to regular intake.
- Tocofersolan is a water-soluble alpha tocopherol preparation that has been developed to provide improved bioavailability for paediatric patients with digestive malabsorption due to congenital chronic cholestasis or hereditary chronic cholestasis.

Multivitamin preparations

- Over-the-counter multivitamin supplement use is widespread but is only justified in children at risk of vitamin D deficiency.

- Children with proven vitamin deficiencies should be treated with defined vitamin preparations.
- Children with insufficient nutritional intake due to restricted and incomplete diets should preferably be treated with a balanced and complete paediatric micronutrient supplement (e.g. Fruitivits®, Seravit®, Phlexyvits®) under supervision of a paediatric dietitian.
  - Acceptance of these supplements can be problematic.
  - Alternatively, a combination of partial micronutrient supplements can be considered to improve palatability.
  - Pharmacists or specialist dietitians should be consulted if administration of micronutrient supplements through a feeding tube is required to avoid complications.

Metabolic disorders

Acute and long-term treatment of genetic metabolic disorders usually requires liaison with regional paediatric metabolic centres. Specialist advice on safe medication can be obtained from a number of specialised pharmacies, and a number of treatment protocols including advice on how to prepare medication used in emergencies can be found on the website of the BIMDG.[4] Many drugs are available as unlicensed specials only. More information on prescribing such drugs can be found on the website of the Pharmaceutical Services Negotiating Committee (PSNC).[1] Prescribing and monitoring of enzyme replacement therapy and of enzyme inhibitors for lysosomal storage disorders is commissioned as a highly specialised service in England and available through individual treatment requests in other parts of the UK.

Drugs used in metabolic disorders

L-carnitine

- L-carnitine is eliminated via renal excretion, and the dose should be adjusted to a reduced glomerular filtration rate (GFR).
- Usual maximum dose is 3×1 g per day.
- The fishy odour that occurs with high doses of L-carnitine may respond to a short course of antibiotic treatment using metronidazole.
- D,L-carnitine preparations should not be used, as they can cause toxic adverse effects.

L-arginine

- IV and oral liquid preparations of L-arginine are available as unlicensed specials.
  - Concentrations vary, depending on manufacturer, and need to be carefully checked to avoid medication errors (see chapter 31).

- Powder sachets are licensed as a food supplement and can be used for the treatment of urea cycle disorders.
- Both L-arginine base or L-arginine hydrochloride can be used, which differ in molecular mass, solubility and taste.
  - Care should be taken to prescribe the most palatable formulation for oral intake and to avoid frequent changes of the preparation in children to ensure long term drug compliance.
  - Dosing intervals are every 6–8 hours, and dose is adjusted to individual requirements.

L-citrulline

- Unlicensed powder and enteral liquid preparations are available from special manufacturers. L-citrulline can be given as an alternative to L-arginine in ornithine transcarbamylase deficiency, carbamoyl phosphate synthetase deficiency or lysinuric protein intolerance.

Carglumic acid

- Carglumic acid (N-carbamoylglutamate) is licensed for treatment of hyperammonaemia due to N-acetylglutamate synthetase deficiency or organic acidaemias.
  - This drug should be available in larger neonatal units or might be carried by retrieval teams to allow immediate emergency treatment of acutely ill children without delay.

Sodium benzoate

- Sodium benzoate has been in use for decades as an unlicensed chemical to treat acute and chronic hyperammonaemia. IV and liquid enteral preparations are available from special manufacturers. The dose for long-term treatment is individually adjusted between 100 and 250 mg/kg per day, with 6–8 hourly dosing. Higher doses are used for emergency management of hyperammonaemia and in the treatment of non-ketotic hyperglycinaemia.

Sodium phenylbutyrate

- Sodium phenylbutyrate (NaPBA) is licensed for the treatment of urea cycle disorders as plain oral granulate (Ammonaps®, 940 mg or 5 mmol of NaPBA/g) for oral or enteral use and also as a taste-masked formulation (Pheburane®, 483 mg or 2.6 mmol of NaPBA/g) for exclusive oral use. The enteral liquid glycerol phenylbutyrate preparation Ravicti® is odourless and contains 6 mmol PBA/mL, an equivalent of 1230 mg NaPBA.
- Sodium phenylbutyrate is available from special manufacturers as an unlicensed chemical for IV use and in liquid and tablet preparations for oral or enteral use.

- The dose for long term treatment of urea cycle disorders is individually adjusted between 100 and 250 mg/kg per day, with 6–8 hourly dosing. Great care should be taken to choose the most suitable formulation and dosing regimen to ensure adherence to treatment.
- Large doses of sodium phenylbutyrate and sodium benzoate can cause nausea, and patients may require IV anti-emetic drugs, e.g. ondansetron, during acute high dose IV therapy. Hypokalaemia and hypernatraemia are frequently observed during high dose treatment with both drugs. Plasma electrolytes should be regularly monitored, and potassium supplements are usually required.
- Advice on acute management of severe hyperammonaemia and on IV dosing of both sodium benzoate and sodium phenylbutyrate is available from the BNFC and from the website of the BIMDG.[4]

Betaine
- Licensed as anhydrous betaine powder for all forms of genetic hyperhomocysteinaemia.
- Liquid and tablet preparations are available from special manufacturers.
- Betaine hydrochloride is less palatable, associated with caustic effects, and should be avoided.
- Betaine supplementation in cystathionine beta synthase (CBS) deficiency – classical homocystinuria – increases methionine plasma concentrations, especially in patients with insufficient dietary protein restriction.
- Patients with methionine plasma concentrations that exceed 1000 µmol/l are at increased risk of cerebral oedema; treatment needs careful monitoring, with betaine dose adjustment as required.

Conclusions

In this chapter we have summarised key principles relevant to prescribing micronutrients, food supplements and medical formula feeds, and introduced agents used in metabolic disorders. Prescribing for complex patients such as those with rare metabolic disorders is fraught with complications, including medication errors or unintended drug interactions. The BNFC and this chapter are resources to aid prescribing and highlight common pitfalls. In many situations, however, there will be limited information available and liaison between primary care, general inpatient care and specialist clinical and pharmacy teams will be required to agree on individualised treatment and monitoring plans.

References

1 Pharmaceutical Services Negotiating Committee. Unlicensed specials and imports. http://psnc.org.uk/dispensing-supply/dispensing-a-prescription/unlicensed-specials-and-imports
2 Saudubray JM *et al.* (eds). *Inborn Metabolic Diseases. Diagnosis and Treatment.* 6th edn. Berlin, Heidelberg: Springer, 2016.
3 Alfadhel M *et al.* Drug treatment of inborn errors of metabolism: a systematic review. *Arch Dis Child* 2013; 98: 454–461.
4 British Inherited Metabolic Diseases Group. Emergency guidelines. www.bimdg.org.uk/site/guidelines.asp

Further recommended reading

The Association of UK Dietitians (BDA). Paediatric Specialist Group. www.bda.uk.com/regionsgroups/groups/paediatric/home
British Inherited Metabolic Disease Group (BIMDG). www.bimdg.org.uk
Metabolic Support UK (formerly known as Climb). https://www.metabolicsupportuk.org/
Galactosaemia Support Group. www.galactosaemia.org
National Society for Phenylketonuria (NSPKU). www.nspku.org

52

Rheumatology

S Sampath, CE Barker and E Baildam

Introduction

This chapter provides an overview of important drugs used in paediatric rheumatology and their common or significant adverse effects. The management of many paediatric rheumatological conditions has changed dramatically in recent years, following the advent of disease modifying anti-rheumatic drugs (DMARDs). As in other areas of paediatrics, informed use of unlicensed or off-label medications is also necessary in paediatric rheumatology,[1,2] and early specialist advice helps to optimise the management of complex cases.

Throughout this chapter, we focus on the aspects of the pharmacology that are important in clinical practice. For further information, including additional details about adverse reactions and drug–drug interactions, please refer to the product details contained in the manufacturer's summary of product characteristics and the *British National Formulary for Children* (or your equivalent national formulary).

The learning objectives of this chapter are:

> to recognise the key factors underpinning the safe and effective use of non-steroidal anti-inflammatory drugs (NSAIDs) and corticosteroids in children with rheumatological conditions
> to understand the role of DMARD therapy and the associated safety issues
> to be familiar with other drugs and drug classes commonly used in paediatric rheumatology.

NSAIDs

NSAIDs inhibit the activity of cyclo-oxygenase enzymes (COX-1 and COX-2) and therefore interfere with prostaglandin synthesis. They are commonly used in juvenile idiopathic arthritis (JIA), where, as well as being analgesic, their anti-inflammatory effects can modify disease activity. Children can be intolerant or non-responsive to one NSAID but respond to another, so serial NSAIDs may be tried. Selective or preferential cyclo-oxygenase-2 inhibitors such as diclofenac can sometimes be used, but since long term safety is unknown, especially regarding cardiovascular toxicity, they should be reserved as second line NSAIDs. The lowest effective dose of NSAID should be prescribed for the shortest period of time to control symptoms, and the need for long term treatment reviewed periodically.

Formulations

NSAIDs are available in a variety of formulations and strengths (solid dose forms such as tablets and capsules, dispersible tablets, melt formulations, granules, liquid preparations, suppositories and topical agents applied to the skin or eye). Some formulations are unlicensed and must be prepared extemporaneously or by a specials manufacturer or are imported into the UK. Slow release preparations are currently available for diclofenac, ibuprofen and indometacin, and may be of value in older children. These formulations should not be manipulated to achieve a smaller dose. Dispersible forms are available for diclofenac and piroxicam. The choice of formulation depends on side-effect profile, taste, potency of the anti-inflammatory effect, frequency of use and duration of action, and should take account of patient preference, the waking day and school day, in addition to the desired therapeutic effect.

Side-effects and cautions

- All NSAIDs may cause gastrointestinal (GI) toxicity. Ibuprofen has the best side-effect profile but the weakest anti-inflammatory effect and the shortest duration of action (4–6 hours). Piroxicam is associated with a high risk of GI toxicity, while indomethacin, diclofenac and naproxen are associated with moderate incidence. Gastro-protection with proton pump inhibitors (PPIs; preferred over histamine H2 receptor antagonists in light of their once-daily regimen) is commonly used, especially if NSAIDs are taken for prolonged periods or along with other medications such as corticosteroids. (Note that the dispersible PPI formulation is often preferred.)
- In adults, NSAID use can be associated with a small increased risk of thrombotic events (myocardial infarction/stroke), independent of baseline cardiovascular risk factors or duration of NSAID use; however, the greatest risk may be in those receiving high doses long term. The risk of these adverse effects in children is unclear.
- Naproxen can cause pseudoporphyria – photosensitive blistering rash and scarring, particularly in fair-skinned individuals; photoprotection is recommended, and treatment must be discontinued if this side-effect

occurs. Renal interstitial nephritis or papillary necrosis is rare. However, NSAIDs should only be used cautiously in patients with pre-existing renal conditions and may be contraindicated, particularly in the context of dehydration.

Drug interactions

Interactions are uncommon. NSAIDs can reduce methotrexate elimination, but this is rarely clinically important at the doses used for immunomodulation in rheumatology.

Practical considerations

Therapeutic regimens should take account of patient preference and capability, the adverse effect profile of the medicine, and lifestyle considerations (such as the waking day and school day). Sugar free preparations of liquid medicines should be specified where possible. Slow release preparations administered in the evenings can help with early morning stiffness. Indometacin has superior anti-inflammatory effects but higher rates of GI upset, and is therefore reserved for difficult systemic onset JIA, severe spondyloarthritis and gout. Higher doses of NSAIDs may be needed in all forms of JIA, especially systemic onset JIA.

All NSAIDs should be given with (or after) food or milk.

Corticosteroids

Corticosteroids remain important and widely used in many paediatric rheumatic disorders. They can be life-saving in serious disease and are commonly used to induce rapid disease remission because of their immediate and powerful anti-inflammatory effects. Prolonged systemic use should be actively minimised, in view of the significant side-effect profile. There are currently no head-to-head trials to direct the route of administration or choice of steroids in remission induction.

Intra-articular corticosteroids

This is the preferred route to deliver steroids to inflamed joints in oligoarticular JIA, with minimal systemic exposure for maximum targeted effect.

Formulations
Triamcinolone hexacetonide is the intra-articular drug of choice (dosages vary according to which joint is being treated). Triamcinolone acetonide can also be used (double the dose of the hexacetonide is required), but has greater

systemic absorption and a shorter duration of action. Methylprednisolone can be used, especially in small joints and tendon sheaths, although the duration of effect may be shorter than for the less soluble triamcinolone hexacetonide.

Side-effects and cautions

Some systemic absorption occurs, and transient facial flushing and Cushingoid effects can be seen. Symptom relief of non-injected joints is reported, again suggesting systemic absorption from the injected joints. Subcutaneous atrophy can occur at the injection site; screening with radiographic contrast-enhanced arthrograms to ensure accurate placement may reduce this. Peri-articular calcification can sometimes be seen, especially with repeated injections or around small joints. With good aseptic technique, septic arthritis following joint injection is extremely rare. Adrenal suppression can occur following intra-articular joint injection, especially if multiple sites are injected at once with a high total steroid dose.

Practical considerations

In young children or when deeper or multiple joints need injecting, general anaesthetic is necessary; older children may tolerate injection under nitrous oxide sedation and local anaesthetic. Even when many joints are injected, there is no total ceiling dose, as it is rare to approach the equivalent of high dose intravenous methylprednisolone. Intra-operative imaging using radiographic contrast medium is recommended for deeper joints and when learning the procedure, to ensure needle placement within the joint. It is not necessary to 'rest the joint' post-injection, and this is impossible to achieve in small children anyway. In tendonitis, steroid injection into the tendon sheath is done with direct imaging; inadvertent injection into the tendon is associated with the possibility of tendon rupture.

Oral, intravenous and intramuscular corticosteroids

Systemic steroids at high doses are used in many paediatric rheumatic diseases, as 'induction therapy'.

Formulations

- Prednisolone enteric-coated tablets have typically been the preferred form; however, a recent review of the evidence failed to show any benefit of gastro-protection compared with the non-enteric-coated forms. Soluble tablets may be required for younger children. In the UK, soluble prednisolone tablets are much more expensive than standard prednisolone tablets or licensed liquid formulations. The most cost-effective dosage form available that delivers the appropriate dose and takes account of the child's capability and preferences should be selected.

- Methylprednisolone is usually given as intravenous pulsed therapy (15–30 mg/kg, maximum dose of 1 g) for severe inflammatory rheumatic disorders, usually administered in 100 mL of 0.9% sodium chloride as an infusion over 1–4 hours. The number of doses administered as part of a pulsed course should be clearly documented. When absorption of oral prednisolone is unreliable and systemic steroids are vital, an intravenous equivalent dose of methylprednisolone is used (1 mg of prednisolone is equivalent to 0.8 mg of methylprednisolone).
- Methylprednisolone acetate is used effectively in intramuscular depot injections to induce remission.

Side-effects and cautions

Common side-effects associated with systemic corticosteroid use include increased facial flushing, metallic taste, slight mood changes, sleep disturbance and hunger; with long term use, Cushingoid changes, striae, adrenal suppression and growth retardation are possible. Less common side-effects include altered conscious states, psychosis and seizures. Hypertension, sweating and flushing can be experienced during pulsed intravenous methylprednisolone infusion and may respond to slowing the rate of the infusion. Perceived pain of deep intramuscular steroid injection currently limits its use to older children, although it has not been studied in early childhood. It is important to remember that steroids are immunosuppressive with additive effects with other immunosuppressive therapies. Paradoxically, some patients are actually allergic to steroids, even though these are used to treat severe allergic reactions.

Drug interactions

Steroids along with NSAIDs will increase the risk of gastritis; hence gastroprotection should be used. Systemic use of steroids can increase ciclosporin levels.

Practical considerations

- Steroid cards or bracelets should be given with any long term prescriptions. Varicella serology status should be assessed before systemic steroid therapy; non-immune children could be immunised if a delay in treatment is possible and should receive aciclovir prophylaxis or treatment in the event of chickenpox exposure or infection. Zoster immune globulin may also be used. Remember the increased risk of measles in the non-immune.
- Methylprednisolone acetate should be administered as a deep intramuscular injection to minimise the chance of subcutaneous atrophy; it can be mixed with 1% lignocaine to minimise pain at the injection site.
- The total daily dose of oral prednisolone is preferably given as a single dose in the morning. In severe conditions, the dose can be split and given

twice a day, but the greater efficacy is associated with greater side-effects and adrenal suppression.

- Vitamin D and calcium supplements should be used to reduce osteoporosis secondary to long term steroid use, with encouragement for increased physical activity, exposure to sunlight and appropriate diet. Bone density should be monitored in long term use.

- Significant immunosuppression should be considered in any child who is taking oral prednisolone as follows: 2 mg/kg/day for > 1 week, 1 mg/kg/day for > 1 month, > 40 mg/day over 1 week or any of the above for > 1 week within last 3 months. Live vaccines (e.g. BCG, MMR, rotavirus, varicella, live attenuated influenza (nasal) vaccine) should be avoided while children are significantly immunosuppressed and until they are off steroids for 3 months. Annual influenza vaccination is recommended.

- Long term oral steroids can cause excessive weight gain; early dietary counselling is recommended.

Drugs that suppress the rheumatic disease process/disease modifying anti-rheumatic drugs (DMARDs)

DMARDs do not provide immediate relief of symptoms, but are used to suppress the rheumatic disease process, thus are proven to be beneficial in improving the long term outcomes. This also translates to reducing long term exposure to corticosteroids and NSAIDs.

Antimalarials/hydroxychloroquine sulfate

In addition to its effect within the antimalarial parasites, hydroxychloroquine sulfate also has immunomodulatory effects, which are likely to be due to effects on the innate immune system. There is strong evidence for the use of hydroxychloroquine sulfate in juvenile-onset systemic lupus erythematosus (SLE), and all patients should receive it during the entire course of the disease. It is less commonly used in JIA, juvenile dermatomyositis, mixed connective tissue disease and scleroderma.

Formulation

Tablets may be halved, crushed or a suspension made. Dispersible forms are available.

Side-effects and cautions

Usually well tolerated. Caution in G6PD deficiency. Rarely, it can precipitate psoriasis and worsen muscle weakness in myasthenia gravis. Ophthalmology assessment at baseline and annually for visual acuity and colour vision is important, although retinopathy is uncommon at low daily doses. Ophthalmic monitoring can also be done at the opticians.

Practical considerations

Doses of 5–6.5 mg/kg (maximum 400 mg) once daily are indicated in juvenile-onset SLE, in most cases of overlap connective tissue diseases, and sometimes in children with JIA who are intolerant to methotrexate and salazopyrin. To avoid excessive dosage in obese children, the dose should be calculated on the basis of ideal body weight.

Drugs affecting the immune response

Azathioprine

Azathioprine is a purine analogue and a prodrug for mercaptopurine, used in vasculitis, juvenile-onset SLE and occasionally JIA.

Formulation

Available as a solid dose (tablet) form; a suspension can be prepared extemporaneously (see chapter 24).[3] The injectable form is very alkaline and irritant to veins, and should be avoided.

Side-effects and cautions

Full blood count (FBC) and liver transaminases should be routinely monitored during therapy. Nausea, vomiting and diarrhoea improve with dose reduction. Dose related bone marrow suppression can manifest itself as fever, sore throat, aphthous ulcers and easy bruising; FBC should be urgently performed, and cytopenias should prompt discontinuation. Azathioprine is teratogenic in animal studies; give appropriate counselling to females of child-bearing age.

Drug interactions

Increased risk of bone marrow suppression when taken with other immunosuppressive therapies, trimethoprim and co-trimoxazole.

Practical considerations

Thiopurine methyltransferase (TPMT) deficiency can result in greater myelosuppression, hence lower doses are required. TPMT should be routinely measured at the start of azathioprine treatment. Patients should avoid live vaccines (see above).

Methotrexate

Methotrexate, a folic acid antagonist, is a widely used DMARD. Its most common use is in JIA and associated uveitis. It is also useful in psoriasis, scleroderma and dermatomyositis. Response to methotrexate is slow and can take around 8 weeks.

Formulation

Available as 2.5 mg and 10 mg tablets which have a similar appearance, leading to a real risk of incorrect dosing if the wrong tablets are inadvertently dispensed. To avoid error with low dose methotrexate, it is recommended that the 2.5 mg strength is prescribed and dispensed. Suspension forms can be made by the hospital pharmacy or specials manufacturers,[3] and concentrations may vary, but 2 mg/mL is the usual concentration. Patients, parents and guardians should be taught to remember the dose in mg as well as the amount in mL and to double-check new prescriptions. A parenteral preparation for subcutaneous injection is available as pre-filled Metoject® pen devices at doses from 7.5 mg to 30 mg. In circumstances where lower doses such as 5 mg are required, these may need to be prepared locally by the hospital pharmacy aseptic unit or procured through a specials manufacturer (see chapter 24). Families can be taught to administer the injections at home. Intravenous use may help in severe intractable disease.

Side-effects and cautions

The most common adverse effects encountered are nausea and vomiting, leading to intolerance. Transient increases in liver transaminases and mouth ulcers are frequent and can be reduced with folic acid prophylaxis (usually 5 mg once weekly on a different day to the methotrexate). Regular monitoring of FBC, liver transaminases, urea and creatinine is needed. The single weekly dose of methotrexate should be stressed and availability of two strengths of methotrexate tablets and potential differences in liquid concentrations should be highlighted, especially if the child receives the medicine from more than one pharmacy.

Methotrexate is teratogenic, so contraceptive counselling should be provided where appropriate. As it is excreted in the urine, care should be taken when handling nappies of very young children on methotrexate, and parents should wear gloves. All patients on liquid or parenteral methotrexate need cytotoxic waste bins. Spillage of liquid methotrexate needs to be dealt with using gloves and should follow procedures for cytotoxic waste disposal.

Drug interactions

NSAIDs can reduce the elimination of methotrexate, but this is rarely clinically important at the doses used for immunomodulation in rheumatology. Folate reductase inhibitors such as trimethoprim can increase methotrexate toxicity. Antibacterials such as penicillins and quinolones can reduce methotrexate excretion.

Practical considerations

The dose of methotrexate is calculated using body surface area, so accurate height and weight are essential for prescribing. Use of anti-emetics like ondansetron melts or films, before and after methotrexate, can improve tolerance, as can the regular use of folic acid. The GI side-effect profile associated with the subcutaneous route is more favourable than that for the oral route. Cytopenias are less common at doses used in paediatric rheumatic diseases but can still be fatal, so regular FBC monitoring is important. Raised transaminases (after excluding other aetiologies) can be managed by omitting some doses or reducing the methotrexate dose and by adding folic acid prophylaxis (see above). Methotrexate can be given in split doses either on the same day or 2 consecutive days to minimise nausea. Play specialists and psychologists may be helpful in anticipatory nausea. Live vaccines should be avoided, as discussed in 'Oral, intravenous and intramuscular corticosteroids' (above).

Cytokine modulators

General principles

Biologics are immunosuppressive agents that modulate cytokine activity.[4] Children can experience increased frequency of typical childhood infections. Biologics can cause reactivation of latent tuberculosis; hence appropriate screening (chest X-ray, Mantoux test or immunological tests such as QuantiFERON® assay) is essential before starting biologics. Biologic therapy should be withheld during serious intercurrent infections. Recommendations regarding avoiding live vaccines remain the same, as outlined in 'Oral, intravenous and intramuscular corticosteroids' (above).

Document accurate weight and height to enable correct dosing. Safety of biologics in pregnancy is not fully known, so appropriate counselling should be provided. When surgery is planned, it is recommended to stop biologic therapy for 2–4 weeks prior to the procedure. Postoperatively, biologics can be restarted if there is no evidence of infection and if wound healing is satisfactory. Topical local anaesthetic preparations and distraction devices can make injections more tolerable. Combining two biologics is generally not recommended. Blood counts, renal function and liver function need monitoring.

- Etanercept: some individuals while on etanercept develop anti-dsDNA antibodies, hence pre-treatment screening for autoantibodies is recommended. Injection site reaction (redness and swelling) is common but improves with time.
- Abatacept, infliximab, tocilizumab and rituximab: allergic reactions (either at the time of infusion or delayed) can be minimised by pre-dosing with hydrocortisone and chlorphenamine maleate.

Sulfasalazine

Sulfasalazine is a prodrug, which bacterial enzymes in the colon convert into the active components sulfapyridine and 5-aminosalicylic acid. Sulfasalazine is recommended in JIA, particularly in patients with the enthesitis related subtype, and also for arthritis associated with inflammatory bowel disease.

Formulation

Available as tablets (regular and enteric-coated) and suspension.

Side-effects and cautions

Intolerance and adverse events are common (seen in up to 50% of patients) and associated with high discontinuation rate. Nausea, dyspepsia and diarrhoea are among the commonest dose related side-effects. Cytopenias are rare but can be fatal. Warn patients about orange urine discoloration and contact lens staining. Assess for G6PD deficiency (risk of haemolytic anaemia). Sulfasalazine is contraindicated when the patient is hypersensitive to sulfonamides, co-trimoxazole or aspirin. Arrange regular monitoring of FBC and liver function tests, as discussed under methotrexate.

Practical considerations

Gradually increase the sulfasalazine total daily dose from 10 mg/kg in first week to 20 mg/kg in second week and 40 mg/kg in third week. Usual maintenance dose is 40–50 mg/kg/day. Maximum dose is 2 g/day (2–12 years) or 3 g/day (12–18 years). The total daily dose is usually administered in two divided doses, with food or after meals.

Other drugs for rheumatic diseases

Vitamin D

The combination of inflammation, pain, reduced activity and use of glucocorticoids in paediatric rheumatic diseases can negatively impact on the ability to achieve peak bone mass. This can be exacerbated by subnormal vitamin D levels, which should be corrected. Refer to the section on vitamin D in chapter 51. Note that different doses should be used if the patient is known to be vitamin D deficient.

Cyclophosphamide

Cyclophosphamide is one of the most potent immunosuppressive therapies in paediatric rheumatology. Intermittent intravenous dosing is preferred (associated with lower cumulative dose and side-effects compared with daily oral dosing). Mesna (sodium 2-mercapto-ethanesulfonate) is co-administered to prevent urothelial toxicity (see chapter 49). Record the cumulative dose. Treatment courses longer than 6 months are rarely required.

Bisphosphonates (pamidronate, risedronate)

Vitamin D levels, serum calcium levels and renal function should be checked prior to initiation of bisphosphonates. A transient rise in body temperature and flu-like symptoms commonly occur with the first infusion of pamidronate, so predosing with paracetamol and ibuprofen is recommended.

Bone hunger can occur in marked vitamin D deficiency, which should be corrected prior to bisphosphonate treatment.

Human normal immunoglobulin

Human normal immunoglobulin (see chapter 56) can be a useful immuno-modulatory and steroid sparing treatment in some paediatric rheumatic diseases such as Kawasaki disease, refractory juvenile dermatomyositis, in vasculitides, systemic JIA and juvenile-onset SLE. It is usually administered intravenously.

Mycophenolate mofetil

Dosage in paediatric rheumatic diseases is $10-20\,mg/kg/dose$ or $600\,mg/m^2/$ dose, twice a day (higher doses are needed in severe vasculitis). The main side-effect is diarrhoea, and is reduced by gradually increasing the dose over a 2- to 4-week period.

Ciclosporin

Bioavailability differs between different preparations, hence preparations should not be changed without monitoring the levels. Monitor trough levels for toxicity. Some patients demonstrate a clinical response at 'sub-therapeutic levels', and may not need dose escalation (see chapter 50).

Iloprost

When used for critical ischaemia associated with severe Raynaud's disease, the infusion is started at a slow rate and increased as tolerated for a set duration, hence there is potential for error during administration. Continuous infusions may be needed in pregangrenous states or in severe pulmonary arterial hypertension. This complex dosing infusion requires a formal infusion regimen agreed with the pharmacy.

Top tips for practice

1 Monitor weight and height regularly and adjust drug dosages accordingly.

2   Long term steroid therapy is associated with many comorbidities, hence active weaning guided by disease activity is important.

3   Assess and address adherence to therapy regularly, particularly during adolescence.

4   Individual therapeutic decisions and monitoring are frequently necessary for optimal outcome in paediatric rheumatic diseases. Hence supervision of therapy by expert physicians and specialist nurses is necessary.

5   When taking the history from an acutely ill child who is prescribed DMARDs, remember to check for the following key information:

- What are the latest blood monitoring results?
- Is an infection present? Are the markers of infection such as C-reactive protein levels likely to be reliable, or are treatments altering them and masking infection?
- What is the patient's immunisation status and infection history, e.g. chickenpox?
- Measure the ferritin as an acute phase protein. High levels may indicate the presence of macrophage activation syndrome or haemophagocytic lymphohistiocytosis, either secondary to an inflammatory disease, or an infection or as part of a drug reaction.

Conclusions

Management of paediatric rheumatic diseases includes adequate symptom control and suppression of disease activity, with induction and maintenance of remission. Regular clinical and blood monitoring is frequently necessary. Inflammatory conditions can run a chronic course and may need prolonged treatment with multiple drugs along with support from a suitable multidisciplinary team.

References

1   General Medical Council. Good practice in prescribing and managing medicines and devices. 2014. www.gmc-uk.org/static/documents/content/Prescribing_guidance.pdf

2   Royal College of Paediatrics and Child Health. The use of unlicensed medicines or licensed medicines for unlicensed applications in paediatric practice. 2013. www.rcpch.ac.uk/system/files/protected/page/The use of unlicensed medicines or licensed medicines.pdf

3   *British National Formulary*. Special-order manufacturers. https://bnf.nice.org.uk/guidance/special-order-manufacturers.html

4   Foster HE, Brogan PA. *Paediatric Rheumatology*. Oxford: Oxford University Press, 2012.

53

Ophthalmology

A Dahlmann-Noor , F Hashmi and J Bloom

Introduction

Eye conditions are common in children. Paediatric practitioners are often the first point of call for families.

The learning objectives of this chapter are:

➤ to understand how to decide when to prescribe topical versus systemic medication
➤ to understand how to choose appropriate anti-infective treatment strategies
➤ to understand when to refer children for specialist assessment and management
➤ to understand the pharmacological principles behind prescribing medications used by eye specialists.

Administration of drugs to the eye

Routes of administration/formulation

- The vast majority of ophthalmic medicines are applied directly onto the surface of the eye and are formulated as drops, gels or ointments.
- For targets deeper inside the eye or in the soft tissues around the eye, oral, intravenous/parenteral and local injections are used to deliver medicines (Figure 1).
- Examples of local injections:
  - Local anaesthetics – into the eyelids, subconjunctival, episcleral, peribulbar or retrobulbar space
  - Botulinum toxin – into extraocular muscles
  - Antibiotics – into anterior chamber ('intracameral') or vitreous cavity ('intravitreal')
  - Chemotherapeutic agents for retinoblastoma – into ophthalmic artery (intra-arterial injection)

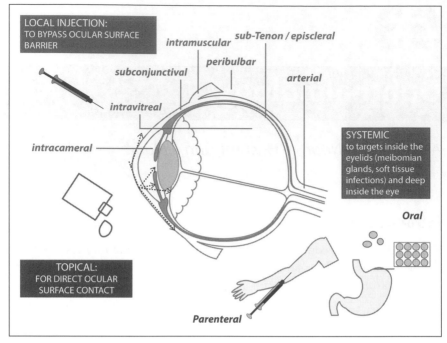

Figure 1 Multiple routes of administration are used to deliver medicines to the eye and periocular tissues.

Eye medication in children

- The formulation of medicines targeting the eye and periocular tissues in children does not differ from adult formulations, e.g. there are no 'paediatric dose' eye drops. However, depending on the child's age, a lower concentration preparation may be preferred.
- Instilling eye drops or eye ointment into children's eyes can be challenging.
  - Therefore, drugs which require less frequent administration (once or twice daily) are preferred by children and their families.
- Reduce systemic absorption by occluding the opening of the lacrimal canaliculi in the medial canthal area after instilling drops (see below).
- Dosage adjustments for intraocular injections can be made, based on the following total volumes of the eye:
  - Adult eye: 6 cm^3 reached by the age of 13 years
  - Eye volume at birth: 2 cm^3
  - At 6 months: 3.4 cm^3
  - At 12 months: 4.5 cm^3
  - At 18 months: 5 cm^3
  - Age 2 years onwards: dose as per adult

- Adult vitreous humour accounts for 4.4 mL (= 4.4 cm^3).
- Dosage adjustments for other ocular medication, e.g. eye drops, may need to take into account the nature of the paediatric eye and its response to the drug itself. For instance, in children the ciliary muscle is more active than in adults, and may require a higher dose of cycloplegic to produce the same response.

Getting the right drug into the right place

Eye drops

- Always wash your hands before and after instillation of eye drops.
- Ask child to tilt the head back or to lie down, which gives the head firm support[1].
- Pull the lower lid down slightly and administer a drop into the conjunctival sac.
- Prevent or reduce systemic absorption by pressing on the medial canthal area during and after application, which occludes the lower lacrimal punctum and prevents drainage of medicines into the tear duct and absorption by the nasal mucosa.
- In infants or very uncooperative children, drops may be applied onto the medial canthal area with the lids closed; the drop will run onto the surface of the eye when the child opens the eye.
- When different eye drops are to be administered at the same time, 5 minutes should be allowed between drops to allow penetration and to avoid washing out the first drop by the next one; excess fluid will be drained via the lower lacrimal punctum into the tear duct.
- When drops and eye ointments are to be administered, the more liquid preparation should be instilled first, followed by the more viscous preparation.

Eye ointment

- Ointments are particularly useful at night or when children are not cooperative with eye drop administration. Ointments are retained in the conjunctival sac for longer than eye drops.
- Application is as for eye drops, into the conjunctival sac, applying a strip of ointment 0.5 to 1 cm in length. As there is less risk of the ointment being washed out into the lacrimal canaliculi, it is not necessary to press on the medial canthus.

Condition specific prescribing

Infectious conjunctivitis

- Bacterial or viral, usually self-limiting, hence avoid treating if possible, to minimise resistance.

- Prescription of topical antibiotics or lubricants may alleviate symptoms of ocular discomfort.
- **Viral conjunctivitis** (intensely red eyes, watery discharge)
  - Topical antibiotics should be avoided if possible but may sometimes be used to treat secondary infection.
- **Bacterial conjunctivitis** (typically with thick white/yellow/green discharge)
  - Antibiotics may marginally speed up resolution; treatment should be deferred, and topical antibiotics only prescribed if symptoms fail to improve spontaneously over a week. Most common choice in the UK is topical chloramphenicol four times daily to 2 hourly, or fusidic acid twice daily.
- Note: **conjunctivitis in newborns** requires urgent specialist assessment and treatment:
  - Example: *Neisseria gonorrhoea* or *Chlamydia trachomatis*
  - Assessment by paediatrician as well as by ophthalmologist
  - Take specific swabs for cultures and sensitivities using appropriate methods prior to starting antimicrobial treatment; send to a laboratory with experience in culturing these microorganisms.
  - Start treatment immediately to prevent perforation of the cornea and blindness.
  - **Gonococcal infection:** typically presents with purulent discharge within the first 5 days of life. Use systemic antibiotics (single intravenous or intramuscular ceftriaxone) and frequent eye surface cleaning with saline. No evidence for efficacy of topical treatment but some add cefuroxime eye drops.
  - **Chlamydial infection:** presents from 3 days to about 2 weeks after birth as red eyes with discharge. Treat with systemic and topical macrolide antibiotics. Note, patients may develop pneumonitis. Refer both parents and/or partners to genitourinary medicine specialists for assessment and treatment.

Allergic conjunctivitis

- **Seasonal allergic conjunctivitis**
  - Typically begins in spring or summer and resolves after a few months.
  - Itchy eyes are a hallmark of allergic eye disease.
  - Treatment: topical antihistamines and mast cell stabilisers. Recent preparations (e.g. olopatadine) require administration twice daily only (more acceptable to families). Use topical lubricants to dilute and wash out chemokines on ocular surface.

- **Severe allergic eye disease associated with atopic conditions such as eczema or asthma, and vernal keratoconjunctivitis**
  - May require additional ocular surface immunosuppression by topical steroids or steroid-sparing agents such as calcineurin inhibitor ciclosporin A.
  - Children treated with steroid eye drops must be monitored by an eye clinic to detect a rise in intraocular pressure or onset of cataract.
  - Prescribe topical mucolytics such as acetylcysteine for mucus that adheres to the cornea.

Blepharitis/blepharokeratoconjunctivitis

- Chronic dysfunction and inflammation of the meibomian glands in the eyelids
- Blepharokeratoconjunctivitis: also involves conjunctiva and cornea
- Treatment:[2]
  - Daily warm lid compresses and lid margin cleaning[3]
  - Age under 12 years: low dose oral macrolides erythromycin or clarithromycin for 3–4 months. More effective and practical than topical medication
  - Age over 12 years: oral tetracycline
  - Reserve topical steroids for cases with corneal involvement; these should be initiated and monitored by a practitioner with experience in ophthalmology.
  - Topical lubricants dilute inflammatory mediators on the ocular surface, helping to soothe irritated eyes.

Preseptal/orbital cellulitis

- Common cause of acute lid swelling in young children
- In young children, the orbital walls are thin; vessels and nerves pierce lamina papyracea between ethmoid sinus and orbit, so infection can spread easily, causing a subperiosteal abscess. Orbital cellulitis can arise from breach of periosteum by infection or seeding into the orbit.
- Extension into brain may result in meningitis or cerebral abscess.
- Treatment:
  - Preseptal cellulitis (apyrexial): oral systemic antibiotic (e.g. co-amoxiclav), with daily review
  - Orbital cellulitis: intravenous antibiotics (e.g. co-amoxiclav)
  - Subperiosteal abscess: ENT (ear, nose and throat) clinical review to consider surgical drainage

Retinopathy of prematurity (ROP)

- Potentially blinding condition
- Established UK screening programme
- Treatment:
  - Conventional: laser photocoagulation of the peripheral immature retina which produces and releases angiogenic growth factors into the vitreous space.
  - New approach, not licensed, systemic adverse effects unknown: intravitreal injection of antibodies against vascular endothelial growth factor (anti-VEGF) – may reduce rate of early treatment failure and allow peripheral retina maturation. ROP may recur, so longer follow-up than conventional laser treatment. Ongoing concerns about dose, timing and potential adverse events.

Infections associated with contact lenses

- Red eye in a contact lens wearer: refer urgently to an ophthalmologist for review, on the same day.
- Two main causes:
  - Overuse: sterile corneal stromal infiltrates, an immunological reaction in the anterior stroma
  - Infection (microbial keratitis): corneal ulcer, which can progress to corneal perforation
    - Workup: retrieval of tissue from the edge of a corneal ulcer for culture and sensitivities
    - High frequency administration of topical quinolone antibiotic, e.g. hourly levofloxacin, ciprofloxacin or moxifloxacin
    - Cycloplegics for symptomatic relief
    - Polihexamide (polyhexamethylene biguanide; PHMB) if acanthamoeba suspected
    - Daily ophthalmic review
    - When safe, topical anti-inflammatory agents.

Pharmacological principles in ophthalmology, and specific drug classes

This section describes the relevant pharmacological principles that should be considered when administering drugs in paediatric eye conditions and the main drug classes used in their management.

Absorption/tissue penetration

- There are various barriers to penetration of drugs into the eye. These may be *desirable* in eye surface inflammation or infection (conjunctivitis, keratitis), as ocular penetration is not required to treat the eye surface, but could cause adverse effects (e.g. steroids causing a rise in intraocular pressure or opacification of the crystalline lens).

- In other situations, these barriers are *undesirable,* e.g. when targeting the iris dilator to induce mydriasis, or the ciliary body to reduce intraocular inflammation or production of aqueous humour, or to paralyse accommodation.
- The physiological barriers and limitations of absorption are summarised in Table 1.

Table 1 Summary of physiological barriers to absorption of drugs administered into the eye

Barrier/limitation	Description
Immediate drainage	The volume of the conjunctival sac is around 10 microlitres, which is only one fifth the volume of a typical eye drop. Hence excess fluid gets drained away via tear duct.
Tear film turnover	Medicines instilled onto the ocular surface are washed out with the tear film.
Tear film composition	Lipophilic, aqueous and mucin layers, so drugs need to cross through hydrophobic and hydrophilic environments. In the first 6 months of life, particularly, a baby's tear film has a much thicker lipid layer, and therefore the transition of a drug across the tear film may differ to that of an adult.
Cornea	
Epithelium	Tight junctions between cells: polar (hydrophilic) molecules pass with difficulty.
Stroma	Consists mainly of extracellular matrix with few interspersed cells: non-polar (lipophilic) molecules pass with difficulty.
Within the eye	
Anterior	Barrier formed by tight junctions in the posterior iris epithelium, combined with the anterior flow of aqueous humour from the ciliary body into the anterior chamber: prevents molecules in the aqueous humour from flowing posteriorly into the vitreous cavity.
Posterior	Internal limiting membrane: prevents the diffusion of large molecules from the vitreous humour into the retina. Hence, for example, bevacizumab may be less likely to reach the systemic circulation and have adverse effects on lung and brain development than ranibizumab, which is smaller.
	Blood–retinal barrier, formed by tight junctions/non-fenestrated capillaries: prevents the penetration of molecules from the choroidal vessels into the retina.

- Barriers described in Table 1 can be disrupted by inflammatory processes:
  - Cytokines and leukocytes can enter the aqueous and vitreous humour (uveitis).
  - Medicines are usually better absorbed by the inflamed eye than when the eye is healthy, leading, e.g., to greater systemic absorption of drugs in conjunctival inflammation, when vessels are dilated and endothelial cell junctions are leaky.

Elimination/excretion

Only a fraction of ocular medication leaves the eye and enters the vascular or lymphatic system, from where it is metabolised and renally or hepatically excreted. This process depends on the administration route.

Drugs that permeate into or are directly administered/injected into:

- Ocular surface – washed out with tears → lacrimal drainage system → highly vascularised nasal mucosa
- Conjunctival epithelium – drained via conjunctival veins and lymph vessels
- Cornea/anterior chamber – follow aqueous drainage pathway → trabecular meshwork → Schlemm's canal or uveoscleral tissue → episcleral veins → ophthalmic veins → cavernous sinus
- Periocular tissues drain into ophthalmic veins
- Choroidal vasculature → vortex veins → ophthalmic veins

Toxicity

Children are more prone to toxicity than adults, because of their smaller body volume and immature metabolisation pathways. Children below the age of 2 years also have a smaller eyeball (see section 'Administration of drugs to the eye', above).

- Common examples of toxicity:
  - Facial flush, dry mouth/skin, drowsiness following administration of antimuscarinics (atropine in amblyopia treatment; cyclopentolate for retinoscopy)
  - Superficial keratitis and, in severe cases, corneal oedema, due to preservatives in eye drops (benzalkonium chloride), which cause disruption of corneal epithelial tight junctions
  - Repeated administration of some drugs, e.g. aminoglycosides, can lead to high corneal epithelial toxicity

Measures of efficacy

Efficacy of ophthalmic medication is assessed based on the drug used and condition being treated.

Criteria used to assess efficacy are shown in Table 2.

Table 2 Criteria used to assess efficacy of ophthalmic medication	
Ocular surface infection and inflammation	Intense conjunctival hyperaemia (redness) and discharge
Corneal conditions	Slit lamp examination: integrity and clarity of epithelium, stroma and endothelium
Intraocular pressure (IOP)	IOP measurements (tonometry) and fundoscopy (optic nerve head changes); in older children, formal visual field assessment
Intraocular inflammation (uveitis)	Visual acuity and slit lamp examination of the aqueous humour in the anterior chamber, the vitreous humour and the retina; ancillary technologies, e.g. optical coherence tomography, to visualise vitreous inflammation and accumulation of fluid under the retina

Drug classes used in ophthalmology

Anti-infective eye preparations

- Treating eye infections is particularly challenging due to the limited anti-infective preparations available for topical or systemic administration or intraocular or periocular injection.
- Choice of agent guided by conjunctival swabs, corneal scraping or biopsy, or extraction of fluid from the anterior or posterior chamber.
- Infections of the ocular surface tissues such as conjunctiva and corneal epithelium and stroma – topical preparations.
- Intraocular infections – injection into the anterior or posterior chamber of the eye, and/or systemic treatment.
- Efficacy of intraocular anti-infective agents may, however, not restore visual function if pathogens or inflammatory changes have destroyed parts of the cellular network of the retina, e.g. in bacterial or fungal endophthalmitis or herpetic acute retinal necrosis.
- Some anti-infectious agents, particularly aminoglycosides, have high corneal epithelial toxicity when administered repeatedly, leading to superficial keratitis.

Bacterial/fungal endophthalmitis

This is a rare infection inside the eye. Most common causes in children are penetrating trauma and eye surgery. Intravitreal and systemic medication is required.

Antibacterials

- Management of endophthalmitis comprises:
  - Vitrectomy to obtain samples for culture

- Intravitreal antibiotics (such as vancomycin and amikacin/ceftazidime); start oral/IV ciprofloxacin, clindamycin, rifampicin concurrently or before vitreous samples can be obtained, as it may take several hours to arrange a vitreous tap under general anaesthesia in a child.
- As soon as culture/sensitivity results are received, tailor oral/IV therapy appropriately.
- Baseline bloods, weight, blood sugar and blood pressure measurements
- Start oral prednisolone and ranitidine the day after intravitreal antibiotics given; do NOT give prednisolone if endophthalmitis is fungal.
- Topical dexamethasone and levofloxacin/moxifloxacin eye drops

Antifungals

- Fungal infection is a rare cause of eye surface infection (keratitis):
  - Usually after trauma involving vegetable/organic matter
  - Identified on cultures from corneal scraping
  - Topical amphotericin B 0.15% or voriconazole 1%
- Fungal infections inside the eye, including endophthalmitis:
  - Intravitreal voriconazole/amphotericin plus oral/intravenous voriconazole or intravenous amphotericin
  - Do not give steroids
  - Occasionally endogenous (spread of systemic fungal infection via blood vessels)

Antivirals

- Herpes simplex virus (HSV): ubiquitous in the general population
- In the eye, can cause recurrent inflammation of the ocular surface, with keratitis and lid or conjunctival inflammation (or both)
- Repeated recurrences can lead to corneal scarring and opacification with loss of vision and growth of blood vessels across the limbus into the peripheral and eventually central cornea.
- Management:
  - Urgent referral to eye clinic
  - Epithelial corneal disease ('dendritic ulcer'): topical aciclovir or ganciclovir
  - Stromal inflammation: topical steroids and aciclovir/ganciclovir under specialist supervision
  - Corneal transplantation (penetrating keratoplasty, PKP) can be attempted to restore vision, but the risk of HSV recurrence in the graft is high
  - Oral aciclovir long-term for recurrent keratitis and after PKP
  - Oral valaciclovir or intravenous aciclovir (depending on age) for acute retinal necrosis (ARN): fulminant inflammation of the retina caused by HSV or varicella zoster virus (VZV)

Anti-inflammatory preparations

Corticosteroids

> Do not administer topical steroids if the cause of ocular inflammation
> is unknown, as they may exacerbate viral and fungal infections.

Initiate and monitor steroids only if experienced in ophthalmology –
otherwise refer to rapid access eye clinic (e.g. for suspected uveitis, severe
blepharokeratoconjunctivitis, flare-up of vernal keratoconjunctivitis).

Administration:

- Topical route: for severe non-infectious ocular surface inflammation,
  uveitis and after eye surgery
- Intraocular or periocular injection for severe uveitis or after surgery
  - Biodegradable intravitreal dexamethasone implant
  - Not licensed for use in children; in autoimmune uveitis, increasingly
    replaced by systemic monoclonal antibody treatment
  - May improve control of inflammation, cystoid macular oedema and
    visual acuity in children with non-infectious posterior uveitis that is
    unresponsive to standard treatment
  - Risk of: migration of the implant into the anterior chamber; raised
    intraocular pressure with optic nerve fibre loss, necessitating glaucoma
    filtration surgery; and crystalline lens opacification
- Injection into the lid for haemangioma; now increasingly replaced by sys-
  temic propranolol and topical timolol maleate 0.1%
- Systemic route, e.g. oral prednisolone: rarely used in ophthalmology.
  Examples are acute exacerbations of vernal keratoconjunctivitis, optic
  neuritis, para-infectious retinitis (except for known fungal infections),
  and keratitis or uveitis not controlled by topical administration; a paediatrician should be involved in patient's care.

Adverse effects:

- *Local:*
  - Rise in intraocular pressure, with subsequent damage of the retinal
    ganglion cell axons (glaucoma): monitoring required
  - Opacification of the crystalline lens (cataract): monitoring required
  - Increased susceptibility of the cornea to infection
  - Induction of corneal collagenolytic enzymes in the cornea: risk of
    corneal thinning and perforation
  - Deposition of crystals under the conjunctiva
- *Systemic* (reported after topical administration in isolated cases): see
  chapter 52.

- *Regional:*
  - Central retinal artery embolisation and blindness following injection of triamcinolone into periorbital haemangioma; treatment with systemic (propranolol) or topical (timolol maleate 0.1%) beta blockers is now increasingly used, with better safety and efficacy than triamcinolone

Consider:

- Prescribing topical steroids with lower corneal penetration, such as loteprednol or fluorometholone, for eye surface inflammation

Other anti-inflammatory preparations

- Mainly used in the treatment of allergic eye disease, which is very common in children (hay fever, allergic conjunctivitis, rhinoconjunctivitis).
- Children and families prefer preparations that only require twice-daily instillation.
- Newer agents such as olopatadine act on several targets in the inflammatory cascade, i.e. act as mast cell stabilisers as well as binding to histamine receptors.
- Prolonged use of preparations containing vasoconstrictors such as xylometazoline can cause rebound hyperaemia (red eye).
- Cytokine modulators:
  - *Systemic:* human monoclonal antibodies against tumour necrosis factor. Adalimumab is licensed as systemic immunomodulatory agent in children with chronic uveitis. It is used when standard therapies have not been successful.
  - *Topical:* ciclosporin A for severe eye surface inflammation.

Mydriatics and cycloplegics

- Nearly exclusively used as topical preparations
- Exception: to induce maximal pupil dilatation, eye surgeons may inject adrenaline into the anterior chamber during operations or give a subconjunctival injection of Mydricaine® (unlicensed preparation of atropine, adrenaline, procaine) or Mydrane® (tropicamide, phenylephrine and lidocaine, not licensed for children)
- With topical use, the onset of action is slower, and the duration of the effect is prolonged in children with darkly pigmented irides, as these agents bind to melanin

Antimuscarinics

- Most commonly used to temporarily paralyse accommodation and allow the objective measurement of refractive errors in children under the age of 7 years (cycloplegic retinoscopy):

- Cyclopentolate 1% eye drops (in children under the age of 3 months, 0.5%), one or two instillations
- Atropine 1% eye drops twice daily on 3 consecutive days prior to the refraction appointment, but not on the day of the test itself
- Other indications:
  - Treatment of amblyopia (atropine 1% twice weekly)
  - Ciliary spasm and anterior uveitis (cyclopentolate 1% up to three times daily to prevent adhesions between iris and lens, 0.5% in children under 3 months)
  - Mydriasis for fundoscopy: tropicamide 1% (in children under the age of 3 months, 0.5%) in conjunction with a sympathomimetic
- Plasma concentrations can reach toxic levels in children, due to their low body weight.
- In children under the age of 3 months use formulations with weaker concentration.
- Children with trisomy 21 may have an increased risk of adverse effects, though reports are anecdotal.
- Adverse effects:
  - *Systemic*: bradycardia followed by tachycardia, palpitations/arrhythmia, dry mouth, flushing of skin, nausea, vomiting, giddiness, altered behaviour, temperature elevation
  - *Local*: photophobia (common), closure of the iridocorneal angle and raised intraocular pressure (very rare in children)

Sympathomimetics

- Induce mydriasis: phenylephrine 2.5% eye drops
- Note that phenylephrine 10% is contraindicated in children, as serious adverse effects (severe hypertension, tachycardia, arrhythmia, coronary artery spasm and myocardial infarction if pre-existing cardiovascular disease)
- Other indication: pharmacological haemostasis in strabismus surgery by inducing vasoconstriction of conjunctival and episcleral vessels: adrenaline (0.01% or 0.1%) eye drops

Treatment of glaucoma

- The following drugs are used to reduce raised intraocular pressure in infantile or juvenile glaucoma or following uveitis or trauma
- Miotics are rarely used in children

Beta blockers

- Reduce aqueous fluid production by the ciliary body
- Contraindications and adverse effects: see chapter 39

- First choice for childhood onset glaucoma, often used whilst definitive surgery is organised or if pressure requires lowering despite surgery
- In children, use beta-blockers with weaker concentration (e.g. timolol 0.25%).

Prostaglandin analogues

- Contraindicated in children with uveitis, aphakia or damaged posterior lens capsule
- Increase uveoscleral outflow of aqueous humour
- Good systemic safety profile
- Local adverse effects: increasing iris and eye lash pigmentation, thickening of lashes, cystoid macular oedema in cases of pre-existing ocular inflammation

Sympathomimetics

- Reduce aqueous fluid production by the ciliary body
- Alpha 2 receptor agonists apraclonidine and brimonidine: not recommended under the age of 12 years
- Apraclonidine:
  - Short-term medication before glaucoma filtration surgery or after laser treatment of the trabecular meshwork or iris
  - Diagnosis of Horner syndrome
- Brimonidine:
  - Age under 2 years: contraindicated
  - Age 2–12 years: use with caution
  - Adverse effects: tiredness, lethargy, drowsiness, fainting attacks, pallor, irritability, ataxia, hypotension, bradycardia, respiratory depression, apnoea

Carbonic anhydrase inhibitors

- Reduce the secretion of aqueous fluid
- Contraindicated in children with known sulfonamide hypersensitivity, hypokalaemia or hyponatraemia
- Oral preparations (acetazolamide) achieve rapid lowering of intraocular pressure
- Topical preparations (dorzolamide, brinzolamide) frequently used in combination with other topical pressure-lowering medications to maintain pressure within a normal range
- Acetazolamide tablets can be crushed (unlicensed) or a specially formulated suspension purchased from commercial providers, to allow oral administration in young children

- Adverse effects: blood disorders, skin rash, metabolic acidosis, growth retardation (linked to metabolic acidosis after systemic acetazolamide)

Local anaesthetics

- Use with caution in premature infants, because following systemic absorption, local anaesthetics undergo hydrolysis by plasma esterases and hepatic metabolism. Although not recommended in premature infants, proxymetacaine and oxybuprocaine are commonly used during screening examinations for retinopathy of prematurity.
- Local adverse effects:
  - Stinging/burning
  - Disruption of corneal epithelial tight junctions, which can cause epithelial loss and stromal oedema; this effect is also used to enhance the corneal penetration of other agents, such as cycloplegics and mydriatics
  - Rarely, an immediate-type hypersensitivity reaction with diffuse corneal epithelial keratitis and necrosis and sloughing of the corneal epithelium
- Systemic adverse effects: hypersensitivity reaction

Miscellaneous ophthalmic preparations

Tear deficiency, ocular lubricants, and astringents

- Wide range of preparations available, differing mainly in viscosity
- Used in dry eye symptoms and also to provide symptomatic relief of inflammation
- Acetylcysteine: used in the presence of abnormal mucus production and adherence of mucus filaments to the cornea, such as in vernal keratoconjunctivitis with corneal plaque or shield ulcer

Ocular diagnostic and perioperative preparations

- Fluorescein
  Topical:
  - To visualise corneal epithelial defects
  Systemic:
  - Systemic use (off-licence in children), usually by intravenous injection, for retinal angiography
  - Use with caution in children with known history of anaphylaxis, atopy, respiratory failure, uncontrolled hypertension, heart failure, kidney or liver disorders

- Adverse events: nausea, vomiting, sneezing, skin itching, extravasation at the injection site, urticaria, vasovagal syncope, pyrexia, bronchospasm, anaphylaxis, cardiac arrest, myocardial infarction and circulatory shock

Drugs affecting metabolic pathways

- Mercaptamine (cysteamine) eye drops are used for corneal crystal deposits in children with cystinosis.

Conclusions

Most children with eye conditions present with conditions affecting the surface of the eye, and a wide range of topical medicines are available which limit the risk of systemic exposure and adverse events. Pain, redness and loss of vision are hallmarks of problems inside the eye and require urgent referral. In acute lid swelling, orbital cellulitis must be ruled out or treated promptly.

References

1   Moorfields Eye Hospital. Administration of eye drops in children and babies. YouTube. Available at: https://www.youtube.com/watch?v=d3wtEWX7HxU [last accessed 5 May 2019].
2   National Institute for Health and Care Excellence (NICE). Blepharitis. 2015. https://cks.nice.org.uk/blepharitis#!scenario [last accessed 5 May 2019].
3   Moorfields Eye Hospital. How to clean the eyelids in children and babies. YouTube. http://youtu.be/eJmWNlMziXM [last accessed 5 May 2019].

54

Ear, nose and throat disorders

C Vaughan, S Paulus and RK Sharma

Introduction

Ear, nose and throat (ENT) disorders are fairly common in children. This is thought to be related to the small size of the individual, increased exposure to upper respiratory tract pathogens through contacts at school, and a developing immune system. It may be compounded in special groups – including children with cleft palate, craniofacial syndromes and genetic disorders (e.g. Down's syndrome).

The learning objectives of this chapter are:

➢ to be able to manage common clinical conditions in ENT
➢ to be aware of likely drug side-effects and complications
➢ to know when to consider specialist referral.

Ear conditions

Ear wax

Wax is normally produced in the ears and is directed outwards by the natural migration of skin (self-cleaning mechanism). Wax accumulation occurs in pathological conditions (cholesteatoma, keratosis obturans) or, more commonly, following the use of cotton buds by parents/carers. The latter pushes the wax inwards and may lead to complete obstruction of the ear canal by impacted wax, which can lead to pain and a reported reduction in hearing.

Management

- Educating carers on avoiding cleaning of ears
- Use of wax softening agents for a few weeks, which include olive oil, sodium bicarbonate or hydrogen peroxide (H_2O_2) drops
  - Sodium bicarbonate and H_2O_2 drops may cause dryness and irritation of the ear canal.

- H_2O_2 drops also cause bubble formation – the child hears sounds like little explosions in the ear.
- Consider referral to ENT for syringing/microsuction if wax remains problematic.

Otitis media

Acute otitis media (AOM) is inflammation of the middle ear, and is very common in children. It is at its highest prevalence between the ages of 3 and 7 years. The Eustachian tube is wider and shorter in children than in adults, making children more prone to infections of the middle ear. Symptoms include pyrexia, ear pain and ear discharge. If bacterial otitis media is left untreated, complications include mastoiditis, meningitis and intracranial spread of infection.

Causative bacterial organisms:

- *Streptococcus pneumoniae*
- *Haemophilus influenzae*
- *Moraxella catarrhalis*

Management

- If symptoms are mild to moderate and present for less than 48 hours, consider supportive treatment, as may be a viral infection, ensuring follow-up is available.
- If symptoms severe or bilateral, provide antibiotics (amoxicillin – also recommended if symptom duration > 48 hours).
- If symptoms persist for > 1 week, consider topical treatment with ciprofloxacin drops only if the ear is discharging, as an adjunct. Systemic absorption is minimal and ciprofloxacin drops are safe to use even in the presence of a tympanic membrane perforation.[1]

Acute mastoiditis

AOM may progress to osteomyelitis and sub-periosteal abscess formation, i.e. acute mastoiditis. These children need admitting for observation. Imaging may be required if there are any focal neurological signs. Treatment is with intravenous (IV) antibiotics and drainage of abscess, with or without (+/−) grommet insertion

Acute otitis externa

Otitis externa is inflammation of the ear canal. Acute otitis externa is uncommon in children by itself, but usually occurs secondary to ear discharge from an otitis media or as part of systemic allergy (eczema) or, rarely, fungal infection (otomycosis). The ear canal is usually oedematous, tender on examination and filled with infective and keratinous debris. During assessment, a swab is helpful to identify the causative organism.

Causative organisms:

- *Pseudomonas aeruginosa*
- *Candida albicans* (fungal)
- *Aspergillus niger* (fungal)
- *Staphylococcus aureus*

Management

- Cleaning of the ear canal is required (if tolerated), by microsuction.
- Treatment is with a topical antibacterial/antifungal agent plus a topical steroid to reduce inflammation.
- Avoid prolonged used of topical steroids due to risk of adrenal suppression.
- See Table 1 below for commonly used topical treatments.

Nasal conditions

Acute sinusitis

Acute sinusitis is an extremely common condition, particularly prevalent during the winter months. Symptoms include nasal discharge, nasal blockage and cough. The illness is usually self-limiting and does not require any medical intervention. Those patients with symptoms persisting for longer than 7–10 days may require medical treatment.[2]

Causative organisms:

- Viral
- *Streptococcus pneumoniae*
- *Haemophilus influenzae*
- *Streptococcus pyogenes*
- *Moraxella catarrhalis*

Management:
- Supportive, if symptoms present for < 10 days (viral aetiology most common).
- If symptoms worsening after 5 days or persist beyond 10 days, consider bacterial sinusitis and treat with amoxicillin.
- Consider use of intranasal steroids if symptoms severe.

Table 1 Common topical agents used to treat paediatric ENT conditions

Topical agent	Indication	Active components	Systemic absorption?	Length of treatment	Age	Contraindications
Aural preparations						
Gentisone HC	Otitis externa, eczema	Gentamycin, hydrocortisone acetate	Hydrocortsone acetate is less readily absorbed than hydrocortisone via the skin, however there is still some systemic absorption.	Usually no more than 2 weeks	Age range not specified	In the presence of a tympanic membrane perforation, do not use for longer than 2 weeks due to ototoxicity of aminoglycosides.[2]
Sofradex	Otitis externa, esp. S.aureus infections	Framycetin, dexamethasone and gramicidin	Framycetin is readily absorbed via inflamed skin and wound edges.	Usually no more than 2 weeks	Age range not specified	In the presence of a tympanic membrane perforation, do not use for longer than 2 weeks due to ototoxicity of aminoglycosides.[2]
Ciprofloxacin (unlicensed) eye drops	Otitis media/otitis externa	Ciprofloxacin	Minimal	Usually no more than 2 weeks	Age range not specified	Hypersensitivity
Betnesol	Otitis externa, eczema, aural polyps	Betamethasone	Minimal from ear canal	Usually no more than 2 weeks	Age range not specified	Untreated/active bacterial fungal infection
Aureocort ointment	Eczema	Triamcinolone, chlortetracy-cline	Minimal		Not licensed for use in children under 8 years	Hypersensitivity
Canesten	Otomycosis	Clotrimazole	Minimal	For at least 2 weeks following resolution of symptoms	Age range not specified	Hypersensitivity

Table 1 (*Continued*)

Topical agent	Indication	Active components	Systemic absorption?	Length of treatment	Age	Contraindications
Nasal preparations						
Beconase	Rhinitis	Beclometasone	Yes – bioavailability 44%	3 months	Licensed for use in children over 6 years	Hypersensitivity
Flixonase	Rhinitis	Fluticasone propionate	Minimal	Indefinite	Licensed for use in children over 4	Hypersensitivity
Avamys	Rhinitis	Fluticasone furoate	Yes – Bioavailability 0.5%	Indefinite	Licensed for use in children over 6	Hypersensitivity
Betnesol	Rhinitis, nasal polyps	Betamethasone	Yes	2 weeks	Age range not specified	Untreated/active bacterial fungal infection
Rhinolast	Allergic rhinitis	Azelastine hydrochlorice	Minimal	Indefinite	Licensed for use in children over 5 years	Hypersensitivity

475

Orbital complications secondary to sinusitis

The ethmoid and maxillary sinuses are present at birth. Direct spread of infection from ethmoidal acute sinusitis can lead to pre-septal cellulitis anteriorly, or post-septal (orbital) cellulitis and abscess formation posteriorly. Early ophthalmology involvement is essential (see chapter 53), as the optic nerve is at risk. In addition to appropriate systemic antibiotics, topical decongestant nasal drops, e.g. paediatric Otrivine®, can be used (not for >2 weeks, as risk of rebound rhinitis). If there is any concern regarding the patient's vision, arrange urgent CT scan and ENT referral if abscess present.

Allergic rhinosinusitis

Allergic rhinosinusitis is an immunoglobulin E (IgE) mediated hypersensitivity reaction that is becoming extremely prevalent in the Western population. Patients may be affected seasonally (i.e. hay fever) or perennially. Common causative allergens include pollen, house dust mites, and cat and dog dander. Patients may be atopic. There is a risk from polypharmacy, as these patients may be on several different steroid modalities, e.g. inhalers, topical drops, nasal sprays and ointments.

Management

- Consider allergy testing (helpful to direct allergen avoidance advice – refer to local guidelines).
- Use topical steroid nasal sprays +/- topical or oral antihistamine.[3]
- Avoid topical decongestants (risk of rebound rhinitis).

Throat conditions

Tonsillitis

Acute tonsillitis is infection of the palatine tonsils. It is very common in childhood. It is thought that up to 50% of infections may be viral. If recurrent tonsillitis is a persistent problem, children may be considered for a tonsillectomy if they meet the Scottish Intercollegiate Guidelines Network (SIGN) guidance.[4]

Causative organisms:

- Respiratory viruses
- Epstein–Barr virus (EBV)
- *Streptococcus pyogenes* (group A *Streptococcus*; GAS)

Assessment of the presence of Centor criteria (fever, tonsillar exudates, no cough, tender anterior cervical lymphadenopathy) can help guide clinicians regarding whether antibiotics are required.

Management

- Ensure adequate hydration and analgesia.
- If antipyretics are needed: paracetamol and/or ibuprofen.
- Consider topical analgesia such as Difflam® in children older than 8 years.
- Consider antibiotics for patients with three or four of the Centor criteria listed above.
- Oral antibiotics covering GAS (e.g. phenoxymethylpenicillin): a 10 day course is usually recommended (note that pharmacies sometimes only provide 1 week's supply at a time, because of the formulation's shelf life).
- Avoid prescribing amoxicillin in tonsillitis, since it may precipitate a maculopapular rash if the patient has Epstein–Barr virus.
- If patient unable to take oral medication, consider admission for IV rehydration and antibiotics.

Quinsy

Quinsy is a peritonsillar collection of pus, secondary to acute tonsillitis. Treatment consists of IV antibiotics (co-amoxiclav) with ENT referral for surgical drainage.

Acute neck abscesses

Children with superficial abscesses will present with a hot, tender, inflamed fluctuant neck swelling. Occasionally children can develop deep space neck abscesses, which are not so obvious clinically but do have the potential for airway compromise.

Causative organisms:

- *Staphylococcus aureus*
- *Streptococcus pyogenes* (GAS)
- *Anaerobes*

Management

- Start a broad spectrum antibiotic with anaerobic cover (e.g. co-amoxiclav: amoxicillin/clavulanate)
- Refer for surgical drainage

- If presentation is more insidious, and abscess/neck lump is non responsive to antibiotics, consider atypical mycobacterial infection (requiring supportive management or complete excision)

Airway disorders

Acute epiglottitis

Acute epiglottitis is a bacterial infection of the throat, which has become uncommon thanks to the use of vaccinations. However, it causes diffuse swelling of the upper airway (supraglottis) and epiglottis, and is considered a dangerous condition due to the impending risk of loss of the airway. It is most commonly seen in children aged between 2 and 6 years of age.

Causative organisms:

- *Haemophilus influenzae* type B

Management
- Avoid distressing the child, due the risk of laryngospasm.
- Intubation is required and a consultant anaesthetist should be contacted.
- Once the airway has been secured, IV access can be obtained.
- IV antibiotics, usually cefotaxime, are given.
- Steroids, usually dexamethasone, are used to reduce inflammation and oedema of the airway. If a prolonged course of steroids is required, careful weaning is essential due to the risk of adrenal suppression.

Acute laryngotracheobronchitis (croup)

An acute viral infection of the upper airway, typically with parainfluenza, can lead to swelling and oedema of the subglottic area. This can lead to the development of stridor and a harsh, barking cough typical of croup. Children with croup differ from those with acute epiglottitis, as they usually do not appear toxic.

Management
- Assess the child. Conservative management may be appropriate if symptoms are not too severe.
- If signs of increased work of breathing, give the following.
  - Steroids (e.g. oral dexamethasone – recommended dose 0.5–1.0 mg/kg body weight), which are beneficial through their anti-inflammatory effect on laryngeal mucosal oedema
  - Adrenaline nebulisers (reserved for moderate to severe croup; beneficial through adrenergic stimulation)
  - Humidified oxygen

- If no improvement, or there are signs that the child is tiring, consider early involvement of paediatric anaesthetist for possible intubation.

Acute stridor

Stridor is defined as noisy breathing caused by partial obstruction of the upper airway, at the level of the larynx or below the larynx. It can be inspiratory, biphasic or expiratory.

Congenital causes

- Laryngomalacia
- Vocal cord palsy
- Subglottic stenosis
- Tracheomalacia

Acquired causes

- Infection (see above)
- Trauma
- Foreign body
- Allergy

Management

- This depends on the underlying cause, the severity of airway compromise, and the severity of symptoms of increased work of breathing.
- Seek early advice from an ENT specialist.
- Consider:
  - Nebulised adrenaline (as with croup)
  - Steroids (dexamethasone/hydrocortisone)
  - Humidified oxygen
  - Heliox, if available; heliox is a mixture of oxygen and helium, and due to its low density increases laminar flow in the airway

Conclusions

- ENT disorders are common in childhood, particularly infections.
- Be aware of local guidelines.
- For common conditions such as AOM, avoid unnecessary antibiotic prescriptions.
- When systemic antibiotics are indicated, use the most narrow spectrum agent when suitable, e.g. amoxicillin (rather than amoxicillin/clavulanate).
- Consider topical treatment if appropriate.
- Abscesses need to be surgically drained.

References

1 Lieberthal AS *et al*. The diagnosis and management of acute otitis media. *Pediatrics* 2013; 131(3): e964–e999.

2 Phillips JS *et al*. Evidence review and ENT-UK consensus report for the use of aminoglycoside-containing ear drops in the presence of an open middle ear. *Clin Otolaryngol* 2007; 32(5): 330–336.

3 Fokkens WJ *et al*. European position paper on rhinosinusitis and nasal polyps. *Rhinology* 2012; 50 (suppl. 23): 1–299.

4 Scottish Intercollegiate Guidelines Network (SIGN). Management of sore throat and indications for tonsillectomy. www.sign.ac.uk/sign-117-management-of-sore-throat-and-indications-for-tonsillectomy.html

55

Medical therapy in dermatology

TEJP Hopmans, M Hennekam, Y Liem and S Pasmans

Introduction

Medical treatments of skin diseases include topical, intralesional and systemic medication. In this chapter we discuss topical therapy in general, anti-inflammatory drugs, anti-infective drugs and the treatment of pruritus.

The learning objectives of this chapter are:

➤ to understand the key principles of topical therapy in paediatric dermatological conditions
➤ to know how to choose appropriate vehicles and quantities
➤ to be familiar with dosage calculation for creams/ointments
➤ to understand the main treatment options for inflammatory diseases of the skin, including both topical and systemic treatments
➤ to recognise the indications for and potential adverse effects of treatment with corticosteroids.

Topical therapy – the basics

The benefits of topical treatment include direct drug delivery to the target site of action and reduced systemic toxicity. Side-effects may still occur, especially when skin absorption is enhanced (see Box 1).[1-4]

Box 1 Situations in which percutaneous absorption is increased[1-7]

- Premature neonates
- Younger children (due to relatively large skin surface in relation to the body mass index)
- Long-term application on large surfaces of skin
- An impaired skin barrier (e.g. burns)

- Treatment in skin regions with thin stratum corneum (e.g. skin of the face, scrotum and eyelids)
- Treatment in body folds
- Treatment under occlusion
- During the use of preparations with increased potency or higher concentrations of active substance
- Specific vehicles (e.g. ointments are more potent than creams)

Base ointments are used for external therapy. They do not contain any specific/targeted pharmacologically active substances and are also used as a vehicle for specific drugs. Preparations that contain a relatively high percentage of water are cooling and drying, as the water evaporates. Fatty ointments protect damaged skin. For the success of topical treatment, not only is the correct drug important but also the correct vehicle. Various bases/vehicles are listed in Box 2.

Box 2 The main bases/vehicles used in dermatological products[1-4,8]

Gel: aqueous emulsion. Suitable for application on face and scalp.
Lotion: liquid vehicle. Lotions have a cooling effect and are often used for application on hairy areas. Shake lotions contain an insoluble powder.
Cream: semi-solid emulsion of oil in water, which the skin quickly absorbs and is therefore comfortable to use.
Ointment: semi-solid grease or oil, containing little or no water. Ointments are suitable for dry lesions. Ointments can be occlusive (sealing; i.e. trapping moisture from the body, thereby increasing absorption through the skin).
Paste: stiff preparations containing high proportions of powder.

Quantities required

In order to apply the right dose (especially concerning corticosteroid), the 'fingertip unit' (FTU) can be used. The amount of cream or ointment that can be applied to the adult terminal phalanx is approximately equal to 0.5 g.[2,9,10]

In practice, the use of the FTU significantly helps to avoid overdosing and underdosing. Table 1 shows how many FTUs per body part are needed. It is important that the patient applies the correct amount of cream or ointment and that the doctor prescribes a sufficient quantity.[1-3,9]

Age	FTUs						Mass (g)
	Face and neck	Arm and hand	Leg and foot	Torso (front)	Torso (back)	Complete body	Complete body per week with application once per day*
3–12 months	1	1	1.5	1	1.5	8.5	30 grams
1–2 years	1.5	1.5	2	2	3	13.5	47 grams
3–5 years	1.5	2	3	3	3.5	18	63 grams
6–10 years	2	2.5	4.5	3.5	5	24.5	86 grams
Adult	2.5	4	8	7	7	40	140 grams

Table 1 Quantifying fingertip units for different age groups of patients[1,2,9,10]

*Amount of cream for seven applications (i.e. application once per day for 1 week) of complete body (FTU complete body × 0.5 g × 7 days).

Treatment of inflammatory diseases

Corticosteroids

- Topical corticosteroid therapy has anti-inflammatory, vasoconstrictive and antimitotic activity.
- Corticosteroid preparations are classified into four classes (see Table 2), each class increasing in efficacy.
- In addition to potency, therapeutic effectiveness is also influenced by:
  - The base in which the corticosteroid is incorporated (ointments are generally more effective than creams, because their occlusive properties support skin penetration)
  - The presence of penetration-promoting substances (e.g. urea, salicylic acid, propylene glycol)
  - The method of application (occlusion enhances penetration)[1-3]

Side-effects: atrophy of the skin, acne-like skin conditions or perioral dermatitis, allergic contact dermatitis or tachyphylaxis. Systemic absorption (dependent on the class of dermatocorticosteroid used) can very rarely lead to adrenal suppression, Cushingoid appearance, growth retardation, increased intraocular pressure and increased risk of cataracts. Excessively rapid withdrawal may lead to an Addisonian crisis (acute adrenal failure, which can be life-threatening). These side-effects are only seen after prolonged and intensive use of the higher classes of dermatocorticosteroids.

Table 2 Corticosteroids classified into four classes[1-3]	
Class	**Common examples**
1 (mild)	Hydrocortisone 1% and 2.5% (Efcortelan®, Mildison®)
2 (moderate)	Clobetasone butyrate 0.05% (Eumovate®), Fludroxycortide 0.0125% (Haelan®)
3 (potent)	Betamethasone valerate 0.1% (Betnovate®), Beclomethasone dipropionate 0.025% (Propaderm®), Fluticasone propionate 0.05% (Cutivate®), Hydrocortisone butyrate 0.1% (Locoid®), Triamcinolone acetonide 0.1% (Adocortyl®), mometasone furoate 0.1% (Elocon®)
4 (very potent)	Clobetasol propionate 0.05% (Dermovate®), Diflucortolone valerate 0.3% (Nerisone forte®).

There remains a generalised 'phobia' of corticosteroids, and optimal use should be promoted to ensure inflammatory skin conditions are not under-treated. Topical corticosteroids should be used appropriately, i.e. sufficient to treat the skin condition, but therapy should not continue on uninflamed skin unless directed (e.g. proactive treatments to prevent flares of atopic eczema). Use of the FTU helps to reduce the risk of side-effects. The use of corticosteroids with a short biological half-life (e.g. fluticasone propionate) is thought to reduce systemic side-effects.[1-3,5,10,11]

Other topical treatments of inflammatory dermatoses

Vitamin D3 derivatives

- Include calcitriol and calcipotriol
- Precise mechanism of action unknown
- Effects thought due to inhibition of keratinocyte proliferation and induction of differentiation
- Used in topical treatment of psoriasis
- Efficacy comparable to class 3 corticosteroids
- Do not cause skin atrophy, in contrast to corticosteroids

Side-effects: irritation, dry skin, urticaria, pruritus, hypercalcaemia. These agents may cause reduced levels of endogenous vitamin D, hence it is advised to monitor vitamin D levels in children. It is preferable not to use these agents on the face and body folds, because of increased risk of irritation.[1-3,12]

Dithranol

- Used in specialist clinical settings for treatment of subacute or chronic psoriasis

- Inactivates various enzymes (e.g. glucose-6-phosphate dehydrogenase), binds to DNA, inhibits mitosis, and induces the formation of free radicals
- Overall, leads to prevention of cell growth and cell proliferation
- When salicylic acid or liquid nitrogen are not sufficiently effective for warts, dithranol is also used in combination with salicylic acid

Side-effects: burning sensation and irritation, temporary purple-brown discoloration of skin/nails/hair, and permanent stains of clothing and bedding (do not wash out). The face and body folds should not be treated. We also recommend avoiding use on the scalp in children. Furthermore, be very careful when using dithranol on the hands, because of the risk of conjunctivitis in case of eye contact; recommend using gloves when applying. During 'short contact therapy' for psoriasis, the therapeutic effect is somewhat reduced, but the therapy leads to less irritation and minimises other adverse effects.[1,2,13]

Coal tar

- Used as treatment for psoriasis of the skin and scalp, chronic eczema and seborrheic dermatitis of the scalp (dandruff)
- Reduces number and size of epidermal cells, and thus the thickness of the epidermis
- Due to side-effects, and because it is not a standardised product, tar preparations are now rarely used

Side-effects: skin irritation, unpleasant odour, skin/hair discoloration, hypersensitivity phenomena, carcinogenic effects, phototoxicity. Do not use on damaged skin; contact with the eyes should also be avoided.[1,2,8,13]

Topical calcineurin inhibitors

- Include pimecrolimus and tacrolimus
- Used in the treatment of resistant atopic dermatitis from 3 years of age
- Inhibit calcium-dependent signal transduction in T-cells and thereby inhibit transcription and synthesis of various cytokines, preventing T-cell activation
- Do not cause skin atrophy (unlike corticosteroids)

Side-effects: long term risks are currently unknown. Often transient skin irritation and burning occur at the start of therapy. Treatment may be associated with a greater risk of herpes infections. Calcineurin inhibitors should not be used in infected eczema and acute viral infections of the skin, and treatment should only be restarted after recovery from infection. Although a causal relationship has not been established, there are rare cases of associated malignancies, including (skin) lymphoma and skin cancer. Neither pimecrolimus nor tacrolimus are licensed for use in children under 2 years of age, and they should not be used during pregnancy or lactation. During treatment, exposure to sunlight (UV radiation) should be minimised.

There is a risk of vaccination failure, therefore it is recommended to vaccinate before the start of treatment or after a treatment free period of 14 days (or 28 with live, attenuated microorganisms).[1,2,11,13]

Systemic agents in inflammatory dermatoses

Prednisone/prednisolone

- Has anti-inflammatory, immunosuppressive and vasoconstrictive effects

Side-effects: adrenal suppression, increased susceptibility to infection, diabetes mellitus, loss of muscle mass, osteoporosis, psychosis, delayed healing of an existing peptic ulcer. Growth of children treated with corticosteroids should be observed, as growth inhibition is a risk[2,13] (see 'Corticosteroids', 'Side-effects and cautions', chapter 52).

Methotrexate

- Folic acid antagonist
- Inhibits nucleic acid synthesis and cell division
- Used in treatment of psoriasis
- Dosage required is significantly lower than for cytostatic therapy; however, treatment lasts much longer.
- Consider serious side-effects and drug–drug interactions.
- During treatment, monitor full blood count and kidney and liver function (at least monthly).
- Given the potential for severe mutagenic and teratogenic effects in both men and women, contraceptive measures should be used up to 3 months after the end of therapy.
- Avoid abrupt discontinuation (as patient may experience more severe psoriasis than at baseline: the rebound phenomenon).
- Do not use in children < 3 years due to insufficient safety/efficacy data.[2,11,12]

Keratolytic drugs

Salicylic acid

- Acts as a keratolytic
- Also has some anti-inflammatory, anti-bacterial and fungicidal activity
- For local application at concentrations of 3–10% in hyperkeratosis and 17% in warts

Side-effects: Irritation may occur with continuous use. After use on large areas of skin and/or under occlusion, systemic symptoms of acute salicylate intoxication can occur. In children, salicylic acid should only be used on small areas of skin (e.g. warts, corns). For large skin areas, choose a maximum concentration of 3%. Use in children < 2 years is not recommended. Caution is advised in children < 4 years. [2,11,12]

Urea

- Hygroscopic and keratolytic
- Loosens the dense structure of the horny layer, thereby improving skin penetration of creams/ointments
- Also holds water, reducing skin dryness
- Can be used in asteatosis (too dry, scaly skin due to water loss), ichthyosis and hyperkeratotic skin disorders

Side-effects: Local irritation (usually transient) especially on the face and damaged/inflamed skin; more common in young children. Use cautiously on the face or damaged skin. Do not use near the eyes.[2,13]

Anti-infective drugs

Antimicrobial agents

There are several antimicrobials that can be used topically; key examples are discussed below.

Fusidic acid

- Narrow spectrum of activity, especially active against Staphylococci, but Streptococci are also sensitive
- Commonly prescribed for impetigo and folliculitis

Mupirocin

- Effective against Staphylococci and Streptococci
- Note, nasal mupirocin is commonly used in methicillin resistant *Staphylococcus aureus* (MRSA) decolonisation protocols, together with chlorhexidine gluconate wash for the skin

Tetracyclines

- Broad spectrum activity against many Gram positive microorganisms (such as *Staphylococcus* and *Streptococcus*) and Gram-negative microorganisms
- Safety and effectiveness not yet established for children < 11 years

Silver sulfadiazine

- Bactericidal, broad spectrum activity
- Covers both Gram positive and Gram negative bacteria

General principles

- Do not use antimicrobial agents for longer than necessary.
- There is a risk of antibiotic resistance, in particular with fusidic acid containing topical treatments.
- Note that oral anti-infective agents are often used in bacterial skin conditions because of the increased effectiveness.

Topical antiseptics: chlorhexidine

- Topical antiseptics can be preferable for prophylaxis against cutaneous infections.
- Chlorhexidine cream is bactericidal.
- Chlorhexidine can be used for bacterial skin infections.
- Broad spectrum of activity against both Gram positive and Gram negative bacteria.
- Not effective against bacterial or fungal spores.
- Damages bacterial cell wall; after cell penetration, causes cytoplasmic coagulation, killing the cell.
- Organic material (pus, blood) reduces the effect.
- Due to skin adhesion, chlorhexidine remains effective for approximately 6 hours after application.
- Note that alcohol also has a disinfecting effect.

Side-effects: (especially with prolonged use or use on mucous membranes or broken skin): irritation, contact dermatitis, urticaria, photosensitivity. Because of the risk of severe irritation or chemical burns, caution should be observed when prescribing chlorhexidine to young children, especially <2 years of age. Specific alerts have recently been issued regarding chlorhexidine use as a skin disinfectant for preterm neonates, which can cause severe chemical burns.[14] In a preparation containing alcohol, it may also cause dry and chapped skin, and pain in the presence of fissures. Furthermore, erythema and oedema can occur. Hypersensitivity reactions are also possible (including anaphylaxis). Contact with eyes, brain, meninges or middle ear (especially in damaged eardrum) should be avoided. Chlorhexidine can stain linen.[1,2,4,11–13]

Antifungals

Antifungals are active against dermatophytes and/or yeasts. Local therapy is often used. In extensive, resistant or frequently recurrent infections, an oral antifungal may be used.

Imidazoles

- Include ketoconazole, miconazole and clotrimazole
- Exert pharmacological effect by altering fungal cell membrane permeability

- Imidazoles often are the drugs of first choice, because of extensive experience
- Effective for most fungal infections in humans (in particular, yeasts and dermatophytes, *Candida* and *Malassezia furfur*)
- Also active against some Gram positive bacteria (although clinical relevance not yet demonstrated)
- In 2013, the European Medicines Agency suspended the marketing authorisation for oral ketoconazole as a treatment for fungal infections, in view of the risk of liver injury, so this agent should no longer be prescribed for this indication.[15]

Terbinafine

- Inhibits sterol synthesis in fungal cell membrane, by inhibiting the enzyme squalene epoxidase
- Thereby causes intracellular squalene accumulation and a lack of ergosterol, resulting in cell death
- Used in tinea capitis, onychomycosis
- Used for other dermatomycoses when imidazoles are insufficiently effective or not tolerated

Side-effects: local reactions such as skin dryness, irritation, burning, allergic reactions, and paradoxical worsening of the index condition. In oral application, the most common side-effects are: gastrointestinal disturbances (including abdominal pain, bloating, nausea and diarrhoea), muscle and joint pain, and skin reactions (e.g. erythema and urticaria). Occasionally a change in (or loss of) taste occurs, which usually resolves within weeks after treatment ends. Rare side-effects include hearing loss, liver function abnormalities, Stevens–Johnson syndrome, anaphylactic reactions and haematological abnormalities. Contraindications: severe renal impairment (creatinine clearance < 30 mL/min) and severe hepatic impairment. There are limited studies on terbinafine use in children, therefore caution is advised in children.

Selenium sulfide (suspension)

- Active against *Malassezia furfur* – a fungus (yeast), part of natural flora of superficial layers of skin and scalp
- Must be used on intact scalp

Side-effects and cautions: local irritation – consider treatment discontinuation. Avoid contact with the eyes or mucous membranes. Selenium can discolour damaged or grey/white hair. There are no studies on selenium sulfide use in children, therefore caution is advised.

Griseofulvin (oral)

- Fungistatic activity against dermatophytes
- Inhibits mitosis and thereby stops fungal cell division

- Concentrated in the keratin (hair and nails, and in superficial layers of skin)
- Protects newly formed cells against dermatophytes
- Main indication in children is tinea capitis (*Microsporum canis*): 6–8 week course shown by randomised studies to be safe and effective in children
- Intake with milk or high fat foods recommended
- Be cautious in renal impairment and blood disorders
- During prolonged therapy, monitor kidney function, liver function and blood counts regularly, every 3–4 weeks

Side-effects: headache, gastrointestinal disturbances, hypersensitivity reactions including urticaria, rash and rarely angioedema. Sometimes fatigue, thirst, dizziness and insomnia. Rarely, lupus-like symptoms or exacerbation of existing systemic lupus erythematosus. In children, griseofulvin can have oestrogenic effects (including gynaecomastia).[1,2,11,12]

Antivirals

Aciclovir

- Blocks viral DNA synthesis
- Active against herpes simplex virus types 1 and 2 (local or systemic treatment)
- Active against varicella zoster virus (systemic only)
- Duration of skin lesions (eruptions) only slightly shortened in some cases and only during the first (primary) genital herpes infection
- Can irritate mucous membranes; avoid contact
- Use oral aciclovir for patients with severe genital herpes infections
- Consider oral administration in immunocompromised patients
- Oral aciclovir is also very important in management of eczema herpeticum
- In immunodeficiency, note potential for resistant viruses

Antiparasitic agents

Permethrin

- Kills both lice and nits
- Is also scabicide
- In lice, causes disruption of sodium ion transport in nerve cell membranes
- Human toxicity is rare, because body quickly converts to non-toxic metabolites (excreted in the urine)

Side-effects: are usually transient skin complaints, which may also be associated with scabies: burning or stinging, erythema, oedema, eczema, skin rashes and itching up to 4 weeks after treatment. There is some resistance to permethrin. No other skin preparations should be used during treatment with a scabicide agent, since they can promote systemic absorption of the scabicide.

Benzyl benzoate

- Kills mites: particularly effective against *Sarcoptes scabiei*
- Does not kills the eggs, therefore less effective than permethrin
- Low toxicity

Lindane

- An insecticide, acaricide (targeting ticks and mites) and scabicide (by the stimulation of the central nervous system of the mite).
- In scabies, lindane kills both mites and eggs.
- In children aged 2 months to 3 years, permethrin is preferable because of the risk of human neurotoxicity caused by accidental ingestion of lindane.

Side-effects: neurotoxicity (see above); skin irritation and contact dermatitis with repeated use. Inhaling lindane vapour may cause headache, nausea, vomiting and irritation of eyes, nose and throat. General caution in children, given increased risk of neurotoxicity compared with adults.

Malathion

- Insecticidal: inhibits cholinesterase
- Used in *Pediculosis capitis* (head lice) and *Pediculosis pubis* (pubic lice)

Side-effects: It has a very unpleasant odour. Sensitisation and hypersensitivity reactions may occur. It may temporarily increase dandruff. Neurological symptoms in young children are possible with frequently repeated use. The safety and effectiveness of malathion is uncertain in children <6 years of age. Note that malathion lotion is flammable.[2,11-13]

Pruritus

The treatment of itch/pruritis is primarily focused on finding the underlying cause (e.g. underlying skin disease, uraemia, liver disease with cholestasis, diabetes, anaemia, hyperthyroidism, hypothyroidism, parasitic infestations, gout, leukaemia or lymphomas). When possible, a therapy targeted towards the primary cause should be started. Symptomatic treatment is also possible. As previously mentioned, preparations containing plenty of water are cooling and drying, because the water evaporates. However, for dry skin, bases containing a lot of water (see Box 2) should be avoided, because they desiccate the skin, which worsens itching. Antipruritic agents, such as 1% levomenthol, cause capillary dilation, resulting in a cooling effect and analgesia. Levomenthol also triggers cold-sensitive neurons, which gives a brief cooling sensation. Local anaesthetics (e.g. lidocaine) sometimes reduce itching, but their effect is marginal. Oral antihistamines are often used, but will only be effective when there is a reaction in which histamine is released.[1,2]

Conclusions

It is important to choose an appropriate vehicle when prescribing for dermatological conditions, and to prescribe adequate amounts. FTUs can be used to estimate the correct amount of cream or ointment. Advocate optimal application of topical corticosteroids, which should be used neither too excessively nor too sparingly. Corticosteroid 'phobia' should be addressed: it should be stressed that these agents are of more benefit than harm when used correctly. In view of the risk of antimicrobial resistance, use anti-infective agents for the minimum possible duration.

References

1   de Groot AC,Toonstra J. Behandeling van huidafwijkingen. In: *Dermatologie en Venereologie in de Praktijk*. Den Haag: Boom Lemma Uitgevers, 2012: 65–81.
2   Zorginstituut Nederland. Farmacotherapeutisch Kompas. The Netherlands. www.farmacotherapeutischkompas.nl
3   Gawkrodger DJ. Basics of medical therapy. In: *Dermatology*. China: Elsevier, 2008: 22–24.
4   McKoy K. Principles of topical dermatologic therapy. In: *Merck Manual*. 2013. www.merckmanuals.com/professional/dermatologic_disorders/principles_of_topical_dermatologic_therapy/principles_of_topical_dermatologic_therapy.html
5   van Velsen SGA *et al*. The self-administered eczema area and severity index in children with moderate to severe atopic dermatitis: better estimation of ad body surface area than severity. *Pediatr Dermatol* 2010; 27(5): 470–475. www.researchgate.net/profile/Suzanne_Pasmans/publication/227667444_The_SelfAdministered_Eczema_Area_and_Severity_Index_in_Children_with_Moderate_to_Severe_Atopic_Dermatitis_Better_Estimation_of_AD_Body_Surface_Area_Than_Severity/links/0fcfd50a3e68ff0ae1000000.pdf
6   Lev-Tov H, Maibach HI. Regional variations in percutaneous absorption. *J Drugs Dermatol* 2012; 11: e48–51.
7   DermNet New Zealand Trust. Topical medications for skin conditions. www.dermnetnz.org/treatments/topical-treatment.html
8   Long CC *et al*. A practical guide to topical therapy in children. *Br J Dermatol* 1998; 138(2): 293–296.
9   UMCUtrecht. Vingertop als maateenheid voor het zalven. www.umcutrecht.nl/getattachment/Ziekenhuis/Ziekte-onderzoek-behandeling/Behandelingen/hormoonzalven-bij-eczeem/Vingertopalsmaateenheidvoorhetzalven.pdf.aspx
10 van Velsen SG *et al*. The potency of clobetasol propionate: serum levels of clobetasol propionate and adrenal function during therapy with 0.05% clobetasol propionate in patients with severe atopic dermatitis. *J Dermatolog Treat* 2012; 23(1): 16–20.
11 Nederlands Kenniscentrum voor Farmacotherapie bij Kinderen (NKFK). Kinderformularium. www.kinderformularium.nl
12 Drugs.com. Information from Drugs.com. www.drugs.com

13   Liem TBY. Geneesmiddelen uit het Handboek kinderdermatologie: nader belicht. In: Oranje AP, de Waard-van der Spek FB. *Handboek Kinderdermatologie,* 2nd edn. Maarssen: Elsevier gezondheidszorg, 2005: 688–756.

14   European Medicines Agency, Pharmacovigilance Risk Assessment Committee. PRAC recommendations on signals. Section 1.2, Chlorhexidine cutaneous solutions – chemical injury including burns when used in skin disinfection in premature infants. 2014. www.ema.europa.eu/docs/en_GB/document_library/PRAC_recommendation_on_signal/2014/09/WC500174026.pdf

15   European Medicines Agency. European Medicines Agency recommends suspension of marketing authorisations for oral ketoconazole. EMA/458028/2013. 2013. www.ema.europa.eu/docs/en_GB/document_library/Press_release/2013/07/WC500146613.pdf

Further recommended reading

Amir J *et al.* Treatment of herpes simplex gingivostomatitis with aciclovir in children: a randomised double blind placebo controlled study. *BMJ* 1997; 314: 1800–1803.

Dhar S *et al.* Systemic side-effects of topical corticosteroids. *Indian J Dermatol* 2014; 59(5): 460–464.

Fuller LC *et al.* British Association of Dermatologists' guidelines for the management of tinea capitis. *Br J Dermatol* 2014; 171(3): 454–463.

Gilbert M. Topical 2% mupirocin versus 2% fusidic acid ointment in the treatment of primary and secondary skin infections. *J Am Acad Dermatol* 1989; 20: 1083–1087.

Kwok CS *et al.* Topical treatments for cutaneous warts. *Br J Dermatol* 2011; 165(2): 233–246.

Livingood CS *et al.* Effect of prolonged griseofulvin administration on liver, hematopoietic system, and kidney. *Arch Dermatol* 1960; 81: 760–765.

Pariser D. Topical corticosteroids and topical calcineurin inhibitors in the treatment of atopic dermatitis: focus on percutaneous absorption. *Am J Ther* 2009; 16: 264–273.

van Geel MJ *et al.* Systemic treatments in paediatric psoriasis: a systematic evidence-based update. *J Eur Acad Dermatol Venerol* 2015; 29(3): 425–237.

White DG *et al.* Topical antibiotics in the treatment of superficial skin infections in general practice – a comparison of mupirocin with sodium fusidate. *J Infect* 1989; 18: 221–229.

56

Immunological products

M Taranto and N Klein

Introduction

Non-specific and disease-specific antibody products are used for children as primary prevention in immunodeficiencies, as treatment of autoinflammatory conditions and as secondary prevention in proven or presumed infection exposure. Immunoglobulin products contain immunoglobulin G (IgG) and are prepared from pools of at least 1000 (up to 50 000) donations of human plasma from healthy donors. As such, immunoglobulin is a limited resource, and judicious use according to proven indications is fundamental. For example, in the UK it is currently imported, due to the possible risk of transmitting variant Creutzfeldt–Jakob disease (vCJD) from British plasma, for which there is no screening test.

The key learning objectives are this chapter are:

➤ to recognise the indications for immunoglobulin products
➤ to identify the recommended specialist consultations prior to immunoglobulin prescription
➤ to understand the main risks, side effects and monitoring of immunoglobulin therapies.

Normal immunoglobulin

Human normal immunoglobulin contains polyclonal IgG antibodies that include antibodies to many microorganisms, such as measles, rubella, varicella and other viruses that are currently prevalent in the general population.

Indications for immunoglobulin

The UK national guideline for the use of immunoglobulin incorporates a colour-coded system to classify indications based on priority to support the regulation of the use of immunoglobulin in times of shortage.[1]

Red indications are assigned to conditions where there is a risk to life without treatment. Blue indications are those for which there is reasonable evidence, but where other treatment options exist. Grey indications are those for which the evidence base is weak. In addition to the UK national guideline,[1] analogous guidelines are available in other countries.

Immunoglobulin for replacement therapy

Primary and secondary antibody deficiency states

There are several primary immunodeficiencies where immunoglobulin replacement is an essential, often lifelong, therapy.[2] They include common variable immunodeficiency, X-linked agammaglobulinaemia and combined immunodeficiencies, including severe combined immunodeficiency.

Patients with long term antibody deficiency states can receive intravenous immunoglobulin (IVIg) or subcutaneous immunoglobulin (SCIg). SCIg has many potential advantages over IVIg. The ease of administration and fewer side-effects allow patients to self-administer their therapy at home. SCIg provides steadier plasma IgG levels, mainly because the frequency of infusions is greater, whereas IVIg is associated with peaks and troughs.

Consultation with an immunologist should establish a diagnosis and an appropriate immunoglobulin replacement plan. In the UK, a generally accepted guide for immunoglobulin dosing in children with a primary immunodeficiency is 0.4–0.6 g/kg of IVIg every 3–4 weeks to provide trough plasma concentrations of about 7–8 g/L. Regular monitoring of clinical outcomes and trough plasma IgG levels is necessary in ongoing dosing adjustments. Larger doses may be required in certain disease states where either the desired trough level is higher, such as in immunodeficiency with bronchiectasis, or the plasma half-life of immunoglobulin is reduced due to consumption or protein loss.

Normal immunoglobulin may also be administered by intramuscular injection for the protection of high risk contacts against viruses such as hepatitis A and measles, and for varicella where varicella specific immunoglobulin is unavailable.

Immunoglobulin for immunomodulation

The other main use for immunoglobulin is for immunomodulation in a variety of autoimmune and autoinflammatory conditions. Immunomodulation effectively means dampening down the immune system through binding to pathogenic antigen targets or 'mopping up' circulating autoantibodies (alloantibodies in the case of some neonatal conditions). IVIg for immunomodulation is generally short term (less than 3 months) and at higher doses – typically 1–2 g/kg per treatment. Dosing recommendations, including frequency and duration of therapy, vary between different indications. For conditions where IVIg is needed for immunomodulation, the relevant subspecialists should be consulted.

The following are some of the 'red' indications for immunoglobulin. Please refer to the National Clinical Guidelines for the complete list of indications for immunoglobulin.

Haematological conditions
- Haemolytic disease of the newborn
- Immune thrombocytopenic purpura

Neurological conditions
- Chronic inflammatory demyelinating polyradiculoneuropathy
- Guillain–Barré syndrome

Other immune mediated inflammatory conditions
- Kawasaki disease
- Toxic epidermal necrolysis
- Stevens–Johnson syndrome

Formulations

- In the UK, IVIg products are available in concentrations ranging between 50 mg/mL and 100 mg/mL, while SCIg products are available in concentrations ranging between 160 mg/mL and 200 mg/mL.
- Immunoglobulin should appear clear and is usually colourless to a light yellow. Do not use an immunoglobulin product if it appears turbid or contains any sediment.
- Storage at 2–8°C is recommended.
- Immunoglobulin products are presented ready for use and do not require reconstitution.
- These products contain no antimicrobial preservative and must be used immediately after opening the vial.
- Vials come in a range of volumes. Where possible, use vials that amount to the dose required and administer the entire vial.
- For regular immunoglobulin replacement, it is best practice not to switch products once commenced on a particular brand, as there is an increased risk of reactions or intolerance to an alternative product.

Administration

- Prior to commencing immunoglobulin therapy, the important tests to be conducted are: full blood count, immunoglobulin trough levels, hepatitis C virus, and renal and liver function; also take serum for long term storage.

- The product, dose, batch numbers and expiry date should always be recorded.
- Bring the product to room temperature.
- IVIg infusions should commence slowly and increase to the maximum rate as per the manufacturer's recommendations. Vital signs should be assessed before each rate increase.
- For SCIg, suitable infusion sites are thighs for infants and young toddlers, or the abdomen for older children. Local anaesthetic cream can be used.
- SCIg is generally infused over 30–90 minutes through one or more sites depending on the age and the amount of subcutaneous tissue of the child.

Pharmacokinetic notes

- IVIg is immediately bioavailable. For SCIg, peak levels are achieved in the recipient's circulation after 3–4 days.
- The plasma half-life for IgG is approximately 3 weeks.
- IgG and IgG complexes are broken down in the reticuloendothelial system.

Adverse effects

Immunoglobulin products are generally well tolerated, and severe reactions are rare. Plasma is processed to inactivate or remove pathogens; however, there remains an immeasurably small risk of transmitting infections.

Hypersensitivity reactions and anaphylaxis

As with many blood products, there is a risk of immune and non-immune mediated hypersensitivity reactions. Mild reactions such as flushing and headache may be rate dependent and may respond to a reduction in the rate of the infusion. For SCIg, swelling and redness at the site of the infusion is normal and disappears around 24 hours after the infusion.

Anaphylaxis is rare. The infusion should be ceased immediately and emergency anaphylaxis management commenced. Human normal immunoglobulin contains a small quantity of immunoglobulin A (IgA). Individuals with IgA deficiency can potentially develop IgA antibodies and have a greater risk of anaphylactic reactions with administration of IgA containing blood components. Some immunoglobulin products contain less IgA than others and could therefore be considered following such cases of anaphylaxis.

Other moderate to severe adverse reactions

Haemolysis: human normal immunoglobulin contains blood group antibodies, which may act as haemolysins by coating erythrocytes. This may result in a positive direct antiglobulin test and, occasionally, haemolytic anaemia.

Thromboembolic events: IVIg infusion may lead to a relative increase in blood viscosity. Rapid infusion should be avoided in patients at increased risk of thromboembolic and renal adverse events. Ensure that patients are well hydrated prior to infusion.

Renal impairment: patients receiving IVIg have an increased risk of renal failure or dysfunction.

Vaccination and serological considerations

Immunoglobulin administration may interfere with the development of an immune response to live attenuated virus vaccines, such as rubella, mumps and varicella, for up to 3 months. Parents should be informed that live attenuated virus vaccines (except for yellow fever vaccine) should not be given during this time.

After injection of immunoglobulin, the transitory rise of the various passively transferred antibodies in the patient's blood may result in misleading positive results in serological testing.

Disease specific immunoglobulins

There are several disease specific immunoglobulins that are indicated for use in circumstances where there is a high risk of infection.[3] These products are usually prepared by cold ethanol fractionation of plasma donated through routine blood bank collections or from plasma of hyperimmunised donors.

The potential side-effects and risks are similar to those for normal immunoglobulin products.

Hepatitis B immunoglobulin

The risk of perinatal transmission of hepatitis B virus (HBV) is up to 90% in infants born to hepatitis B e antigen (HBeAg) positive women, with the majority of these infants being at risk of chronic infection. Hepatitis B immunoglobulin (HBIG) administered in conjunction with the hepatitis B vaccine can prevent up to 90% of perinatal infections in high risk infants.

Dosing and administration notes

- In the UK, HBIG is available in 200 or 500 unit vials at a concentration of 100 units/mL for intramuscular administration.
- It is recommended that HBIG be administered in combination with the hepatitis B vaccine as soon as possible, but not later than 48 hours after birth in high risk babies or exposure in the case of older children. These injections should be administered at different sites.
- Should administration of HBIG be required within 4 weeks following HBV vaccination, then revaccination should be performed 3–4 months later.

Rabies immunoglobulin

Rabies is an invariably fatal zoonotic disease caused by exposure to saliva or nerve tissue of an animal infected with rabies virus or other lyssaviruses. Specific human rabies immunoglobulin (HRIG) administered in conjunction with the rabies vaccine is indicated following exposure of an unimmunised child to an animal in or from a country where the risk of rabies is high. Consultation with an infectious diseases physician is recommended before use.

Dosing and administration notes

- The dose of HRIG is 20 IU/kg for all ages.
- The site of wounds should be washed with soapy water, and appropriate anaesthetic used prior to infiltration of HRIG in and around all wounds, using as much of the calculated dose as possible. This is done to provide localised anti-rabies antibody protection. If infiltration of the whole volume is not possible or the wound has healed, the remainder of the HRIG should be administered intramuscularly at a site away from the rabies vaccine injection site.
- For wounds to fingers and hands, a fine gauge needle should be used to gently infiltrate HRIG, being careful not to cause adjacent tissue to turn pale.
- If the wounds are severe and the calculated volume of HRIG is inadequate for complete infiltration of all wounds (e.g. extensive dog bites in a young child), the HRIG should be diluted in saline to make up an adequate volume for the careful infiltration of all wounds.
- HRIG should not be used if 8 days or more have elapsed since the first dose of vaccine, as the HRIG may interfere with the immune response to the vaccine.
- HRIG is generally supplied in vials with a minimum titre of 150 units/mL. It is important to note that the potency of different batches, even within the same manufacturer, can vary, and must therefore be confirmed in order to provide the required dose on each individual case.

Tetanus immunoglobulin

Tetanus immunoglobulin (TIG) is indicated for all cases of clinical tetanus. It is also used for the management of tetanus-prone wounds in high risk cases, patients with humoral immunodeficiency, or where booster immunisations are not up to date. High risk is regarded as heavy contamination with material likely to contain tetanus spores and/or extensive devitalised tissue.

Dosing and administration notes

- In the UK, TIG is primarily available as 1 mL ampoules containing 250 units for intramuscular injection.

- The dose for post-exposure prevention is 250 units, or 500 units if more than 24 hours have elapsed or there is risk of heavy contamination following burns.
- For cases of clinical tetanus, the intramuscular dose is 150 units/kg, which should be administered across multiple sites. An intravenous preparation for administration at a dose of 5000–10 000 units by slow infusion is also available. Consultation with an infectious disease physician is recommended.
- Clinicians should remember to also administer the tetanus vaccine in patients whose immunisations are not up to date, and to consider the need for antibiotics.
- TIG provides immediate protection that lasts for a period of 3–4 weeks.

Varicella zoster immunoglobulin

Varicella zoster immunoglobulin (VZIG) prophylaxis is recommended for individuals who fulfil all of the following three criteria:

- Significant exposure to varicella zoster virus (VZV), either as chickenpox or herpes zoster (considerations for the definition of a significant exposure include the type of VZV infection in the index case, the timing of exposure in relation to the onset of rash in the index case, and the closeness and duration of contact).
- A clinical condition that increases the risk of severe varicella. This includes immunosuppressed patients, neonates and pregnant women (refer to national guidelines for specific recommendations).
- No detectable antibodies to VZV (note that VZIG is not necessary in an immunocompromised VZV contact who has proven recent evidence of detectable antibodies).

VZIG has no proven use in the treatment of established varicella or VZV infection.

Dosing and administration notes
- VZIG is available in 250 mg 2–3 mL vials, containing a minimum potency of 100 IU/mL, for intramuscular injection.
- The UK recommended dosage for VZIG is age banded:
  - 0–5 years, 250 mg (one vial)
  - 6–10 years, 500 mg (two vials)
  - 11–14 years, 750 mg (three vials)
  - 15 years or over, 1000 mg (four vials)
- VZIG should be given as early as possible in the incubation period (within 96 hours of exposure), but may have some efficacy if administered up to 10 days post exposure.

- In the case of a second exposure after 3 weeks, a further dose is required.
- In contacts where intramuscular injections are contraindicated, intravenous normal immunoglobulin can be used at a dose of 0.2 g/kg instead to produce serum VZV antibody levels equivalent to those achieved with VZIG.

Conclusions

Guidelines for immunoglobulin use regulate its supply so that it is available for critical indications. Specialist consultation should be sought prior to immunoglobulin prescription. Immunoglobulin therapy is generally well tolerated, but appropriate training and knowledge is required to ensure safe administration and monitoring.

References

1 Department of Health. *Clinical Guidelines for Immunoglobulin Use*, 2nd edition update (updated 15 November 2011). London: Department of Health, 2011. www.gov.uk/government/publications/clinical-guidelines-for-immunoglobulin-use-second-edition-update
2 Immune Deficiency Foundation. Immunoglobulin therapy & other medical therapies for antibody deficiencies. http://primaryimmune.org/treatment-information/immunoglobulin-therapy
3 Department of Health. *Immunisation against infectious disease* (the Green Book) (last updated 2 September 2014). London: Public Health England. www.gov.uk/government/collections/immunisation-against-infectious-disease-the-green-book

57

Prescribing vaccines: an overview

CP O'Sullivan and PT Heath

Introduction

The age at which childhood vaccinations are given is guided by the national immunisation schedule of the country the children live in. Immunisation schedules recommend vaccines at particular ages based on the age specific risk of a disease and the way the child's immune system will respond to the vaccine. The schedule also indicates when booster doses, which are given to provide continued protection, should be given. Subsequent vaccinations are recommended when appropriate for the child's circumstances (e.g. for travel).[1]

The learning objectives of this chapter are:

➤ to recognise the key features of the current UK vaccination schedule
➤ to understand that certain patient groups have specific vaccination requirements and/or contraindications, including immunocompromised children, children with HIV and premature infants
➤ to be aware of adverse reactions to vaccines, including programme related and vaccine related adverse events following immunisation.

UK vaccination schedule:

At the time of writing, the UK immunisation schedule (summarised in Table 1) recommends:

- three infant doses of the diphtheria, tetanus, pertussis, polio, *Haemophilus influenzae* type b and hepatitis B vaccine (DTaP/IPV/Hib/HepB), given at 2, 3 and 4 months
- two doses of the pneumococcal conjugate vaccine, given at 2 and 4 months
- two doses of the oral rotavirus vaccine
- two doses of Bexsero® (known as the meningitis B vaccine), given at 2 and 4 months
- one dose of the live vaccine against measles, mumps and rubella (MMR), given within 1 month of the first birthday

Table 1 UK routine immunisation schedule for children (date: July 2017)

Age due	Diseases protected against	Vaccine given and trade name		Usual site
8 weeks old	Diphtheria, tetanus, pertussis (whooping cough), polio, *Haemophilus influenzae* type b (Hib), and HepB	DTaP/IPV/Hib/HepB	Infanrix Hexa	Thigh
	Pneumococcal (13 serotypes)	Pneumococcal conjugate vaccine (PCV)	Prevenar 13	Thigh
	Meningococcal group B (MenB)	MenB	Bexsero	Left thigh
	Rotavirus gastroenteritis	Rotavirus	Rotarix	By mouth
12 weeks old	Diphtheria, tetanus, pertussis (whooping cough), polio, *Haemophilus influenzae* type b (Hib), and HepB	DTaP/IPV/Hib/HepB	Infanrix Hexa	Thigh
	Rotavirus	Rotavirus	Rotarix	By mouth
16 weeks old	Diphtheria, tetanus, pertussis (whooping cough), polio, *Haemophilus influenzae* type b (Hib), and HepB	DTaP/IPV/Hib/HepB	Infanrix Hexa	Thigh
	MenB	MenB	Bexsero	Left thigh
	Pneumococcal (13 serotypes)	PCV	Prevenar 13	Thigh

Table 1 (*Continued*)

Age due	Diseases protected against	Vaccine given and trade name		Usual site
1 year old	Hib and MenC	Hib/MenC booster	Menitorix	Upper arm/thigh
	Pneumococcal (13 serotypes)	PCV booster	Prevenar 13	Upper arm/thigh
	Measles, mumps and rubella (German measles)	MMR	MMR VaxPRO or Priorix	Upper arm/thigh
	MenB	MenB booster	Bexsero	Left thigh
2–8 years old (including children in school years 1, 2 and 3)	Influenza (each year from September)	Live attenuated influenza vaccine	Fluenz Tetra	Both nostrils
3 years, 4 months old	Diphtheria, tetanus, pertussis and polio	DTaP/IPV	Infanrix IPV or Repevax	Upper arm
	Measles, mumps and rubella	MMR (check first dose given)	MMR VaxPRO3 or Priorix	Upper arm
Girls aged 12–13 years	Cervical cancer caused by human papillomavirus (HPV) types 16 and 18 (and genital warts caused by types 6 and 11)	HPV (two doses 6–24 months apart)	Gardasil	Upper arm
14 years old (school year 9)	Tetanus, diphtheria and polio	Td/IPV (check MMR status)	Revaxis	Upper arm
	Meningococcal groups A, C, W, and Y disease	MenACWY	Nimenrix or Menveo	Upper arm

Boosters are given at these points:

- In the second year of life – of the Hib/MenC, meningitis B vaccine and pneumococcal conjugate vaccines
- From 3 years, 4 months – of the diphtheria, tetanus, pertussis and polio vaccines, and the MMR
- In the mid teens – for tetanus, diphtheria and polio (Td/IPV) and MenC, as part of the MenACWY conjugate vaccine

The intranasal influenza vaccine is being phased in over several years for the 2–17 years age group. The human papilloma virus vaccine is recommended for girls at age 12–14 years: two doses 6 months apart. The varicella vaccination is not on the UK schedule but if given (e.g. in a non-NHS setting), there are two doses.

There are special circumstances in which the vaccines are given not as per the routine schedule but where suitable for those children. There is guidance available (via Public Health England) on catch-up schedules for children who have incomplete immunisation histories.

Special populations with specific vaccine needs

Some patient groups have different vaccine requirements and/or contraindications, the most important of which are outlined below.

Immunocompromised children

The vaccination of immunocompromised children is a complex area, because while such children potentially benefit the most from the protection offered, they face two possible problems with vaccinations: they may not mount as good an immune response as immunocompetent children and, with live vaccines, they may develop a severe infection from the vaccine strain.[2]

Children who receive bone marrow transplants, and in some situations those who receive chemotherapy (cancer drugs), may lose their natural or immunisation derived antibodies and need to be considered for re-immunisation.

Expert advice should be sought when vaccinating immunocompromised children, but the principles to follow are:

- They should receive all recommended non-live vaccinations as per the immunisation schedule.
- They may require additional doses of vaccines they have had previously (if they have responded less well than non-immunocompromised children).
- They may require additional (non-live) vaccines.
- Family members may require immunisation to reduce potential exposure of the children.

- Live vaccines should be avoided in the following immunosuppressed children:
  - Those with evidence of severe primary immunodeficiency
  - Those being treated with immunosuppressive chemotherapy or radiotherapy
  - Those who have completed treatment with immunosuppressive chemotherapy or radiotherapy in the past 6 months
  - Those who are on immunosuppressive therapy following a solid organ transplant
  - Those who have received a bone marrow transplant, until at least 12 months after all immunosuppressive therapy is finished (potentially longer if the child has developed graft versus host disease)
  - Those who are receiving systemic high dose steroids, until at least 3 months after the treatment has stopped. For the purposes of the postponement of vaccination, high dose steroids would be defined as prednisolone orally or rectally at a daily dose of 2 mg/kg/day for at least 1 week or 1 mg/kg/day for 1 month
  - Those receiving other immunosuppressive drugs (e.g. ciclosporin or azathioprine), either alone or with steroids, until at least 6 months after the treatment(s) have stopped
  - Those who were exposed to immunosuppressive treatment from the mother, either during pregnancy or via breastfeeding, until a postnatal effect on their immune status remains possible. If this has been *in utero* exposure to tumour necrosis factor alpha (TNFα) antagonists or other biological medicines, this period should be at least 6 months
- Immunisation should be either carried out before immunosuppression occurs or deferred until an improvement in immunity has been seen.
- Vaccines should ideally be given at least 2 weeks before commencement of immunosuppressive treatment.
- Re-immunisation should be considered after treatment is complete and the child has recovered.
- More than 2 weeks between vaccination and commencement of immunosuppressive therapy is preferable with live vaccines; however, the advantages of delaying treatment need to be weighed against the not insignificant disadvantages.

Children with HIV

Children with HIV can receive some live vaccines. Current guidance is that they can receive:

- Rotavirus vaccine
- Live attenuated intranasal influenza vaccine if they are over 2 years old and their infection is stable

- MMR if they are over 1 year old, unless they are severely immunosuppressed, i.e.:
  - CD4 % < 15 (any age) or
  - CD4 count < 750 cells/mm^3 (< 12 months)
  - CD4 count < 500 cells/mm^3 (1–5 years)
  - CD4 count < 200 cells/mm^3 (> 6 years)
- If they are under 18 months old, they should have two doses of MMR at least 3 months apart. If they are over 18 months, the doses should be at least 1 month apart.
- Varicella vaccine if they are varicella immunoglobulin G (IgG) seronegative, over 1 year of age, and not severely immunosuppressed (as above). The two doses should be 1–2 months apart. There should be a 1 month gap between the MMR and varicella vaccines.

If immunocompromised children have suspected or confirmed HIV, they should not receive the BCG vaccine. It can be given to HIV negative children and infants born to HIV positive mothers but who are at low risk of mother to child transmission.

Premature infants

Due to the benefit of vaccinations for this at-risk group, premature infants should not have their vaccinations and boosters delayed or omitted: they should receive them at the normal chronological age.

The likelihood of desaturation, apnoea and bradycardia following vaccination is increased in the extremely premature (those born at ≤ 28 weeks' gestation); if they are in hospital at the time of their first immunisations, they should be monitored for the following 48–72 hours for these events. If such events occur, the second immunisations should also be given to the baby as a monitored inpatient. If the baby is at home at 2 months and receiving immunisations in the community, he or she does not require any post-immunisation monitoring.

Rotavirus vaccination should be considered even if the infant is still a neonatal intensive care unit inpatient. Respiratory syncytial virus (RSV) immunoprophylaxis prior to the infant's first RSV season should also be considered in appropriate circumstances.

Other medical conditions

Certain medical conditions and medications increase the child's risk of specific infectious diseases. Children who suffer from such conditions or are receiving such treatments require additional protection.

The following vaccines are recommended in these circumstances.

- Asplenia or splenic dysfunction:
  - Hib/meningococcal C conjugate, meningococcal B, meningococcal ACWY

- Influenza
- Pneumococcal conjugate
- Cochlear implants:
  - Pneumococcal
- Complement disorders:
  - Hib/meningococcal C conjugate, meningococcal B, meningococcal ACWY
  - Pneumococcal conjugate
- Chronic cardiac and respiratory conditions:
  - Influenza
  - Pneumococcal conjugate
- Chronic renal conditions (including those children on haemodialysis):
  - Hepatitis B
  - Influenza
  - Pneumococcal conjugate
- Chronic liver conditions:
  - Hepatitis A
  - Hepatitis B
  - Influenza
  - Pneumococcal conjugate
- Chronic neurological conditions:
  - Influenza
  - Pneumococcal conjugate
- Diabetes mellitus:
  - Influenza
  - Pneumococcal conjugate
- Haemophilia:
    Note: subcutaneous rather than intramuscular administration of vaccines is recommended in order to minimise the possibility of bleeding into the muscle.
  - Hepatitis A
  - Hepatitis B

Maternal vaccination

Mothers may be offered vaccines during pregnancy to either protect themselves from relevant infection(s) antenatally or to protect their infant in the early postnatal period.[3]

In response to the 2012 pertussis (whooping cough) outbreak, the UK Department of Health introduced a maternal vaccination programme. A pertussis-containing vaccine is recommended for women from week 20 of their pregnancy. The aim is to maximise the transplacental antibodies transferred and therefore passively protect the infant in the pre-immunisation months. The influenza vaccination is also offered to women during pregnancy.

There was 60.7% uptake of pertussis vaccination in England in March 2016, and 31.8% uptake of influenza vaccination in 2015.

Vaccine contraindications

Almost all children can be vaccinated with all vaccines without safety concerns. Vaccination is contraindicated or should be deferred in very few situations.

Vaccines are contraindicated in children who have had a confirmed anaphylactic reaction to a previous dose of a vaccine containing the same antigens as, or a component (e.g. neomycin) of, the vaccine in question. Immunosuppression (see above) and pregnancy are contraindications to live vaccines.

Expert advice should be sought before administering an influenza vaccine to a child with egg allergy, as they may be at increased risk of allergic reaction with these vaccines. Children with a confirmed anaphylactic reaction to egg should not receive the yellow fever vaccine.

The tip cap and rubber plunger of some syringes may contain latex proteins, as may the stoppers of some vaccine vials. It is theoretically possible that these latex proteins may cause allergic reactions in those with latex allergy. Although the risk, if such a risk exists, is extremely small, the precautionary measure of not giving vaccines from latex-containing syringes or vials should be taken in those with a history of an anaphylactic reaction to latex, unless the benefit of vaccination outweighs the risk of allergic reaction.

Adverse reactions

There are some predictable side-effects of vaccines; most of these are mild and self-resolving. However, it is not always possible to predict who might suffer from more serious side-effects (adverse events) following a vaccine.

The World Health Organization (WHO) classifies adverse events following immunisation (AEFI) into four main categories. These are:

- Programme related
- Vaccine induced
- Coincidental
- Unknown

AEFIs may be true adverse events that are related to the vaccine, the way it is administered, or to an underlying medical condition of the child. AEFIs may also be coincidental events whose occurrence is not related to the vaccine.

Programme related AEFIs

These are adverse events caused by practices in the storage, distribution, preparation and administration of the vaccine – i.e. the vaccination programme rather than the vaccine itself.

Examples of such practices are:

- Incorrect storage of vaccine or diluent
- Contaminated vaccine or diluent
- Incorrect preparation (e.g. mixing, diluent used, amount of diluent used) of the vaccine
- Incorrect vaccine administration (e.g. incorrect dose, route, site, technique)
- Use of vaccines beyond their expiry date
- Storage of reconstituted vaccines beyond the recommended time frame

Vaccine induced AEFIs

These are events caused by a particular vaccine or its components. They may be direct effects; they may also be due to an underlying medical condition or an idiosyncratic response of the patient.

Local reactions (e.g. swelling at the vaccination site) and fever in the 48 hours following the DTaP/IPV/Hib vaccine would be an example of a direct vaccine induced AEFI.

Local reactions such as pain, swelling and erythema at the injection site occur commonly and should be anticipated. They are usually mild, they are not allergic in nature, and they do not contraindicate further doses of immunisation with the same vaccine or vaccines containing the same antigens.

Parents should be given advice about these more common vaccine induced AEFIs and how to manage them should they occur. Advice should be given on use and dose of paracetamol or ibuprofen to treat a post-immunisation fever or any discomfort caused by local reactions. National Institute for Health and Care Excellence (NICE) guidelines on feverish illness in children can be referred to. While ibuprofen and paracetamol can reduce distress and discomfort, there is no evidence that prophylactic use of antipyretics prevents febrile convulsions. There is evidence that such use of antipyretics may reduce the antibody responses to some vaccines. For these reasons, giving antipyretics to prevent a post-vaccination fever is not currently recommended, with the exception of the MenB vaccine, for which studies have shown that antibody responses are not suppressed but fever is reduced.

Immune-mediated and neurological vaccine induced AEFIs occur much more rarely than local reactions. Seizures, idiopathic thrombocytopaenic purpura and allergic reactions (including anaphylaxis) are examples of these. For example, anaphylaxis post vaccination (in a child with no allergy history) would be an idiosyncratic vaccine induced AEFI.

Coincidental AEFIs

These are events that are not true adverse reactions to the vaccine, but are linked to the vaccination because of the timing of their occurrence. For an AEFI to be described as coincidental, it needs to be clear that the event would have occurred even if the child had not been immunised.

Anaphylaxis

All health professionals administering immunisations must have training in the resuscitation of a patient experiencing anaphylaxis. Any location where immunisations are taking place must have an algorithm or protocol for the management of anaphylaxis and an anaphylaxis pack.

Conclusions

Vaccinations are an essential part of child health. It is important to use up-to-date resources to provide age appropriate vaccinations and the correct information to parents or colleagues dealing with more complex situations.

References

1   Department of Health. *Immunisation against infectious disease* (the Green Book) (last updated 2 September 2014). London: Public Health England. www.gov.uk/government/collections/immunisation-against-infectious-disease-the-green-book
2   Pinto MV *et al*. Immunisation of the immunocompromised child. *J Infect* 2016; 72 (Suppl): S13–S22.
3   Marchant A *et al*. Maternal immunisation: collaborating with mother nature. *Lancet Infect Dis* 2017; 17(7): e197–e208.

Further recommended reading

NHS Choices. Vaccinations. www.nhs.uk/Conditions/vaccinations/Pages/vaccination-schedule-age-checklist.aspx
Public Health England. www.gov.uk/government/organisations/public-health-england

58

Sedation and anaesthesia

R Sunderland and C Davison

Introduction

This chapter focuses on premedication and perioperative drugs used for sedation and anaesthesia that have an implication for patients on the ward. It will not discuss the use of drugs for inducing and maintaining general anaesthesia.

The learning objectives of this chapter are:

➢ to understand key drugs used for procedural sedation and premedication
➢ to recognise specific diseases with implications for patients undergoing anaesthesia
➢ to understand the preparation and post-anaesthetic care of patients.

Drugs for procedural sedation and premedication

General anaesthesia induces a state of hypnosis and can lead to airway obstruction, loss of protective reflexes and hypoventilation, putting patients at risk of aspiration and hypoxia; it is for this reason that children must be starved prior to the administration of anaesthesia.[1] Current guidelines recommend the following starvation times.

- Clear fluids: 1 hour
- Breast milk: 4 hours
- Food and milk: 6 hours

Children often require sedation to facilitate non-painful investigations and painful procedures. Sedated children are at risk of losing their airway reflexes and thus should be starved as for general anaesthesia.

While oral sedation is relatively easy to administer, the interpatient variability makes the depth of sedation difficult to titrate. Intravenous sedation may be easier to titrate to effect; however, it requires specialist training and equipment to deal with the potential complications. It should be stressed that all these sedative drugs have the potential to cause respiratory and cardiovascular compromise, and should only be administered in the constant presence of an appropriately trained healthcare professional. Pulse oximetry, heart rate and blood pressure should be monitored continuously, and resuscitation equipment must be available to allow airway support. End-tidal carbon dioxide can be monitored by nasal cannulae or a face mask, and it is recommended that this is carried out during deep sedation. Supplemental oxygen should be considered for all children undergoing procedural sedation.[2]

Commonly used drugs for procedural sedation are described below.

Chloral hydrate

Chloral hydrate has been used as an oral and rectal sedative in children for many years; however, it is currently not licensed for sedation for painless procedures in the UK. It is metabolised to an active metabolite, trichloroethanol, which is excreted in the bile and urine and thus should be used with caution in liver or renal failure. It accumulates on prolonged use, and so this should be avoided. It can precipitate respiratory depression, coma, gastritis and acute porphyria. Repeated doses may lead to tolerance and dependence, which may result in withdrawal symptoms on abrupt cessation. The oral liquid preparation is best diluted with juice to mask the unpleasant taste.[3]

Benzodiazepines

Benzodiazepines can be given to patients for sedation for painless procedures or as premedication prior to general anaesthesia. Midazolam, the most commonly used benzodiazepine used for this purpose, can be administered by a variety of routes depending on clinical need. The intravenous preparation can be given orally; however, it is bitter and should be diluted with a sweet beverage to mask this taste.[3] The timing of midazolam prior to the procedure depends on the route of administration.

- Oral: 30–40 minutes
- Buccal: 3–5 minutes
- Intramuscular: 15 minutes
- Rectal: 15–30 minutes
- Intravenous: 1.5–5 minutes

Intravenous midazolam should be titrated carefully and at least 5 minutes should be allowed between boluses to avoid respiratory depression. Flumazenil should be readily available to treat overdose. Some children may have a paradoxical reaction to midazolam causing agitation.

Ketamine

Ketamine has analgesic properties and therefore can be used as sedation prior to painful procedures. The racemic preparation is most commonly used, although (S)-ketamine is available, which has approximately twice the potency and a shorter elimination time. The main contraindications to ketamine include any conditions where excessive sympathomimetic stimulation may be deleterious for the patient, such as severe cardiovascular disease, and caution is traditionally advised in patients with raised intracranial pressure. Ketamine can be administered by a variety of routes, including the oral use of the intravenous preparation diluted in a beverage palatable to the child.[4] Intravenous ketamine can cause excessive secretions, therefore pretreatment with intravenous glycopyrronium bromide is suggested to decrease the risk of laryngospasm and potential airway obstruction. A single dose of ketamine can be used as the sole agent for a procedure of short duration (less than 30 minutes) or as premedication or an induction agent for general anaesthesia. The recovery from ketamine may be complicated by auditory and visual hallucinations, which may be reduced by the concomitant use of a benzodiazepine. A concern about the deleterious effect of ketamine on the developing brain of primates has led many to avoid its use in the neonatal and infant population.[5]

Entonox

Entonox (nitrous oxide and oxygen, 50 : 50) can be used as inhalational sedation for painful procedures. Entonox is readily available in premixed cylinders and is delivered through a demand valve via a mouthpiece or face mask. Therefore is it only suitable for children who can comprehend and cooperate with this technique – usually those over 5 years-old. Positioning of the delivery system by parents or carers should be avoided, as this could lead to excessive administration and subsequent loss of consciousness. Nitrous oxide can diffuse into air-containing spaces causing them to expand, therefore Entonox should not be used where gas may be trapped in the patient's body, e.g. if the patient has pneumothorax, intestinal obstruction, abdominal distension or pneumocephalus (e.g. post craniectomy), or following middle ear procedures.

Propofol

Propofol is a potent intravenous sedative and anaesthetic agent and should only be used by appropriately trained and equipped individuals.

Specific diseases with anaesthetic implications

Malignant hyperthermia

- Rare condition (associated with ryanodine receptor gene RYR1) which puts patients at risk of a life-threatening hypermetabolic reaction during general anaesthesia[6]
- Mortality 2–3% with modern treatment (previously 70–80%)
- Triggered by suxamethonium and volatile anaesthetic agents
- Suspect in patients with family history of unexplained death under anaesthesia or previous suspicious reaction to anaesthesia
- Patients may have undergone previous uneventful anaesthesia
- Associated with central core disease (autosomal dominant mutation in the RYR1 gene), King–Denborough syndrome and Evans myopathy
- Clinical reaction is variable in severity and identified by unexplained or unexpected:
  - rigidity of the jaw muscles
  - increasing tachycardia
  - tachypnoea or increase in end-tidal carbon dioxide
  - hyperthermia
  - worsening metabolic acidosis and increases in serum levels of potassium, creatine kinase and myoglobin.
- Treatment:
  - Call anaesthetist/critical care team
  - Dantrolene – titrated to response (may require repeated doses)
  - Active cooling and supportive measures
- Safe anaesthesia is possible avoiding triggers and using 'clean' anaesthetic equipment and total intravenous anaesthesia techniques.

Suxamethonium apnoea

- Suxamethonium is a depolarising neuromuscular blocking drug normally metabolised by plasma cholinesterase within 2–6 minutes.[7]
- Suxamethonium apnoea is a rare condition in which the clinical effect of suxamethonium is prolonged, leading to inadequate respiration.
- Inherited condition: the levels of plasma cholinesterase are reduced.
  - Several variations of the normal enzyme
  - Incidence varies by ethnic group
- Acquired disease: plasma cholinesterase activity is decreased. Occurs in:
  - pregnancy
  - hypothyroidism
  - liver disease

- renal disease
- carcinomatosis
- cardiopulmonary bypass
- treatment with anticholinesterases
- treatment with monoamine oxidase inhibitors
- methotrexate therapy.
- Clinical effect can last 30 minutes to several hours.
- Supportive measures and sedation are required until adequate respiratory function returns.

Duchenne muscular dystrophy

- Incidence of 1 in 3500 live male births (X-linked recessive disorder)[8]
- At risk of hyperkalaemia and rhabdomyolysis associated with anaesthesia; case reports of cardiac arrest following anaesthesia
- Children with Duchenne muscular dystrophy who are < 8 years old most at risk.
- Can occur in recovery room post anaesthetic.
- Avoid suxamethonium and volatile anaesthetic agents.
- Total intravenous anaesthesia is the preferred technique.

Mitochondrial myopathies

- Heterogeneous group of conditions with variable clinical manifestations, including muscle weakness.[8]
- Theoretical risk of propofol infusion syndrome if total intravenous anaesthesia is used.
- Propofol infusion syndrome manifests as lipaemia, metabolic acidosis, renal and liver failure.
- Regional anaesthetic techniques and remifentanil infusion to minimise dose of propofol

Renal dysfunction

Caution should be exercised in using repeated doses or infusions of any drugs if their accumulation may cause deleterious effects, such as morphine and pethidine.

Obesity

- Increasing problem in the paediatric population.[9]
- Preferably use short-acting volatile anaesthetic agents (desflurane or sevoflurane) to reduce respiratory complications.

- Weak and moderately lipophilic drugs, such as non-depolarising neuro-muscular blocking agents, should be dosed to lean body weight (LBW), i.e. ideal body weight (IBW) plus 20%.[10]
- Succinylcholine should be calculated using total body weight.[10]
- Paracetamol should be dosed to IBW to avoid toxicity.[10]
- In very obese patients, LBW may not be accurate, therefore bispectral index (BIS) monitoring may be a helpful guide to the adequate depth of anaesthesia.[9]

Preparation and post-anaesthetic care of patients

Anaesthesia and long term medications

The basic rule is to continue all medications, with the exception of the following.

- Insulin: use locally agreed hospital guidelines for diabetics undergoing surgery.
- Angiotensin converting enzyme (ACE) inhibitors: many anaesthetists will want these omitted on day of surgery due to hypotensive effects in combination with inhalational anaesthetics.
- Aspirin: the antiplatelet function can cause perioperative bleeding; there must be consultation with the surgeon and anaesthetist and consideration given to stopping it 7–10 days prior to surgery.
- Any concerns regarding other medications should be discussed with the child's anaesthetist.

Despite children being 'nil by mouth', they can have regular medication or analgesia given with a sip of water prior to anaesthesia.

Post-anaesthesia implications

Children less than 46 weeks' gestational age are at risk of apnoeas for 24 hours post anaesthesia, thus must be monitored for 24 hours as an inpatient; if a child is preterm, this may need to be extended to a post-conception age of 60 weeks.[11]

Post-anaesthesia delirium

This is a recognised phenomenon, most commonly seen with anaesthetic techniques using sevoflurane in children receiving no other sedative or opioid drugs.[12] The child may be inconsolable, and the delirium may last up to 40 minutes; it is important to rule out postoperative pain as a cause of the child's distress.

Comorbidities and sedation

Any child with significant comorbidities (such as severe cardiac, respiratory, renal or hepatic disease) should only be sedated by healthcare professionals with appropriate expertise.

Local anaesthetic toxicity

The following children are at risk:[13]

- Patients with regional anaesthetic catheters *in situ*, e.g. epidurals or local anaesthetic blocks for pain relief
- Small infants receiving topical anaesthesia, especially in areas of high bioavailability such as mucus membranes
- Patients receiving inadvertent intravenous administration of local anaesthetic
- Children administered excessive doses of local anaesthetic

Symptoms and signs:

- Perioral numbness
- Dizziness
- Agitation
- Seizures
- Arrhythmias, including bradycardia and cardiac arrest

Treatment: call for help and provide standard cardiorespiratory support following the airway-breathing-chest Compressions (A-B-C) approach.

In cardiac arrest secondary to local anaesthetic toxicity, intravenous administration of a lipid solution such as Intralipid® 20% is recommended, and this should be readily available wherever local anaesthetic toxicity may occur. If there is no response to the initial bolus dose, this may be repeated twice more and followed by an infusion. It should be noted that recovery from local anaesthetic induced cardiac arrest may take over 1 hour and require prolonged resuscitative efforts. Intralipid may be considered prior to cardiac arrest in the severely compromised child.

Unexplained cardiorespiratory arrest

In the event of sudden unexplained cardiorespiratory arrest in a child post anaesthetic, the differential diagnosis should include the inadvertent administration of a potent anaesthetic drug during flushing of an indwelling intravenous catheter. Those children most at risk include:

- neonates and infants
- children with extensions on their intravascular catheters
- children with central venous catheters, especially if tunnelled.

Treatment should include immediate and appropriate cardiorespiratory support while the likely cause is sought. Anaesthetic drugs that are most likely to be responsible include:

- Opioids – remifentanil given via infusion in theatre may leave some residual drug in the line and lead to an unintended bolus when flushing the intravascular catheter. A potent respiratory depressant, it may lead to apnoea, hypoxia and pinpoint pupils. Treatment is with respiratory support; also consider giving naloxone, although remifentanil is relatively short acting.
- Neuromuscular blocking drugs – these may cause a dose dependent impairment of respiratory function from hypoventilation to respiratory arrest. Treatment is with respiratory support and sedation or anaesthesia (to reduce post-traumatic stress of 'awareness') until the neuromuscular blocking agent wears off. Duration of support will be dependent on the agent used and may be reduced by appropriate use of a reversal agent such as neostigmine or abolished in the case of rocuronium with the specific antagonist sugamadex.[3]

Conclusions

Many of the drugs used for premedication or procedural sedation can be administered via multiple routes but may be potent cardiorespiratory depressants. Therefore, they should only be used by those with appropriate training and equipment. These drugs should be used cautiously in patients with severe comorbidities. Malignant hyperpyrexia and suxamethonium apnoea, while both being rare, are two conditions with specific pharmacogenetic implications for anaesthetic drugs.

References

1 Thomas M *et al*. Association of Paediatric Anaesthetists of Great Britain and Ireland Consensus statement on clear fluids fasting for elective pediatric general anesthesia. *Paediatr Anaesth* 2018; 28(5): 411–414.
2 NICE. Sedation in under 19s: using sedation for diagnostic and therapeutic procedures (clinical guideline CG112). NICE, 2010. http://guidance.nice.org.uk/CG112
3 Paediatric Formulary Committee. BNF for Children 2013–2014. London: BMJ Group, Pharmaceutical Press and RCPCH Publications, 2013.
4 Cunnington PMD. Management of the uncooperative frightened child. In: Bingham R *et al*. (eds). *Textbook of Paediatric Anaesthesia*, 3rd edn. London: Hodder Arnold, 2008: 369–381.
5 Slikker W *et al*. Ketamine-induced neuronal cell death in the perinatal rhesus monkey. *Toxicol Sci* 2007; 98(1): 145–158.
6 Halsall PJ, Hopkins PM. Malignant hyperthermia. *BJA: CEACCP Reviews* 2003; 3: 5–9.
7 Sinclair RCF, Faleiro RJ. Delayed recovery of consciousness after anaesthesia. *BJA: CEACCP Reviews* 2006; 6: 114–118.

8   Ragoonanan V, Russell W. Anaesthesia for children with neuromuscular disease. *BJA: CEACCP Reviews* 2010; 10: 143–147.

9   Owen J, John R. Childhood obesity and the anaesthetist. *BJA: CEACCP Reviews* 2012; 12: 169–175.

10 De Baerdemaeker LEC *et al*. Pharmacokinetic in obese patients. *BJA: CEACCP Reviews* 2004; 4: 152–155.

11 Gormley SMC, Crean PM. Basic principles of anaesthesia for neonates and infants. *BJA: CEACCP Reviews* 2001; 1: 130–133.

12 Reduque LL, Verghese ST. Paediatric emergence delirium. *BJA: CEACCP Reviews* 2013; 13: 39–41.

13 Christie LE *et al*. Local anaesthetic systemic toxicity. *Contin Educ Anaesth Crit Care Pain* 2015; 15(3): 136–142.

59

Palliative care

E Harrop and N Christiansen

Introduction

Palliative care for children is defined as an active and total approach to care, embracing physical, emotional, social and spiritual elements. In contrast with adult palliative medicine, oncology diagnoses make up only a small proportion of cases, with over 300 conditions recognised among the paediatric palliative population.[1] This leads to a wide range of complex symptoms, which may also be difficult to recognise and manage, particularly in very young and non-verbal children.

The learning objectives of this chapter are:

> to understand that pharmacological treatment is only one aspect of palliative care
> to know common symptoms encountered in children during palliative treatment and how to manage them
> to recognise key drug administration challenges and solutions in this setting, including the use of enteral feeding tubes, subcutaneous syringe drivers, buccal/sublingual and transdermal administration routes.

Background

Palliative care focuses on enhancements to the quality of life for the child and support for the family. It includes the management of distressing symptoms, provision of respite, and care after bereavement.

The National Institute for Health and Care Excellence (NICE) in the UK produced guidance entitled 'End of life care for infants, children, and young people with life limiting conditions: planning and management' (NG61) in December 2016, which offers additional evidence-based guidance on a number of the topics covered in this chapter; although designed for a UK audience, its relevance is broad.[1] Paediatric palliative care management plans should, when feasible, be devised by a multidisciplinary team and shared in the form of symptom management plans, in order to facilitate consistent patient-centred care. The care plan should involve the appropriate healthcare professionals from primary, secondary and tertiary services. Effective and clear communication is therefore essential to ensure safe prescribing and supply of medication. This is particularly important as often not all those involved in the patient's care are familiar with drugs and doses used in palliative care.

Prescribing in this setting also involves frequent use of unlicensed or off-label medication (see chapter 28).[2] There are also numerous challenges to optimise prescribing for children in a palliative context, which include:

- the wide range of underlying diseases, many of which are individually rare diseases
- the limited evidence base available for many of the therapeutic interventions[3,4]
- the need to care for the child in his or her choice of setting (home, hospice, hospital)[4]
- medication regimens that often have to be administered by non-medical carers[4]
- the use of routes of administration that are less commonly encountered in general paediatrics (such as oral transmucosal, transdermal and subcutaneous infusion).[3,4]

Management of specific symptoms

Gastrointestinal

Poor oral intake

The key to successful management of reduced eating and drinking in children approaching the end of life is usually to identify and (where possible) treat any underlying cause, examples of which include:

- poorly controlled pain
- anxiety
- nausea
- mouth pain, e.g. oral thrush
- low mood
- reflux
- environmental factors
- cancer cachexia.

Once these are addressed (where possible), the child should be encouraged to eat and drink if able. If enteral tube feeding or intravenous support is offered, this should be regularly reviewed to ensure that it remains in the child's best interest.[1]

Mouth care

Good mouth and lip care can significantly improve quality of life for children who are no longer able to tolerate adequate fluid intake. This can involve keeping the mouth moist (safe use of mouth-care sponges, sips of fluid, ice chips (possibly flavoured), introducing different tastes to the mouth), treatment of oral thrush, management of dry lips (avoid paraffin based products if oxygen is in use), humidifying oxygen, and managing bleeding.

Nausea and vomiting

Precipitating causes need to be considered. Examples include:

- uncontrolled pain
- anxiety
- infection (e.g. urinary tract)
- drugs
- biochemical/metabolic
- bowel obstruction.

Environmental measures must be considered in concert with pharmacological approaches (avoiding strong smells, removing leftover food promptly, offering small blander meals). In raised intracranial pressure, cyclizine is useful first line treatment and may be supplemented by transdermal hyoscine. Dexamethasone may also have a role (e.g. in the case of oedema secondary to brain tumours; see below). Children receiving chemotherapy are often given supportive anti-emetic care, including ondansetron and metoclopramide (which is now not recommended for any other indication in children, and only short term). The prokinetic anti-emetic domperidone is associated with a small risk of serious cardiac side-effects (MHRA warning April 2014 – see https://www.gov.uk/drug-safety-update/domperidone-risks-of-cardiac-side-effects). Its use in palliative care is excluded from the recommendations in the MHRA warning, but caution should be exercised. Domperidone can, however, be particularly useful in cases where poor gastrointestinal motility is contributing to nausea and vomiting. Levomepromazine and haloperidol are both helpful where anxiety is a feature. Levomepromazine is the most broad spectrum but can be more sedating. There is some reported experience of using levomepromazine via the oral transmucosal route.[3] Otherwise, if the enteral route is not possible, intravenous doses are often used during chemotherapy, and subcutaneous infusions are common practice in end of life care.

Constipation

The management of constipation in palliative care should include consideration of underlying causes, and these should be addressed specifically where possible. Examples include:

- inactivity
- neurological dysfunction
- metabolic disturbance
- poor intake
- fear of opening bowels
- drug causes.

A sensible first line choice in most settings would be a macrogol. If the volumes needed are not tolerated, sodium docusate can provide a useful alternative. Rectal measures may be needed in addition, although the use of the rectal route in usually contraindicated in paediatric oncology patients on treatment. It is important to co-prescribe a laxative for children needing long term opiates. The role of methylnaltrexone in paediatric palliative care remains unclear, as constipation is often multifactorial, and the administration requires subcutaneous injection.[3]

Gastrointestinal pain

It is important to consider possible underlying causes, as targeted treatment may be available.

- Reflux (feed thickeners first line; consider proton pump inhibitors or H_2 antagonists, and prokinetics only if severe)
- Gastrointestinal bleeding/gastritis (sucralfate)
- Colicky pain (hyoscine butylbromide)
- Pain related to autonomic gut failure
- Visceral hyperalgesia (gabapentin can be helpful; ketamine may be used by specialists in some cases)

In many of the above, feeding may need to be replaced with dioralyte feeds followed by slow regrading (if tolerated). In gut failure, using a partially hydrolysed/hydrolysed feed may be of benefit in some cases.

Respiratory

Dyspnoea

Considering the underlying cause is important, as specific treatments may relieve symptoms. Causes include:[1]

- obstruction
- bronchospasm (steroids, bronchodilators)

- infection (antibiotic use for symptom relief, rather than only for curative intent)
- anaemia (transfusion – if still within goals of care)
- anxiety (reassure; consider anxiolytics)
- environmental factors (temperature, humidity, positioning).

Low dose morphine (usually at around half the analgesic dose) can bring relief of breathlessness. Buccal midazolam can also be useful for sudden onset breathlessness, particularly if associated with anxiety. There are, of course, also numerous non-pharmacological strategies suitable for older children, including guided imaging and 'square breathing'.

Excessive respiratory secretions

Difficulty managing secretions is often due to bulbar difficulties rather than increased volume. Despite this, reducing volume and increasing viscosity can aid their management. Hyoscine hydrobromide can be used in the form of transdermal patches or can be included in a continuous subcutaneous infusion. Glycopyrronium bromide may also be useful, as it can be administered enterally, titrated to effect, and does not cross the blood–brain barrier. Caution should be exercised to avoid over-thickening, which may lead to mucus plug formation.

Neurological

Convulsions

It is important to consider the underlying/contributing causes for seizures, which may include:

- raised intracranial pressure (see below)
- metabolic disturbance
- infection/fever
- poorly controlled epilepsy
- sleep deprivation
- drug reactions
- excessive environmental stimulation
- constipation (in children with brittle epilepsy).

The Advanced Paediatric Life Support (APLS) guidance on emergency management of seizures is appropriate for acute prolonged seizures/ convulsive status epilepticus. Buccal midazolam would therefore be the first line treatment in most cases, usually repeated and then followed by rectal paraldehyde. The subsequent role of intravenous interventions with escalation to intensive care would depend on the particular clinical situation. Enteral or subcutaneous loading with phenobarbitone can be used in some settings to regain control in the face of uncontrolled fits, when hospital admission does not meet goals of care. This can then (if needed) be followed by continuous subcutaneous infusion of phenobarbitone. Subcutaneous options for end of life seizure control also include clonazepam and midazolam.[1] The child's neurologist generally ought to make changes to the child's long term background antiepileptic medication (in all but absolute end of life situations, where medication is being rationalised). There are times when using a short or medium term course of clobazam can be helpful to redress control during intercurrent illness or in the case of girls whose hormonal changes affect their control. In children and young people who are approaching the end of life, it is important to be aware that abnormal movements (such as dystonic spasms) might be mistaken for seizures. If in doubt, specialist advice should be sought.[1]

Raised intracranial pressure

Oedema around an inoperable brain tumour may be reduced by the use of pulses of dexamethasone. There is little evidence to support particular dose regimens, but the Association of Paediatric Palliative Medicine (APPM) formulary gives guidance based on two small retrospective studies.[3] It is important to understand that the benefits are likely to be less with each successive course, and that a washout period is needed to minimise side-effects. In situations where there is felt to be obstruction of cerebrospinal fluid flow and neurosurgery is no longer in the child's best interest, a trial of acetazolamide therapy may be helpful[3] (this should be done in discussion with the child's oncologist and is likely to involve review of the most recent neuroimaging available).

Restlessness/confusion/agitation

It is important to exclude uncontrolled pain or other treatable symptoms. Anxiety, frustration, primary cerebral irritability, hypoxia or drug side-effects are leading causes. Haloperidol can be useful for hallucinations/agitation, midazolam buccally for anxiety (half the seizure dose), levomepromazine is useful particularly if nausea is associated or in terminal care (as it may be sedative). There is also a considerable role for environmental/non-pharmacological measures. It should be noted that for children and young people with a neurological disability who are approaching the end of life, the signs and symptoms of agitation or delirium can be mistaken for the signs and symptoms of seizures or dystonia.[1]

Sleep disturbances

Once again the underlying cause is key, as it is important not to just sedate children who are sleepless because of unresolved symptoms (e.g. pain, nausea). In children with organic brain disease, melatonin may be very useful in restoring circadian rhythms. There are various protocols relating to its use; if children can swallow, there is a sustained release preparation of granules that can be suspended in puree (but not in liquid). This can be used alone or in combination with immediate release preparations. Otherwise the immediate release preparation can go down a gastrostomy tube, and the dose can be repeated if the child is awake again before 2–3am. If there is concern about nocturnal hallucination, haloperidol is helpful. Chloral hydrate remains a good sedative in other situations.

Muscle spasm/dystonia

It is helpful to differentiate these from seizures or movement disorder if possible. In cases of persistently increased tone, muscle relaxant drugs such as baclofen may be prescribed regularly (often by a neurologist). Acute wind-up episodes of spasm clusters may respond well to buccal midazolam rescue, at a lower dose than that used in status epilepticus. If this is needed more than just occasionally, there may be a role for regular use of longer acting benzodiazepines. Gabapentin has been shown to improve the quality of life of children who experience dystonia.[5] Management of severe dystonia/status dystonicus should include a paediatric neurologist and may involve the use of other drugs such as clonidine.

Pain

(See chapter 60.) Pain in the context of paediatric palliative care is often complex and multifactorial, making it challenging to assess, particularly in non-verbal patients. Examples of cryptic causes include:[1]

- gastrointestinal pain (e.g. associated with diarrhoea or constipation)
- bladder pain (e.g. caused by urinary retention)
- bone pain (e.g. associated with metabolic diseases)
- headache (e.g. caused by raised intracranial pressure)
- neuropathic pain (e.g. associated with cancer)
- musculoskeletal pain (particularly if the child has neurological disabilities)
- dental pain.

In most cases, initial interventions for pain should follow a stepwise approach using simple analgesics such as paracetamol or ibuprofen, followed by a low dose opiate, as described in World Health Organization (WHO) guidance.[6] The use of codeine is no longer recommended in children, following safety concerns; therefore, if simple analgesia proves inadequate, low dose morphine therapy may be needed next. Morphine therapy is usually initiated in opiate-naive patients using a standard release preparation of morphine at a modest dose. Provision should be made for a suitable breakthrough dose alongside regular doses. Once the patient's opiate requirement has been titrated in this way, a longer acting preparation may be substituted with additional doses of a standard release preparation remaining available as required for breakthrough pain. Additional doses may also be offered pre-emptively (anticipatory doses) in children and young people who have pain at predictable times (e.g. when dressings are being changed or when being moved and handled).[1] These anticipatory doses should not be included when calculating the required daily background dose of analgesia. If treatment with a specific opioid does not give adequate pain relief, or if it causes unacceptable side-effects, an alternative opioid preparation should be considered.[1] Non-pharmacological measures (e.g. massage, hot/cold compresses and distraction) should also be offered.

Neuropathic pain

Children who respond poorly to conventional analgesia may be experiencing neuropathic pain. This can be difficult to manage and usually benefits from the input of a specialist team. Adjunctive medication may be used, with examples including antiepileptic drugs (gabapentin) or tricyclic antidepressants (amitriptyline), or sometimes ketamine (usually with specialist support). Rotation of opioid background analgesia to methadone can be helpful, but should not be done without specialist support, as the half-life is long and unpredictable (particularly in children).[1]

Haematological

Bleeding

It is important to acknowledge honestly where there may be risk of catastrophic haemorrhage, as simple measures such as dark bedding or towels may minimise the distress. Mucosal bleeding can be treated with tranexamic acid (topical or as mouthwash) or with local application of 1 : 1000 adrenaline.[3]

Dermatological

Pruritus

Good skin care is actually the most important treatment in most situations. For itch secondary to opiates, ondansetron or cimetidine are useful. In itch related to hypersensitivity, chlorphenamine may help.

Administration challenges – getting the right drug to the right place

Drug administration via enteral feeding tubes

Complex paediatric patients are often reliant on administration of medication via enteral feeding tubes, and the same is true for palliative patients.

When considering the administration of medication through a tube, it is important to consider a number of factors.

- Tube placement: this is particularly important in the case of tubes placed in the jejunum, as it may affect the absorption profile of the drug.
- Size of the tube: the smaller the lumen of the tube and the longer the tube, the more likely it is to block, so close attention should be paid to the drug preparation prescribed, and effective flushing is essential.
- Formulation: a number of factors need to be taken into account when choosing the drug formulation to be prescribed. Although in most cases liquids are preferable, some preparations may have a high viscosity and require dilution prior to administration. Although most ordinary release tablets can be crushed and dispersed in water before administration, this should be a last resort, as, especially if part doses are prescribed, this can result in significant dose variation. Modified release and enteric coated preparations must not be crushed; this would alter the pharmacokinetics and in some cases could result in increased toxicity and death. In palliative care, this issue is frequently encountered with morphine modified release preparations, and it is important to check brand specific details. For example, MST Continus® granules may be given via 6 and 8 Fr NG tubes; however, the NG tube must be flushed well to ensure no granules remain in the NG tube and cause blockage.
- Detailed and drug specific advice is available in the *Handbook of Drug Administration via Enteral Feeding Tubes*.[7]

Continuous subcutaneous syringe driver infusions

Administration of medication via a pump can allow a continuous, steady state infusion of medication to very vulnerable patients in a community setting. This is particularly useful if the child cannot swallow and access through feeding tubes is limited. Contrary to common belief, the syringe driver is an option in a number of indications, not only for the final stage of life.

Indications can be:

- Persistent nausea and vomiting
- Severe dysphagia
- Intestinal obstruction
- Reduced level of consciousness
- Poor absorption
- Patient preference

In the UK, most services now use a McKinley T34 pump, which has up-to-date safety features. Older pumps such as Grasby syringe drivers are no longer recommended.[8]

Multiple drugs may be combined in the infusion and it may, therefore, be possible to offer treatment for multiple symptoms with a single pump.

When given subcutaneously, some drugs may be preferable, e.g. if they are more soluble or require smaller doses, hence allow for smaller volumes to be infused. One such example is diamorphine, which in some cases may be preferred over morphine.

When combining two or more drugs in a syringe driver, it is important to consider the physical and chemical stability of the drugs (see chapter 32). Various factors such as pH of the solution, concentration of the drug or potential chemical reactions between drugs and/or excipients influence the stability of such mixtures. Absence of visible crystallisation or turbidity does not automatically mean the solution is stable, as there may be degradation of the drug which is not visible. There are a number of very useful information resources available to assess compatibility, although in some cases information is only based on observational data relating to physical compatibility rather than chemical compatibility.

- *Handbook of Injectable Drugs*[9]
- Stability at www.stabilis.org
- *Palliative Care Formulary*[3]
- *The Syringe Driver*[10]
- Syringe driver survey data on www.palliativecare.com[11]

Despite an increasing amount of compatibility data becoming available, there may be situations where data are not available, particularly in paediatrics. In such cases, if the solution is clear it may be appropriate to administer and monitor the patient closely for clinical outcome – however, only if there are no alternate drugs or routes available.

Although mixing drugs in an infusion creates a new (unlicensed) product, the National Prescribing Centre allows mixing of medicines prior to administration in appropriate settings, including palliative care.[12] More detailed information on the use of syringe drivers is available in *The Syringe Driver*.[11]

Buccal and sublingual administration

Sublingual and buccal administration of medication provides a route that is non-invasive and independent of enteral absorption. It is relatively simple to teach to non-medical carers and gives fast onset of action. This makes it very attractive for the rapid treatment of breakthrough symptoms. Buccal doses are likely to differ from oral doses, as this route avoids first-pass metabolism.

There are some commercially available preparations, including buccal midazolam (Buccolam®), licensed for use in prolonged seizures, and fentanyl preparation, in sizes suitable for older children. Please note that the prefilled Buccolam® syringes are not graduated, so are not suitable to administer doses other than the one stated on the packaging. There is emerging off-licence experience of using parenteral preparations of other opiates (morphine/diamorphine) via the buccal route; some guidance is available in the APPM formulary.[3]

Transdermal administration

Transdermal delivery systems (TDDS) or patches of hyoscine hydrobromide are relatively commonly used in paediatrics for the management of secretions. Fentanyl and buprenorphine patches are also available, and can be very useful for the management of stable pain in palliative care. Children often require different doses than are commercially available, as the patch size is usually governed by adult dosing. Alteration of the patch, e.g. by cutting, may be an option to achieve the desired dose; however, it must be borne in mind that not all patches can be safely cut.

TDDS can be divided into different designs: the membrane controlled reservoir design (see Figure 1) and the matrix design (see Figure 2).[13] A reservoir patch holds the drug in a gel or solution, and delivery is determined by a rate-controlling membrane between the drug reservoir and the skin.

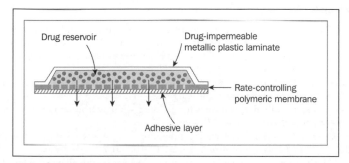

Figure 1 Reservoir patch cross-section

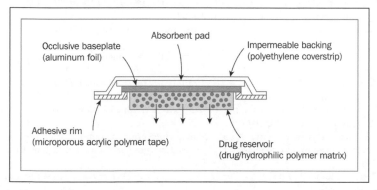

Figure 2 Matrix patch cross-section

In a matrix patch the drug is incorporated in an adhesive polymer matrix, with the dose being dependant on the amount of drug within the matrix and the surface area of the patch in contact with the skin.

Reservoir patches cannot be cut, as any damage to the membrane results in a sudden increase in drug release onto the skin and hence may lead to overdose. Matrix patches, however, can be cut, as the drug dose delivered is proportional to the surface in contact with the skin, e.g. half the patch will deliver half the dose.

Conclusions

The management of children in a palliative care setting requires input from the whole multidisciplinary team, to support both the pharmacological and non-pharmacological aspects of patient care. Prescribing in this context may sometimes involve unfamiliar drugs administered via unfamiliar routes. Ensure that individual cases are discussed with clinical specialists and pharmacists as required, to improve the safety and efficacy of the drugs used, and provide good quality medicines information to patients and their families to help them achieve the maximum therapeutic benefit.

References

1   NICE. End of life care for infants, children, and young people with life limiting conditions: planning and management (NICE guideline NG61). NICE, December 2016.
2   MHRA. Off-label or unlicensed use of medicines: prescribers' responsibilities. Drugs Safety Update April 2009; 2(9): 6.
3   Association of Paediatric Palliative Medicine. *The Association of Paediatric Palliative Medicine Master Formulary*, 4th edn. 2017.
4   Jamieson L *et al*. Palliative medicines for children – a new frontier in paediatric research. *Pharm Pharmacol* 2017; 69(4): 377–383.
5   Lion NY *et al*. Gabapentin can significantly improve dystonia severity and quality of life in children. *Eur J Paediatr Neurol* 2016; 20(1): 100–107.
6   World Health Organization (WHO). WHO Guidelines on the pharmacological treatment of persisting pain in children with medical illnesses. Geneva: WHO, 2010.
7   White R, Bradnam V. *Handbook of Drug Administration via Enteral Feeding Tubes*, 3rd edn. London: Pharmaceutical Press, 2015.
8   NHS National Patient Safety Agency. Safer ambulatory syringe drivers (NPSA/2010/RRR019).
9   Trissel LA. *Handbook on Injectable Drugs*, 17th edn. American Society of Health-System Pharmacists, 2012.
10 Dickman A *et al*. *The Syringe Driver: Continuous subcutaneous infusions in palliative care*. 4th edn. Oxford: Oxford University Press, 2016.
11 Twycross R, Wilcock A. *Palliative Care Formulary*, 4th edn. Nottingham: Palliativedrugs.com Ltd, 2011.
12 National Prescribing Centre. Mixing of medicines prior to administration in clinical practice – responding to legislative changes. Liverpool: National Prescribing Centre, 2010.
13 Perrie Y, Rades T. *FASTtrack Pharmaceutics – Drug Delivery and Targeting*. London: Pharmaceutical Press, 2012.

60

Pain management

A Lo, U Sigg and J Challands

Introduction

High quality pain management requires a multidisciplinary approach, involving medical, pharmacy and nursing staff with additional support from other healthcare professionals, including play specialists, psychologists, physiotherapists and occupational therapists. Organisational aspects include the availability of comprehensive guidelines for the assessment of pain, drug prescriptions, treatment algorithms and options, monitoring requirements, management of adverse effects and patient information. Effective pain management is not only a humanitarian matter but aims to improve quality of care by preventing complications and promoting recovery and rehabilitation.[1]

The learning objectives of this chapter are:

> to understand the key aspects of pain assessment in children
> to recognise the core options for procedural pain relief
> to know the main agents for systemic analgesia in children, with their respective advantages and disadvantages.

Pain assessment

Effective paediatric pain management is intrinsically linked to effective pain assessment. Assessment forms a vital baseline to gain knowledge of the wider issues of the child's pain experience. This knowledge base needs to take into consideration the child's physical, cognitive, physiological and psychological stages of development, as well as how the child may react to the stress of pain.[2] Improvement in pain management has been associated with regular pain assessments.[3]

It has been recognised that paediatric pain assessment is still commonly inadequate. Several recommendations have therefore been made, which include:

- Pain should be anticipated at all times.
- Self-reporting is the ideal approach wherever possible; if a child is unable to self-report, an appropriate behavioural or composite tool should be used. Parental opinion is helpful.
- Pain should not be judged relying on isolated indicators. Changes in behaviour, appearance, activity levels and vital signs could be indicators of pain.
- The use of valid pain assessment tools is strongly recommended.

There is no universally suitable pain assessment tool available, as requirements vary with the child's age and developmental stage (see Table 1), and the type and the cause of pain (e.g. procedural, postoperative, medical, sickle cell or cancer pain). Several tools incorporate self-reporting, physiological and behavioural/observational parameters with the aim of providing more comprehensive measurements.[4] A number of scales have been developed for neonates, infants and children with cognitive impairment, where communication barriers contribute to inadequate pain assessment and management.[5]

Procedural pain

- Many diagnostic and therapeutic procedures cause pain, distress and anxiety. This is a routine event in children with chronic illness. The key to high quality procedural pain management is preparation, planning and communication with the child and family. Pain and memory of initial procedures are known to affect the pain and distress associated with subsequent procedures.[5]
- Children and infants of all ages, including neonates, are capable of feeling pain; consequently, emphasis should be on non-pharmacological measures whenever possible supplemented by pharmacological approaches.[4] Sedation alone is not an adequate alternative to analgesia.[2] Sedation (see chapter 58), strong opioids or general anaesthesia should be contemplated for complex and invasive procedures.[4]
- Procedural pain can be from mild to severe. Pharmacological use needs to be tailored to this.
- In infants and older children, topical local anaesthetics (e.g. EMLA®, Ametop®) have demonstrated high efficacy for venepuncture and cannulation.[4] Vapocoolant sprays, e.g. ethyl chloride spray, are also used.[7]
- Among neonates, heel lancing for blood sampling is a frequent intervention causing pain. This pain can be reduced by utilising a spring-loaded

Table 1 Pain scales algorithm (adapted from Royal College of Nursing (2009) Recognition and Assessment of Acute Pain in Children)[6]

Self-reporting tools		Behavioural tools					
Children and young people		Children < 3 years and neonates		Children > 3 years without cognitive impairment		Children with cognitive impairment	
Peri-procedural pain	Postoperative pain	Peri-procedural pain	Postoperative pain	Peri-procedural pain	Postoperative pain	Peri-procedural pain	Postoperative pain
Faces (Wong Baker)	Colour analogue scale	COMFORT	COMFORT / FLACC (excluding neonates)	COMFORT	COMFORT	Paediatric pain profile (PPP)	Paediatric pain profile (PPP)
Poker chip tool	Faces (6 graded scale by Bieri)	Premature infant pain profile (PIPP)	CHEOPS (excluding neonates)	CHEOPS	CHEOPS	Non-communicating children's pain checklist revised	FLACC
Word descriptor scale	Visual analogue scale (self-rated)	University of Wisconsin pain scale (excluding neonates)	CRIES (suitable for preterm neonates)	FLACC	FLACC		Non-communicating children's pain checklist post-op
	Oucher		Pain assessment tool (PAT) (suitable for preterm neonates)				

device, improved technique, heel massage, 24% sucrose and breast feeding.[8,9] Topical local anaesthetics alone are insufficient.[10] Useful non-pharmacological measures for neonates include tactile stimulation, non-nutritive sucking, swaddling/facilitated tucking and 'kangaroo care'.[4] The analgesic effect of sucrose appears to be related to its sweet taste. The effect of sucrose seems to diminish with age.[11,12]

- Nitrous oxide, an anaesthetic gas with analgesic, sedative and anxiolytic properties, is an efficient option, providing analgesia for procedural pain with minimal side-effects. Adverse effects are caused by absorption into air filled spaces (see chapter 58). Frequent use may cause vitamin B12 deficiency, therefore close haematological monitoring is recommended. Entonox® can successfully reduce pain associated with venous cannulation, dressing changes, suture removals, pin site cleaning, X-ray procedures, physiotherapy, and wound pack and drain removal.

- Oral morphine, intranasal or oromucosal fentanyl, intranasal diamorphine, ketamine and local anaesthetics are also used for procedural pain. Additionally, children benefit from non-pharmacological strategies. Suitable psychological and preparatory measures should be offered to all children; involvement of play therapists is beneficial.[4] There is strong supporting evidence for distraction, guided imagery and hypnosis for needle related pain and distress.[13] Music, massage and virtual reality games are known to reduce pain scores in children undergoing burns dressing changes.[5]

Local anaesthetics

Local anaesthetics reversibly block influx of sodium through ion channels, thereby blocking conduction along nerve fibres. Various local anaesthetics are available with ranges of onset, potency, duration of effect and toxicity. Continuous infusion and repeated bolus administration can lead to drug accumulation. Dosing guidelines are to be followed, especially in neonates, where there is reduced hepatic clearance of amide local anaesthetics and reduced protein binding capacity. All local anaesthetic injections are to be administered slowly to detect accidental intravascular injection.

- Formulations are available for: topical application to skin or mucosa, local instillation and infiltration, peripheral nerve or plexus blockade, and epidural and subarachnoid administration. Vasoconstrictors (e.g. adrenaline) can be added to reduce the systemic absorption rate, thereby prolonging the anaesthetic effect.

- Lidocaine (lignocaine) is used for surface and infiltration anaesthesia and regional nerve blocks. Its rapid onset of action (within minutes) is beneficial. Rapid absorption following topical mucosal application may cause unwanted systemic effects. Various formulations for topical lidocaine

Table 2 Local anaesthetics, with maximum safe dosage in 4 hours		
Drug	Maximum safe dose in 4 hours	
Lidocaine	3 mg/kg	With adrenaline: 7 mg/kg
Bupivacaine	2 mg/kg	With adrenaline: 2.5 mg/kg
Levobupivacaine	2 mg/kg	With adrenaline: 2.5 mg/kg

applications are available: eye drops, ointments for anaesthesia of the skin and mucosa, gels for anaesthesia of the urinary tract, topical solutions or sprays for surface analgesia for mucous membranes in mouth, throat and upper gastrointestinal tract, and transdermal application via a lidocaine patch.[4]

- Bupivacaine is known for its slow onset characteristics and long duration of action, with a half-life of 1.5–5.5 hours in adults and 8 hours in neonates. Levobupivacaine is equipotent but less cardiotoxic. Both solutions are used for infiltration anaesthesia and regional nerve blocks. Solutions of lower concentration are associated with a low incidence of motor block.[4] Example dose limits for these local anaesthetics are shown in Table 2.

- Prilocaine and lidocaine are used in the eutectic mixture of local anaesthetics (EMLA®). The cream is applied under an occlusive dressing to the skin to produce analgesia for procedural pain from venepuncture, cannulation (venous and arterial), lumbar puncture and minor dermatological procedures, among others. EMLA® is used in neonates but in single doses and with caution, as excessive absorption from multiple applications and higher doses may cause methaemoglobinaemia.

- Tetracaine (Ametop®, amethocaine) is used for procedural pain similarly to EMLA®. Ametop® was found to be more effective than EMLA® with a more rapid onset. Mild erythema at the application site is common, and no action is required. Ametop® is administered in reduced doses in neonates.

- A topical local anaesthetic gel containing lidocaine, adrenaline and tetracaine, LAT® is effective for suturing skin and scalp lacerations.

- Absorption of tetracaine from mucous membranes is rapid. Adverse reactions can occur from high systemic toxicity, which may be fatal. Application to inflamed, traumatised or highly vascular surfaces is contraindicated.

Regional analgesia

Peripheral nerve blocks are effective and safe for the management of procedural, perioperative and injury related acute pain. In children, single shot caudal analgesia is widely used for intraoperative and postoperative analgesia for lower abdominal, perineal and lower limb surgery.[2] Safety and high success rates have been demonstrated with caudal bupivacaine, levobupivacaine and ropivacaine. Continuous epidural infusions are effective and safe for postoperative analgesia in children of all ages as long as appropriate doses and equipment are being used by experienced practitioners, and adequate monitoring and management of complications is provided by trained staff. Trainee doctors should seek senior advice about epidurals. Co-administration of local anaesthetics and opioids is beneficial where extensive analgesia is required (e.g. major abdominal surgery, spinal surgery).[4]

Systemic analgesia

Refer to World Health Organization (WHO) pain treatment guidelines[14] and follow a stepwise approach. Pain medication should be administered at regular intervals for persisting pain, with additional 'rescue doses' for breakthrough pain.[14] When pain episodes are intermittent and unpredictable, analgesia on an as-required basis should be provided.

All analgesia should be administered by the simplest, most effective and least painful route. Intramuscular injections are to be avoided, with the oral route preferred wherever possible.[14]

Paracetamol

Paracetamol is effective for mild and moderate pain. The dose required for analgesia is greater than for antipyretic effect.[4] Paracetamol is administered as the sole agent or in combination with non-selective non-steroidal anti-inflammatory drugs (NSAIDs) and may be useful as an adjunct to other treatments for more severe pain. An opioid sparing effect has been observed.

Risk factors for paracetamol hepatotoxicity are hepatic disease, paracetamol overdose, chronic paracetamol use, a nutritionally compromised status or abnormal gastrointestinal function.[14] Acute toxicity is unlikely to occur when dosing regimens are adhered to. Early features of paracetamol poisoning are non-specific (nausea and vomiting). Untreated, an overdose can be fatal.

The route of administration affects the bioavailability of paracetamol. Oral doses are subject to first-pass hepatic metabolism of 10–40%; peak plasma concentrations are reached in approximately 30 minutes. Rectal administration is associated with slower and more erratic absorption, and loading doses may be required to achieve therapeutic effect. Intravenous (IV) injection provides increased dosing accuracy with less absorption variability and more rapid onset.

Non-steroidal anti-inflammatory drugs

NSAIDs are effective for mild to moderate pain, especially for postoperative, trauma and inflammatory condition related pain. It is commonly used for childhood aches, bumps and fever. NSAIDs should be avoided in neonates. Analgesia, antipyretic and anti-inflammatory activities are known. See chapter 52 for further details of NSAIDs. Note that administration of aspirin for pain is contraindicated in children under 16 due to aspirin's association with Reye's syndrome. Oral and rectal preparations are available, but side-effects can occur with all routes of administration.

Opioids

Opioids are routinely used to treat moderate to severe pain, whether due to medical or surgical causes, and can be administered by many routes. Initial doses of opioid should be based on age, weight and clinical status of the child and then titrated against the individual's response.

Routine and regular assessment of pain severity, analgesic response and the incidence of side-effects (nausea and vomiting, itching, respiratory depression and sedation) is essential, with adjustment of opioid treatment accordingly. Side-effects must be treated promptly. Unlike paracetamol and NSAIDs, opioid analgesics have no upper dosage limit, because there is no 'ceiling' analgesic effect. The appropriate dose is the dose that produces pain relief for the individual child. Opioid use may cause constipation and tolerance. Patients should have a laxative prescribed. Opioid treatment for longer than 10 days may result in withdrawal symptoms on cessation. This must be looked for and a slow wean initiated with the help of the acute pain team.

Severe pain can be safely and effectively managed with opioid infusions, which may be delivered by nurse controlled analgesia (NCA), patient controlled analgesia (PCA) or continuous infusion. There must be clear protocols in place for infusion rates, monitoring, staff education and treatment of side-effects. NCA and PCA offer greater flexibility than a continuous infusion. NCA is used in younger children and those with cognitive or physical special needs. It combines a background infusion with the facility for additional nurse-given boluses, usually available every 20 minutes. PCA is used in children 5 years and over who can understand the concept of using the button to give themselves a bolus when in pain and to facilitate movement. The background infusion rate is low, but the bolus is available every 5 minutes if needed.

Morphine

Morphine is the most commonly used opioid for severe pain in children. It may be prescribed by many routes, but most commonly it is given by the oral and IV route in children. Morphine is usually the drug of choice for NCA, PCA and continuous infusion. Other routes include subcutaneous (SC), rectal, epidural and intrathecal. Morphine is metabolised in the liver to the active metabolite morphine 6-glucuronide, which is excreted by the kidneys, and the inactive metabolite morphine 3-glucuronide. The clearance of morphine is reduced and half-life prolonged in neonates and infants, as the glucuronidation pathways are immature. Care must be taken with dosage for neonates, infants and children with renal impairment, as the active metabolite may accumulate. Only severe liver failure is likely to affect morphine clearance.

Codeine

Codeine is a weak opioid and a prodrug. Conversion to morphine by CYP2D6 is required for analgesia. Codeine has been used for moderate pain in children for years, but has a wide range of efficacy from none to overdose. The Medicines and Healthcare Products Regulatory Agency (MHRA) currently only recommends codeine to be used to relieve acute moderate pain in children older than 12 years and only if the pain cannot be relieved by other analgesia such as paracetamol or ibuprofen alone. Codeine is now contraindicated in all children aged 0–18 years who undergo tonsillectomy or adenoidectomy (or both) for obstructive sleep apnoea and all patients of any age known to be CYP2D6 ultrarapid metabolisers. IV administration must be avoided due to the risk of severe hypotension. The addition of codeine to paracetamol may improve analgesia for postoperative pain. Codeine is less effective than ibuprofen for acute musculoskeletal pain in children.

Fentanyl

Fentanyl is a synthetic opioid that has rapid onset and high potency and is short acting. It is used mainly in anaesthesia and postoperative pain by NCA, PCA or epidural administration. It is also used in some emergency departments for treatment of severe acute pain by the intranasal route. Due to its high lipophilicity, it can also be administered transdermally – an approach that is utilised in palliative care and, rarely, for chronic pain. Fentanyl's plasma redistribution contributes to its rapid offset of action. It is metabolised to inactive metabolites, and clearance in neonates is only 70–80% of adult levels. If fentanyl is infused for an extended period, the half-life effect can be prolonged.

Oxycodone

Oxycodone is increasingly used in children. In infants over 6 months of age, the pharmacokinetic profile of oxycodone is similar to that in adults. It is particularly used in its oral short acting and modified release formulations for palliative care and chronic pain. It is occasionally used in NCA, PCA and in the management of sickle cell pain where morphine has been ineffective.

Diamorphine

Diamorphine is used in the emergency department via the intranasal route to achieve rapid control of acute severe pain.[4]

Tramadol

Tramadol produces analgesia by two mechanisms: an opioid effect and an enhancement of serotonergic and adrenergic pathways. It is used for treatment of moderate pain. The role and optimum dose of tramadol in children needs clarifying. IV and oral formulations are available, but there is no paediatric concentration suitable for giving in small oral doses accurately.[5] The side-effects of tramadol are similar to those of opioids, with similar or reduced rates of nausea and vomiting (10–40%), sedation and fatigue, but less constipation and pruritus, and no reports of respiratory depression in children.

Ketamine

(See also the information on ketamine in chapter 58.) Ketamine hydrochloride is a non-competitive antagonist of NMDA (N-methyl-D-aspartate) receptors. It can be administered via almost any route. Oral ketamine is subject to the significant first-pass effect of hepatic metabolism. Onset of analgesia varies depending on the route of administration. Onset is within minutes when administered by the SC or IV routes, and 30 minutes following oral administration. It is used for procedural pain, premedication, anaesthesia and co-analgesia with IV opioids for severe pain. Its main benefit is that it preserves cardiovascular stability, spontaneous respiration and protective airway reflexes at routinely prescribed doses. Ketamine increases blood pressure and heart rate. It also exerts a high incidence of psychotomimetic side-effects (e.g. drowsiness, alterations in body image and mood, floating sensations, vivid dreams, hallucinations and delirium). These symptoms can be managed with a quiet room and a benzodiazepine.

Conclusions

This chapter summarises the key features of effective pain relief in children. High quality pain management should always form a central part of good clinical care, and this should start with an age appropriate pain assessment, when feasible. In complex cases, paediatric pharmacists can give individualised advice, and specialist pain teams, where available, can support case management by the multidisciplinary team.

References

1 The Royal College of Anaesthetists. Acute Pain Services. *Guidance on the Provision of Anaesthesia Services for Acute Pain Management.* 2010.
2 Howard RF *et al.* Association of Paediatric Anaesthetists: Good Practice in Postoperative and Procedural Pain. *Pediatr Anesth* 2008; 18(Suppl. 1): 14–18.
3 Hicks CL *et al.* The Faces Pain Scale revised: towards a common metric in pain measurement. *Pain* 2001; 93(2): 173–183.
4 Association of Paediatric Anaesthetists of Great Britain and Ireland (APA). Good practice in postoperative and procedural pain management. *Pediatr Anesth* 2012; 22(Suppl. 1): 1–79.
5 Schug SA *et al.* (eds). *Acute Pain Management: Scientific Evidence*, 4th edn. Melbourne: Australian and New Zealand College of Anaesthetists and Faculty of Pain Medicine, 2015.
6 Royal College of Nursing. Clinical Practice Guidelines: *The Recognition and Assessment of Acute Pain in Children.* London: Royal College of Nursing, 2009. www.rcn.org.uk/professional-development/publications/pub-003542
7 Davies EH, Molloy A. Comparison of ethyl chloride spray with topical anaesthetic in children experiencing venepuncture. *Paediatr Nurs* 2006; 18(3): 39–43.
8 Shah V *et al.* Evaluation of a new lancet device (BD QuikHeel) on pain response and success of procedure in term neonates. *Arch Pediatr Adolesc Med* 2003; 157: 1075–1078.
9 Shah P *et al.* Breastfeeding or breast milk for procedural pain in neonates. *Cochrane Database Syst Rev* 2006; 3: CD004950.
10 Jain A, Rutter N. Does topical amethocaine gel reduce the pain of venepuncture in newborn infants? A randomised double blind controlled trial. *Arch Dis Child Fetal Neonatal Ed* 2000; 83(3): F207–F210.
11 Lefrak L *et al.* Sucrose analgesia: identifying potentially better practices. *Pediatrics* 2006; 118(Suppl. 2): S197–S202.
12 Slater R *et al.* Oral sucrose as an analgesic drug for procedural pain in newborn infants: a randomised controlled trial. *Lancet* 2010; 376(9748): 1225–1232.
13 Uman LS *et al.* Psychological interventions for needle-related procedural pain and distress in children and adolescents. *Cochrane Database Syst Rev* 2013; 18(4): CD005179.
14 World Health Organization. Persisting pain in children package: *WHO Guidelines on the Pharmacological Treatment of Persisting Pain in Children with Medical Illnesses.* 2012.

Further recommended reading

Arana JV *et al.* Treatment with paracetamol in infants. *Acta Anaesthesiol Scandinavica* 2001; 45(1): 20–29.
Blonk MI *et al.* Use of oral ketamine in chronic pain management: a review. *Eur J Pain* 2010; 14(5): 466–472.
BMJ Group. *British National Formulary for Children (BNFC).* London, 2016/17.
Borland M *et al.* A randomized controlled trial comparing intranasal fentanyl to intravenous morphine for managing acute pain in children in the emergency department. *Ann Emerg Med* 2007; 49(3): 335–340.
Bruce E, Franck L. Self-administered nitrous oxide (Entonox) for the management of procedural pain. *Paediatr Nurs* 2000; 12: 15–19.
Capici F *et al.* Randomized controlled trial of duration of analgesia following intravenous or rectal acetaminophen after adenotonsillectomy in children. *Br J Anaesth* 2008; 100(2): 251–255.
Chaudhary WA *et al.* Ketamine as an adjuvant to opioids for cancer pain management. *Anaesth Pain Intensive Care* 2012; 16(1): 174–178.

Dolansky G *et al*. What is the evidence for the safety and efficacy of using ketamine in children? *Paediatr Child Health* 2008; 13(4): 307–308.

Ecoffey C *et al*. Epidemiology and morbidity of regional anesthesia in children: a follow-up one-year prospective survey of the French-Language Society of Paediatric Anaesthesiologists (ADARPEF). *Pediatric Anesthesia* 2010; 20(12): 1061–1069.

Eidelman A *et al*. Topical anaesthetics for repair of dermal laceration. *Cochrane Database Syst Rev* 2005; 10: CD005364.

El-Tahtawy A *et al*. Population pharmacokinetics of oxycodone in children 6 months to 7 years old. *J Clin Pharmacol* 2006; 46(4): 433–442.

Giaufre G *et al*. Epidemiology and morbidity of regional anesthesia in children: a one-year prospective survey of the French-Language Society of Pediatric Anesthesiologists. *Anesth Analg* 1996; 83(5): 904–912.

Ivani G *et al*. Comparison of racemic bupivacaine, ropivacaine, and levo-bupivacaine for pediatric caudal anesthesia: Effects on Postoperative Analgesia and Motor Block. *Reg Anesth Pain Med* 2002; 27(2): 157–161.

Korpela R *et al*. Morphine-sparing effect of acetaminophen in pediatric daycase surgery. *Anesthesiology* 1999; 91(2): 442d–447.

Llewellyn N, Moriarty A. The national pediatric epidural audit. *Pediatr Anesth* 2007; 17: 520–533.

Moriarty A. Pediatric epidural analgesia. *Pediatr Anesth* 2012; 22: 51–55.

61

Drugs and pharmacology in paediatric intensive care

N Kleiber, A Wignell and SN de Wildt

Introduction

Drug dosing in the critically ill child is a real challenge, as we must take into account the effect of acute illness and the treatment modalities' impact on drug pharmacokinetics (PK) and pharmacodynamics (PD), in addition to developmental pharmacology. Current knowledge is insufficient to set dosing guidelines representing the wide diversity of situations found in intensive care units (ICUs). Here we introduce the general principles governing PK and PD in the critically ill child and describe the main continuous medications used.

The learning objectives of this chapter are:

➤ to recognise the pathophysiological changes that occur in critical illness
➤ to know that these changes can affect both PK and PD
➤ to understand how these alterations can influence optimal dosing of drugs in ICUs.

PK and PD in the critically ill child

PK and PD changes in critically ill children can be due to either intrinsic factors related to the patient's condition or to treatment modalities (e.g. extracorporeal membrane oxygenation, therapeutic hypothermia, haemofiltration).

The effects of critical illness on PK are summarised in Figure 1. Changes in drug absorption are illustrated by the effect of illness on gut absorption (lower right) and first-pass metabolism (lower left). Volume of distribution (V_d) is affected by albumin binding (upper right) and features of critical illness and treatment modalities (listed in the square representing peripheral compartment). The liver is the main organ of drug metabolism, and kidneys (upper left) are the main excretory organ. Changes are represented by

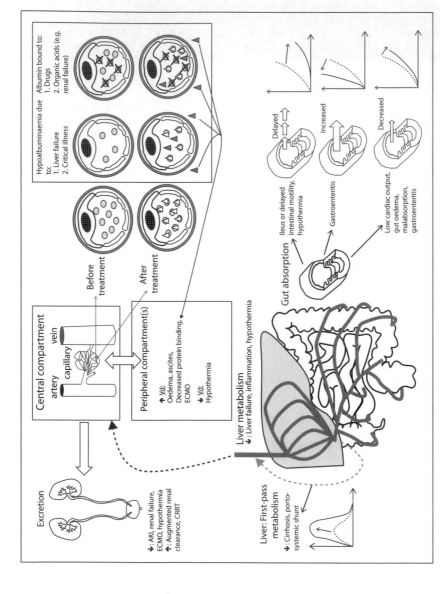

Figure 1 Illustration of the effect of critical illness on drug pharmacokinetics

an arrow (↑ increase; ↓ decrease) and a graphical representation of drug concentration over time, with a dashed line representing PK in a healthy patient and the solid line representing the change induced by critical illness.

Intrinsic factors related to the patient

Intrinsic factors linked to the patient's illness, such as inflammation or organ disease/failure, can alter pharmacology in numerous ways.

Absorption

Intestinal absorption
- Intestinal absorption is dependent on the drug's chemical properties, gastric and intestinal motility and the amount of blood flow to the gastrointestinal tract.
- Many conditions influence absorption.
  - Ileus or decreased intestinal motility often present with shock, sepsis and various gastrointestinal conditions and may result in delayed absorption and thereby delayed effect.[1]
  - Malabsorption and gastroenteritis may increase or decrease absorption and thereby systemic concentrations.
  - Low cardiac output: blood flow to the gut decreases and gut oedema impairs absorption, resulting in lower systemic concentrations of the parent drug.[2]
  - Inflammation, through regulation of drug metabolism and transporter activity, influences gut absorption.[3]

Therefore, in the unstable patient and in situations where absorption is uncertain, intravenous (IV) formulations should be favoured.[4]

First-pass metabolism
- In patients with cirrhosis, the liver is bypassed by extensive portosystemic shunts.
- Drugs with extensive first-pass metabolism may have increased oral bioavailability.
  - This leads to a risk of overdose (e.g. propranolol, morphine).[1,2]

Distribution

The main factors affecting distribution in the critically ill are described below.

Albumin
- A decrease in the amount of unbound albumin leads to:
  - an increase in the free concentration of the drug: if the drug is active, its effect can be enhanced because more free drug is available for receptor binding (e.g. phenytoin)

- an increased apparent V_d: the drugs usually bound to albumin disperse into the tissue and decrease the relative concentration in blood for the same total amount.
- This situation is typically found in the following situations.
  - Renal failure (organic acids compete with drugs for binding albumin)
  - Hypoalbuminaemia (common in critical illness or liver failure)[4]
  - Polypharmacy (drugs compete for albumin-binding sites)

Change in total body water
- Oedema and ascites were found to increase the V_d of hydrophilic drugs (e.g. aminoglycosides), which distribute in the total body water.[5]

Change in blood flow
- Normally, it takes around 30 seconds for blood to flow from a peripheral vein to the arterial circulation.
- When heart function is severely impaired, cardiovascular stability is fragile and distribution in the circulatory system can be significantly delayed.
- Careful titration of cardiodepressant drugs (i.e. virtually all analgesic sedative drugs) is therefore needed.
- Sudden collapse may occur if insufficient time is permitted for distribution.

Metabolism
- The liver is the main organ of drug metabolism.
- Drug metabolites are generally inactive but can also be as active as, or sometimes even more potent than, the parent drug (midazolam, morphine).
- The impact of liver disease on drug clearance is determined by the extraction ratio (ER; fraction of drug extracted by the liver).
  - High clearance 'flow limited' drugs: for drugs with near complete extraction (ER approximately 1, e.g. propofol), decreased liver blood flow leads to decreased metabolism.
  - Low clearance 'capacity limited' drugs: for partially extracted drugs (ER significantly less than 1), reduced liver metabolic capacity is the main determinant of the amount of drug metabolised.
- The impact of acute liver failure on drug metabolism is difficult to predict.
- Alterations in hepatic drug metabolism do not correlate with the alterations in standard liver function tests.[6]
- Systemic inflammation also impacts on liver metabolism.
  - Proinflammatory cytokines induce downregulation of expression of most CYP450 enzymes.
  - This results in decreased drug clearance and increased plasma levels of substrates, with risk of adverse effects (e.g. midazolam, theophylline).

Excretion

- Glomerular filtration is the main renal drug elimination pathway.
- Creatinine clearance is currently used to guide the dosage of renally excreted drugs.
- Glomerular filtration rate (GFR) may serve as a marker of tubular damage.
- In the absence of a practical marker of tubular function, GFR is also used to guide dosing of drugs dependent on renal tubular function (morphine, cephalosporins).
- Usually doses need to be modified when GFR is $< 30-40$ mL/min/1.73 m^2.
- Creatinine clearance measurement in patients with low muscle mass warrants caution.
  - As creatinine production is proportional to the muscle mass, the measurement may overestimate GFR.
- Some drugs have active metabolites that accumulate in renal failure (e.g. one of morphine's metabolites, M 6-G, is more potent than morphine).
- In patients with decreased GFR, maintenance dosage can be adjusted by increasing the dosing interval or by decreasing the dose.
  - Dosing guidelines are available,[7] and expert advice from clinical pharmacists is recommended.
- Conversely, augmented renal clearance (ARC; supranormal GFR) is increasingly recognised in paediatric intensive care unit (PICU) patients.[8–10]
  - ARC leads to increased drug clearance, with risk of underdosing renally excreted drugs.
  - Subtherapeutic levels of, for example, antimicrobial treatment could potentially have devastating consequences.[11]

Extrinsic factors related to the treatment of the patient

A number of external treatment modalities, discussed below, can also affect PK and PD in an ICU.

Extracorporeal membrane oxygenation

Distribution

- For most drugs, V_d increases (secondary to the volume added and adsorption to the circuit).
- Lipophilic drugs (midazolam, fentanyl) are more adsorbed than hydrophilic drugs (morphine, gentamicin, cefotaxime), therefore blood concentrations may be lower.
  - Hence, at extracorporeal membrane oxygenation (ECMO) initiation, expect an increase in (lipophilic) drug requirement.
- Subsequently, steady state levels are mainly affected by clearance and dose rate.[12]

- PK alterations also depend on the ECMO circuit type and priming solution composition.

Clearance

- In general, clearance in patients on ECMO is lower (0–50% decrease).
- Sedatives and analgesics are titrated to effect, generally requiring higher doses (at ECMO initiation).
- Antibiotics are also affected.
- Cautious dosing and monitoring of highly toxic agents (e.g. gentamicin) is advised.
- Dose adjustments are usually not necessary for beta-lactams.
- At the time of writing, there are no paediatric ECMO dosing guidelines.

Hypothermia

Absorption

- Hypothermia decreases the rate of absorption.
- Therapeutic hypothermia is often used in patients with decreased intestinal motility (secondary to cardiac arrest or asphyxia), further increasing unpredictability of oral absorption.
- Therefore IV drug administration is preferable, giving more reliable absorption than oral.

Distribution

- Volume of distribution alters due to:
  - redistribution of blood flow
  - changes in blood pH
  - hypothermia induced changes in physicochemical properties of drugs (e.g. protein binding).
- V_d can increase or decrease depending on drug properties, risking underdosing and overdosing, respectively.[13]

Metabolism

- Decreased enzymatic rate at low temperature decreases drug elimination via hepatic metabolism (e.g. risk of morphine accumulation in neonates).
- Low temperature delays the action of prodrugs (slows transformation into active compounds).

Excretion

- Decreased liver metabolism and renal clearance leads to accumulation risk.
- Decrease maintenance doses, especially for non-clinically titrable drugs and low therapeutic index medications.

Pharmacodynamics:

- EC50 is the drug concentration that produces half-maximal response.
- EC50 can increase or decrease with cooling, depending on the drug.

- For example, morphine's EC50 increases; higher drug levels are needed for same effect.
- The opposite happens for inotropic drugs (effects may be increased).
- Consequently, PK changes can sometimes match PD in particular situations (e.g. drug has increased levels, but these higher levels are needed to produce same effect).[13]
- During rewarming following hypothermia, PK and PD parameters should normalise.
  - Care must be taken to adapt medication dosing accordingly.

Cardiopulmonary bypass and combined effect of ECMO and hypothermia

- Cardiopulmonary bypass is used to preserve perfusion during heart surgery.
- Combines use of an extracorporeal circuit – similar to ECMO – and hypothermia (which preserves organ function).
  - Applied for a shorter period
  - Rewarming initiated within a few hours
- ECMO combined with hypothermia is mainly used for neuroprotection after cardiac arrest.
- In the absence of adult/paediatric data, changes can only be speculated based on cardiopulmonary bypass literature and knowledge regarding each modality.

Distribution

- When bypass or ECMO is combined with hypothermia, need to account for opposite effects on V_d.
- ECMO or bypass initiation causes V_d to increase (especially lipophilic drugs; see above).
- Hypothermia decreases V_d, but only to a limited degree compared with ECMO related increase.

Metabolism and excretion

- Drug clearance will be lower when ECMO or bypass is combined with hypothermia.
- Haemofiltration, often concomitantly used, also affects elimination.
  - Smaller (< 500 Da), hydrosoluble and poorly protein bound drugs will be significantly eliminated.
  - Drugs that are not filtered will be concentrated.

Continuous renal replacement therapy

- Continuous renal replacement therapy (CRRT) has a major impact on drug clearance.[14,15]
- Continuous haemofiltration is based on the principle of hydrostatic pressure to drive fluid through a filter.
  - Filtered plasma is called ultrafiltrate.

- Continuous haemodialysis uses passive diffusion through a membrane for substrate removal.
  - Dialysed plasma is called dialysate.
- Haemodiafiltration uses both the above principles of haemofiltration and haemodialysis.
- Current paediatric CRRT dosing guidelines are mostly derived from adult studies.

To gauge the expected amount of drug that CRRT will remove, consider the following.

Volume of distribution (V_d)

- The higher the V_d, the less likely it is that a drug will be cleared by CRRT, because it is mainly concentrated in extravascular compartments unavailable for CRRT.
- Drugs with a V_d exceeding 0.7 L/kg that are more lipophilic and concentrated in adipose tissues are less likely to be cleared.
  - For example, CRRT is ineffective for digoxin poisoning (V_d of 7.3 L/kg).

Sieving coefficient (Sc)

- This coefficient represents the degree to which a particular membrane allows the passage of a solute.
- Sc is measured as the ratio of solute concentration in the ultrafiltrate to the solute concentration in the plasma (Sc = 1 means that 100% of solute will be removed; Sc = 0 means no solute is removed).
- The major determinants of the drug Sc are:
  - the degree of protein binding: Sc can be estimated by Sc = 1 − protein binding
    - It gives a quick estimate of the expected amount of drug removal.
  - drug−membrane interactions: passage through the membrane is determined by:
    - membrane pore size: allow molecules up to a certain size to pass through (usually 20 kDa)
    - molecular charge.

Amount of ultrafiltrate or dialysate

- This is prescribed by the clinician and is the principal determinant of drug removal.

Continuous medication used in PICU

- Medication administered by continuous infusion allows easy titration and stable plasma levels.

- It takes on average 3–5 half-lives for a drug to reach steady state.
  - Short half-lives thus enable quick titration to the effective concentration (e.g. inotropes, some antihypertensives).
  - Long half-lives mean a loading dose may be needed to reach therapeutic plasma concentrations more quickly (e.g. milrinone, morphine, midazolam).
- It also takes 3–5 half-lives for a drug to be largely cleared from the body.

Cardioactive and vasoactive drugs

- Cardioactive and vasoactive drugs are commonly used in PICU for treatment of low cardiac output syndrome (LCOS).
- LCOS can result from sepsis or cardiogenic shock and needs to be prevented after cardiac surgery.
- Conventional inotropic agents (adrenaline, noradrenaline, dopamine and dobutamine) stimulate different adrenergic receptors and therefore differ in their relative:
  - positive inotropic effect (β1 receptor effect of increased contractility)
  - peripheral vasoconstrictive (α receptor) effect
  - vasodilatory properties (β2 receptor).
- Newer agents include milrinone, an inhibitor of phosphodiesterase type 3, and levosimendan, a calcium sensitiser agent that increases troponin C sensitivity to calcium.
- Agent selection is dictated by patient haemodynamics and physician's preference.
  - In warm septic shock, vasodilation will be countered by noradrenaline.
  - In contrast, in cold shock, adrenaline or dopamine will be preferred.[16]
- Table 1 summarises the effects of cardioactive and vasoactive drugs, derived from adult studies.
- Milrinone has been shown to decrease the occurrence of LCOS diagnosed clinically.
- The lack of comparative effectiveness studies of different agents for LCOS prevention leads to large differences in practice.[16]
- For LCOS prevention and treatment, vasodilating agents are frequently added to cardioactive drugs to reduce afterload on the myocardium once blood pressure has been restored towards normal.
  - Arteriolar and venodilator agents lacking inotropic negative effect are recommended (e.g. sodium nitroprusside, phentolamine).
- Antihypertensive agents with inotropic negative properties (e.g. nicardipine and esmolol) are used for treating hypertension with preserved heart function.

Table 1 Effects of cardioactive and vasoactive drugs, derived from adult studies

Two useful formulas to keep in mind when titrating cardio- and vasoactive drugs
Mean BP $\cong$ CO * SVR. Good blood pressure (BP) doesn't always reflect good CO (cardiac output)
CO = HR * Stroke volume. Note time for filling is needed to ensure stroke volume.

Agent		Receptor	HR	Inotropy	SVR	
Dopamine	<10 mcg/kg/min	β > α	↑	↑↑	↑	
	>10 mcg/kg/min	α > β	↑	=	↑↑	CO can decrease
Dobutamine		β	↑↑	↑↑	↓	More arrhythmias
Adrenaline	< ≈ 0.2 mcg/kg/min	β > α	↑	↑↑	↑	
	> ≈ 0.2 mcg/kg/min	α > β	↑		↑↑	CO can decrease
Noradrenaline		α ≫ β	↑	↑	↑↑↑	Good choice in vasoplegic patient
Milrinone		PDE-3 inhibitor	=	↑↑	↓	
Levosimendan		Calcium sensitiser	=	↑↑	↓	Vasodilation can cause decrease in BP. Caution if borderline BP.

The doses of dopamine and adrenaline inducing more vasoconstriction are approximate, and should be correlated with the overall clinical picture.

Sedatives and analgesics

- Analgesics are targeted to relieve pain.
- Sedatives serve to calm the patient in the stressful PICU environment and facilitate care (e.g. mechanical ventilation, nursing care).
- Pain relief is most commonly achieved with continuous infusion of opiates (fentanyl or morphine) and sedation with benzodiazepines (midazolam, lorazepam).
  - Both opiates and benzodiazepines induce respiratory depression.
- Alpha-agonists (clonidine and dexmedetomidine) have both sedative and analgesic properties.
  - They induce bradycardia instead of respiratory depression.
- Propofol has sedative and hypnotic properties.
  - Propofol has a strong cardiodepressant effect, hampering its use in the haemodynamically unstable child.
  - Propofol has a very short recovery time on discontinuation, which facilitates weaning of long acting sedatives around the time of extubation.

- Propofol is officially contraindicated in children <16 years due the risk of lethal propofol infusion syndrome.
  - Nevertheless, its unique properties motivate some to use it even in small children, and adverse effects may be less common than feared.[17]
- Optimum sedation levels leading to better clinical outcomes are yet to be determined.
  - Oversedation increases the risk of tolerance, withdrawal and delirium and prolongs the duration of intubation.
  - A way of avoiding oversedation is to proceed to daily sedation interruption.
  - Another way of decreasing medications that depress ventilation is to use alternatives such as paracetamol, clonidine or dexmedetomidine.
- Virtually all available sedatives and analgesic medications are neurotoxic in animal models.
- Human studies are still scarce and the data are conflicting.
- Improvement of neurological outcome is a significant concern in PICU.
- Analgesics and sedatives play a significant role, which requires further research.

PICU dosing in practice

Between the areas of uncertainty introduced, some overarching general principles apply when prescribing in the PICU (see Table 2).

- Drugs that can be titrated to effect (e.g. sedatives and inotropes) can be dosed clinically.
- Knowledge of the drugs' properties in a particular situation guides the choice of the right agent (e.g. morphine is adsorbed less than fentanyl in children on ECMO, and therefore should be favoured) or the timely titration of the dose (decrease sedatives in hypothermia).
- Care must be taken to avoid every unnecessary medication, especially in critical illness with organ involvement.
- Favouring medication that is not inactivated by the liver or metabolised through a single step decreases the potential for adverse reactions.
- Frequent monitoring of serum levels of narrow therapeutic index medications (e.g. aminophylline, anticonvulsants, cardiac glycosides, aminoglycosides) is recommended when the clinical condition changes or after use of particular treatment modalities (ECMO, hypothermia).
- IV formulations should be favoured if there is uncertain absorption or the drug is not titrable to effect.

Table 2 The main continuous medications used in the PICU for sedation and analgesia, treatment of low cardiac output and hypertension

	Mechanism of action/site of action	Relevant pharmacokinetic characteristics	Contraindications/toxicity (and therapeutic drug monitoring (TDM) if relevant) Important/common drug interactions
Morphine	μ receptor agonist	Liver metabolism into M3G and M6G (the latter is more potent than morphine); they are excreted by kidneys and therefore may accumulate with renal failure. Morphine clearance decreases with postnatal age < 10 days. Not ideal for painful procedures: peak of action 20 minutes.	Can cause respiratory depression.
Fentanyl	μ receptor agonist Synthetic opioid, 100 times more potent than morphine Anaesthetic agent	Metabolised by the liver by CYP450 3A4 into inactive metabolites. Compared with morphine: easier titration in renal failure (no active metabolite). Quick peak of action: ideal for short painful procedures. Context sensitive half-life: the longer the infusion, the longer the time taken to clear.	Can cause respiratory depression. Can cause chest wall rigidity +/− associated laryngospasm inducing ineffective ventilation, and desaturation (treatment options: naloxone, neuromuscular blocking agent, intubation).
Remifentanil	μ receptor agonist Compared with fentanyl: equipotent, quicker onset of action Anaesthetic agent	Metabolised by plasma esterases. Elimination is independent of hepatic metabolism or renal excretion. Short offset even after long infusion.	Can cause respiratory depression.
Midazolam	GABA receptor agonist Anxiolytic and amnesic agent	Extensive hepatic metabolism by CYP 3A => primary metabolite 1-OH midazolam is equipotent to midazolam. The 1-OH midazolam glucuronide (weak sedative effect) accumulates with renal failure. Large V_d and low Sc, therefore no dosing adjustment is expected on CRRT.	Can cause respiratory depression. Avoid bolus of midazolam in haemodynamically compromised patient (hypotension). Many interactions with CYP3A4 inducing or inhibiting agents: careful titration to effect.
Clonidine	α-adrenergic receptor Sedative and analgesic properties Specificity for α-2 receptors: α-2:α-1 = 200:1	Increased half-life with renal failure Half-life: neonates, 18 h; children, 9 h; healthy adult, 12–16 h; adult with renal disease: 41 h	Bradyarrhythmia No clinically significant respiratory depression

Table 2 (Continued)

	Mechanism of action/site of action	Relevant pharmacokinetic characteristics	Contraindications/toxicity (and therapeutic drug monitoring (TDM) if relevant) Important/common drug interactions
Dexmedetomidine	α-adrenergic receptor Sedative and analgesic properties More specific than clonidine for α-2 receptors (α-2 : α-1 = 1600 : 1)	Liver metabolism Neonatal clearance 40% of adult value; at 1 year, 85% of adult clearance Half-life: 2.4 h (children)	Bradyarrhythmia No clinically significant respiratory depression
Propofol	Alkylphenol with sedative and hypnotic properties; not well defined mechanism of action	Rapid onset and short duration of sedation on discontinuation, and facilitates weaning of long acting sedative around the time of extubation, and neurologic evaluation of patient with traumatic brain injury. Unaffected by renal and hepatic dysfunction. The US Food and Drug Administration (FDA) recommends maximum rate of 4 mg/kg/h for a maximum 48 hours.	Contraindicated in haemodynamically unstable child: can cause profound hypotension and collapse. Risk of propofol infusion syndrome (PRIS) (clinical and biological signs: metabolic acidosis, elevated liver enzymes, lipaemia, rhabdomyolysis, etc.), which can be fatal. Any suspicion of PRIS should lead to an immediate interruption of propofol infusion, but despite discontinuation, death can ensue.
Sodium nitroprusside	Nitric oxide liberation during rapid metabolic breakdown => peripheral vasodilator. No negative inotropic effect: safe with decreased heart function or after cardiac surgery.	Very easy titration: abrupt discontinuation or downward titration if hypotension with very quick response on BP. 1. Converted into cyanide in blood and tissues. 2. Liver: cyanide converted to thiocyanate (risk of cyanide accumulation in liver failure) 3. Thiocyanate renally excreted (risk of accumulation in renal failure).	Signs of cyanide toxicity: cellular dysoxia from mitochondrial dysfunction; lactic acidosis with high mixed venous saturation, hypotension, tachycardia, shock, coma, death. Measure cyanide level if liver dysfunction. Signs of thiocyanate toxicity: confusion, psychosis, coma, death. Determination of blood levels are advised if infusion > 3 days or renal impairment.
Esmolol	β- blocker with β1 selectivity/site of action: AV, SA node	Very quick onset of action. Easy titration. Higher rate of clearance in neonates compared with older children. No accumulation with liver or renal failure (metabolised in blood by esterase). Some formulations contain ethanol and propy ene glycol.	Contraindication: sinus bradycardia, heart block, uncompensated heart failure (negative inotropic effect) Caution: reactive airway disease

Table 2 (Continued)

	Mechanism of action/site of action	Relevant pharmacokinetic characteristics	Contraindications/toxicity (and therapeutic drug monitoring (TDM) if relevant) Important/common drug interactions
Nicardipine	Slow calcium channel blocker => decreased myocardial and vascular smooth muscle cell Calcium concentration => less calcium available for contractility => vasodilation => decreased BP	Extensive hepatic metabolism by CYP 450 isoenzyme (CYP 3A4) => many interactions (with CYP3A inducers or inhibitors).	If cardiac failure, be aware of negative inotropic effect. Contraindicated if significant obstruction of systemic circulation (e.g. coarctation of the aorta).
Labetalol	Antagonist of α1 and β-adrenergic receptor	Long half-life (3–5 hours). Titration should be slow. Metabolised by hepatic glucuronidation.	Contraindicated in cardiac failure, due to negative inotropic effect. Risk of bronchospasm in asthmatic patient.
Hydralazine	Direct arteriolar vasodilator with unknown precise mechanism Combined positive inotropic and chronotropic stimulation of the heart => increased cardiac output Particularly useful in children with underlying hypertension on multiple medication	Extensive first-pass effect with oral administration: 10–30% of oral bioavailability depending on acetylator status. Onset of action: 10 minutes.	Contraindication: dissecting aortic aneurysms, mitral valve rheumatic disease (increase of stroke volume can worsen dissection or regurgitation), significant coronary artery disease (risk of ischaemia). Adverse effect with long term use: drug induced lupus like syndrome. Concomitant use of monoamine oxidase inhibitors may cause profound hypotension.
Phenoxybenzamine, phentolamine	Systemic vasodilators by α-adrenergic blockade. Used in catecholamine induced hypertension (e.g. pheochromocytoma) or for afterload reduction after cardiac surgery Phentolamine: competitive reversible antagonist Phenoxybenzamine: irreversible	Once α-blockade is achieved, if needed β-blockade can be done to counteract tachycardia.	Suspect overdosage if signs of sympathetic nervous system blockade: vomiting, marked tachycardia, hypotension shock. Treatment of overdose: noradrenaline. Note: adrenaline is contraindicated (because α-receptors are blocked and adrenaline will cause selective β-adrenergic stimulation and will further increase hypotension).

Table 2 (Continued)

	Mechanism of action/site of action	Relevant pharmacokinetic characteristics	Contraindications/toxicity (and therapeutic drug monitoring (TDM) if relevant) Important/common drug interactions
Dopamine	α1, α2, β1>β2 adrenergic receptor agonist, dopaminergic receptors increased contractility, increased BP Precursor of noradrenaline	Precursor of noradrenaline. Very easy titration. Short half-life.	At high doses, may lower cardiac output by marked vasoconstriction.
Dobutamine	β1> β2, α1 adrenergic receptor agonist leading to increased contractility and HR, and vasodilation	Very easy titration. Short half-life. Tachycardia not uncommon.	Can decrease BP by vasodilation.
Adrenaline	α1, β1, β2 adrenergic receptor agonist Multiple indications: In bolus: cardiac arrest, extremely low BP or symptomatic bradycardia, anaphylactic reaction Infusion: shock, bronchospasm (if no more selective β2 agonist available)	Very easy titration. Short half-life.	At high doses may lower cardiac output by marked vasoconstriction. Can increase lactates at high dose (can be misinterpreted as anaerobic metabolism due to shock).
Noradrenaline	α ≫ β1 adrenergic receptor agonist Ideal drug for warm shock	Very easy titration. Short half-life.	Vasoconstriction can increase BP without affecting cardiac output or decrease cardiac output.
Milrinone	Phosphodiesterase inhibitor class 3 Lusitropic properties: improvement in diastolic function (and properties listed in Table 1)	Excreted unchanged: accumulation with renal failure. Relatively long half-life (slow titration and bolus dose may be needed to quickly reach steady state).	Can cause hypotension by decrease in vascular resistance. Do not give if borderline BP.
Levosimendan	Calcium sensitising drug: interacts with troponin C and increases its sensitivity to calcium => increased efficiency of contractile apparatus of myocytes	Hepatic metabolism. Infusion given over several hours. Loading can be given at the beginning of infusion but can lead to significant vasodilation and hypotension. Effect lasts for many days.	Can cause hypotension by decrease in vascular resistance. Do not give if borderline BP.

Conclusions

Our understanding of PK and PD in the PICU has improved significantly over recent years. This chapter gives an overview of this complex field. Despite the recent advances, our knowledge is not yet sufficient to allow adequate titration of drugs. Dosing guidelines that incorporate the complexity of critical illness are unlikely to be achieved in the near future. In the meantime, understanding the key principles covered above should help PICU clinicians to develop useful insights when prescribing.

References

1   Zuppa AF, Barrett JS. Pharmacokinetics and pharmacodynamics in the critically ill child. *Pediatr Clin North Am* 2008; 55(3): 735–755.

2   Shammas FV, Dickstein K. Clinical pharmacokinetics in heart failure. An updated review. *Clin Pharmacokinet* 1988; 15(2): 94–113.

3   Cressman AM *et al*. Inflammation-mediated changes in drug transporter expression/activity: implications for therapeutic drug response. *Expert Rev Clin Pharmacol* 2012; 5(1): 69–89.

4   Krishnan V, Murray P. Pharmacologic issues in the critically ill. *Clin Chest Med* 2003; 24(4): 671–688.

5   Daschner M. Drug dosage in children with reduced renal function. *Pediatr Nephrol* 2005; 20(12): 1675–1686.

6   Verbeeck RK. Pharmacokinetics and dosage adjustment in patients with hepatic dysfunction. *Eur J Clin Pharmacol* 2008; 64(12): 1147–1161.

7   University of Louisville Kidney Disease Program. Pediatric Drugs. Available at: https://kdpnet.kdp.louisville.edu/drugbook/pediatric/

8   De Cock PA *et al*. Augmented renal clearance implies a need for increased amoxicillin-clavulanic acid dosing in critically ill children. *Antimicrob Agents Chemother* 2015; 59(11): 7027–7035.

9   Avedissian SN *et al*. Augmented renal clearance using population-based pharmacokinetic modeling in critically ill pediatric patients. *Pediatr Crit Care Med* 2017; 18(9): e388–e394.

10 Hirai K *et al*. Augmented renal clearance in pediatric patients with febrile neutropenia associated with vancomycin clearance. *Ther Drug Monit* 2016; 38(3): 393–397.

11 Claus BO *et al*. Augmented renal clearance is a common finding with worse clinical outcome in critically ill patients receiving antimicrobial therapy. *J Crit Care* 2013; 28(5): 695–700.

12 Wildschut ED *et al*. Pharmacotherapy in neonatal and pediatric extracorporeal membrane oxygenation (ECMO). *Curr Drug Metab* 2012; 13(6): 767–777.

13 Wildschut ED *et al*. The impact of extracorporeal life support and hypothermia on drug disposition in critically ill infants and children. *Pediatr Clin North Am* 2012; 59(5): 1183–1204.

14 Zuppa AF. Understanding renal replacement therapy and dosing of drugs in pediatric patients with kidney disease. *J Clin Pharmacol* 2012; 52(1 Suppl): 134S–140S.

15 Schetz M. Drug dosing in continuous renal replacement therapy: general rules. *Curr Opin Crit Care* 2007; 13(6): 645–651.

16 Vogt W, Laer S. Treatment for paediatric low cardiac output syndrome: results from the European EuLoCOS-Paed survey. *Arch Dis Child* 2011; 96(12): 1180–1186.

17 Koriyama H *et al*. Is propofol a friend or a foe of the pediatric intensivist? Description of propofol use in a PICU*. *Pediatr Crit Care Med* 2014; 15(2): e66–71.

Further recommended reading

Abraham WT *et al*. In-hospital mortality in patients with acute decompensated heart failure requiring intravenous vasoactive medications: an analysis from the Acute Decompensated Heart Failure National Registry (ADHERE). *J Am Coll Cardiol* 2005; 46(1): 57–64.

Admiraal R *et al*. Towards evidence-based dosing regimens in children on the basis of population pharmacokinetic pharmacodynamic modelling. *Arch Dis Child* 2014; 99(3): 267–272.

Ahsman MJ *et al*. Pharmacokinetics of cefotaxime and desacetylcefotaxime in infants during extracorporeal membrane oxygenation. *Antimicrob Agents Chemother* 2010; 54(5): 1734–1741.

Ceelie I *et al*. Effect of intravenous paracetamol on postoperative morphine requirements in neonates and infants undergoing major noncardiac surgery: a randomized controlled trial. *JAMA* 2013; 309(2): 149–154.

Chandar J, Zilleruelo G. Hypertensive crisis in children. *Pediatr Nephrol* 2012; 27(5): 741–751.

Choi G *et al*. Principles of antibacterial dosing in continuous renal replacement therapy. *Crit Care Med* 2009; 37(7): 2268–2282.

Claus BO *et al*. Augmented renal clearance is a common finding with worse clinical outcome in critically ill patients receiving antimicrobial therapy. *J Crit Care* 2013; 28(5): 695–700.

Cressman AM *et al*. Inflammation-mediated changes in drug transporter expression/activity: implications for therapeutic drug response. *Expert Rev Clin Pharmacol* 2012; 5(1): 69–89.

Daschner M. Drug dosage in children with reduced renal function. *Pediatr Nephrol* 2005; 20(12): 1675–1686.

De Cock PA *et al*. Augmented renal clearance implies a need for increased amoxicillin/clavulanic acid dosing in critically ill children. *Antimicrob Agents Chemother* 2015; 59(11): 7027–7035.

de Graaf J *et al*. Does neonatal morphine use affect neuropsychological outcomes at 8 to 9 years of age? *Pain* 2013; 154(3): 449–458.

Dellinger RP *et al*. Surviving Sepsis Campaign: international guidelines for management of severe sepsis and septic shock, 2012. *Int Care Med* 2013; 39(2): 165–228.

Francis GS *et al*. Inotropes. *J Am Coll Cardiol* 2014; 63(20): 2069–2078.

Gillies M *et al*. Bench-to-bedside review: Inotropic drug therapy after adult cardiac surgery – a systematic literature review. *Crit Care* 2005; 9(3): 266–279.

Gupta K *et al*. Randomized controlled trial of interrupted versus continuous sedative infusions in ventilated children. *Pediatr Crit Care Med* 2012; 13(2): 131–135.

Hoffman TM *et al*. Efficacy and safety of milrinone in preventing low cardiac output syndrome in infants and children after corrective surgery for congenital heart disease. *Circulation* 2003; 107(7): 996–1002.

Hunseler C *et al*. Continuous infusion of clonidine in ventilated newborns and infants: a randomized controlled trial. *Pediatr Crit Care Med* 2014; 15(6): 511–522.

Knibbe CA *et al*. Morphine glucuronidation in preterm neonates, infants and children younger than 3 years. *Clin Pharmacokinet* 2009; 48(6): 371–385.

Koriyama H *et al*. Is propofol a friend or a foe of the pediatric intensivist? Description of propofol use in a PICU*. *Pediatr Crit Care Med* 2014; 15(2): e66–e71.

Krekels EH *et al*. Evidence-based morphine dosing for postoperative neonates and infants. *Clin Pharmacokinet* 2014; 53(6): 553–563.

Krishnan V, Murray P. Pharmacologic issues in the critically ill. *Clin Chest Med* 2003; 24(4): 671–688.

Latifi S *et al*. Pharmacology of inotropic agents in infants and children. *Prog Pediatr Cardiol* 2000; 12(1): 57–79.

Munoz R (ed.). *Handbook of Pediatric Cardiovascular Drugs*. London: Springer, 2008.

Ogawa R *et al*. Clinical pharmacokinetics of drugs in patients with heart failure: an update (part 1, drugs administered intravenously). *Clin Pharmacokinet* 2013; 52(3): 169–185.

Olsen EA, Brambrink AM. Anesthetic neurotoxicity in the newborn and infant. *Curr Opin Anaesthesiol* 2013; 26(5): 535–542.

Petrovic V *et al*. Regulation of drug transporters during infection and inflammation. *Mol Interv* 2007; 7(2): 99–111.

Pichot C *et al*. Dexmedetomidine and clonidine: from second- to first-line sedative agents in the critical care setting? *J Intensive Care Med* 2012; 27(4): 219–237.

Potts AL *et al*. Dexmedetomidine pharmacokinetics in pediatric intensive care – a pooled analysis. *Pediatr Anaesth* 2009; 19(11): 1119–1129.

Potts AL *et al*. Clonidine disposition in children; a population analysis. *Paediatr Anaesth* 2007; 17(10): 924–933.

Roka A *et al*. Elevated morphine concentrations in neonates treated with morphine and prolonged hypothermia for hypoxic ischemic encephalopathy. *Pediatrics* 2008; 121(4): e844–e849.

Schetz M. Drug dosing in continuous renal replacement therapy: general rules. *Curr Opin Crit Care* 2007; 13(6): 645–651.

Shammas FV, Dickstein K. Clinical pharmacokinetics in heart failure. An updated review. *Clin Pharmacokinet* 1988; 15(2): 94–113.

Thomas CA. Drug treatment of hypertensive crisis in children. *Paediatr Drugs* 2011; 13(5): 281–290.

Udy AA *et al*. Augmented renal clearance in the ICU: results of a multicenter observational study of renal function in critically ill patients with normal plasma creatinine concentrations*. *Crit Care Med* 2014; 42(3): 520–527.

Udy AA *et al*. Augmented renal clearance in the Intensive Care Unit: an illustrative case series. *Int J Antimicrob Agents* 2010; 35(6): 606–608.

Udy AA *et al*. Augmented renal clearance: implications for antibacterial dosing in the critically ill. *Clin Pharmacokinet* 2010; 49(1): 1–16.

van den Broek MP *et al*. Effects of hypothermia on pharmacokinetics and pharmacodynamics: a systematic review of preclinical and clinical studies. *Clin Pharmacokinet* 2010; 49(5): 277–294.

van Saet A *et al*. The effect of adult and pediatric cardiopulmonary bypass on pharmacokinetic and pharmacodynamic parameters. *Curr Clin Pharmacol* 2013; 8(4): 297–318.

van Zellem L *et al*. Analgesia-sedation in PICU and neurological outcome: a secondary analysis of long-term neuropsychological follow-up in meningococcal septic shock survivors*. *Pediatr Crit Care Med* 2014; 15(3): 189–196.

Veldhoen ES *et al*. Monitoring biochemical parameters as an early sign of propofol infusion syndrome: false feeling of security. *Pediatr Crit Care Med* 2009; 10(2): e19–e21.

Verbeeck RK, Musuamba FT. Pharmacokinetics and dosage adjustment in patients with renal dysfunction. *Eur J Clin Pharmacol* 2009; 65(8): 757–773.

Verbeeck RK. Pharmacokinetics and dosage adjustment in patients with hepatic dysfunction. *Eur J Clin Pharmacol* 2008; 64(12): 1147–1161.

Verlaat CW *et al*. Randomized controlled trial of daily interruption of sedatives in critically ill children. *Pediatr Anaesth* 2014; 24(2): 151–156.

Vet NJ *et al*. The effect of inflammation on drug metabolism: a focus on pediatrics. *Drug Discov Today* 2011; 16(9–10): 435–442.

Vet NJ *et al*. Optimal sedation in pediatric intensive care patients: a systematic review. *Int Care Med* 2013; 39(9): 1524–1534.

Vogt W, Laer S. Prevention for pediatric low cardiac output syndrome: results from the European survey EuLoCOS-Paed. *Pediatr Anaesth* 2011; 21(12): 1176–1184.

Vogt W, Laer S. Treatment for paediatric low cardiac output syndrome: results from the European EuLoCOS-Paed survey. *Arch Dis Child* 2011; 96(12): 1180–1186.

Wildschut ED *et al*. Determinants of drug absorption in different ECMO circuits. *Int Care Med* 2010; 36(12): 2109–2016.

Wildschut ED *et al*. Pharmacotherapy in neonatal and pediatric extracorporeal membrane oxygenation (ECMO). *Curr Drug Metab* 2012; 13(6): 767–777.

Wildschut ED *et al*. Effect of hypothermia and extracorporeal life support on drug disposition in neonates. *Semin Fetal Neonatal Med* 2013; 18(1): 23–27.

Wildschut ED *et al.* The impact of extracorporeal life support and hypothermia on drug disposition in critically ill infants and children. *Pediatr Clin North Am* 2012; 59(5): 1183–1204.

Xie HG *et al.* Clonidine clearance matures rapidly during the early postnatal period: a population pharmacokinetic analysis in newborns with neonatal abstinence syndrome. *J Clin Pharmacol* 2011; 51(4): 502–511.

Zanelli S *et al.* Physiologic and pharmacologic considerations for hypothermia therapy in neonates. *J Perinatol* 2011; 31(6): 377–386.

Zuppa AF, Barrett JS. Pharmacokinetics and pharmacodynamics in the critically ill child. *Pediatr Clin North Am* 2008; 55(3): 735–755, xii.

Zuppa AF. Understanding renal replacement therapy and dosing of drugs in pediatric patients with kidney disease. *J Clin Pharmacol* 2012; 52(1 Suppl): 134S–140S.

Index

Note: Abbreviations used in index subentries, are listed within the index e.g. PICUs (paediatric intensive care units).
Page numbers suffixed by '*f*' refer to figures, whilst those suffixed by '*t*' refer to tables. Likewise, those suffixed by '*b*' refer to boxes.